with chapters by
LARRY I. LIPSHULTZ, M.D.,
GEORGE M. GRUNERT, M.D.,
and
SHERRY M. WILSON, M.S.W.

An Owl Book
HENRY HOLT AND COMPANY
New York

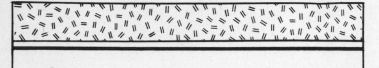

In Pursuit of Fertility

SECOND EDITION

*A FERTILITY EXPERT TELLS YOU
HOW TO GET PREGNANT*

ROBERT R. FRANKLIN, M.D.,
and
DOROTHY KAY BROCKMAN

Henry Holt and Company, Inc.
Publishers since 1866
115 West 18th Street
New York, New York 10011

Henry Holt® is a registered trademark
of Henry Holt and Company, Inc.

Library of Congress Cataloging-in-Publication Data
Franklin, Robert R.
In pursuit of fertility: a fertility expert tells you how to get
pregnant / Robert R. Franklin and Dorothy Kay Brockman;
with chapters by Larry I. Lipschultz, George M. Grunert,
and Sherry M. Wilson.—2nd ed.
p.   cm.
"An Owl book."
Includes bibliographical references and index.
1. Infertility—Popular works.   2. Fertility, Human—Popular
works.   I. Brockman, Dorothy.   II. Title.
RC889.F73   1990   95-24961
616.6'92—dc20   CIP

ISBN 0-8050-4181-8 (An Owl Book: pbk.)

Henry Holt books are available for special promotions
and premiums. For details contact: Director, Special Markets.

First published in hardcover in 1990 by
Henry Holt and Company, Inc.

First Owl Book Edition—1991
Second Owl Book Edition—1995

Printed in the United States of America
All first editions are printed on acid-free paper.∞

10   9   8   7   6   5   4   3   2   1
(pbk.)

Contents

Foreword

For millions of men and women, starting a family is a long and distressing process. At least one in twelve couples of childbearing age in the U.S. is infertile—that is, they are unable to conceive after one year of unprotected intercourse—and the problem is growing. These people, many of whom have postponed childbirth to further their education and careers, need expert answers concerning the diagnosis and treatment of infertility. No longer do infertility patients merely say to their gynecologist, "Let's get pregnant." Couples want to know what is wrong and how their doctors are going to help solve their problems. Today's woman wants to know how her body works. She deserves in-depth information about how her reproductive system functions and how she can protect her health and enhance her fertility. To answer these questions, she may seek a physician who is interested in infertility—a doctor who has kept up with the latest advances in this complicated and ever-changing field.

If you are an infertility patient, the relationship between you and your doctor is a special one. Your physician needs to spend some time with you to help you through this difficult period in your life. It is important for you to be able to sit down together and discuss your problems. You deserve his or her total concentration during every visit, and you must make certain that your symptoms are clearly understood. But even though your doctor is a good listener and wants to do the best job possible, sometimes you may leave the office with unanswered questions. At times, all of us in the health care field are frustrated by our inability to answer our patients' questions as thoroughly as we would like. Understanding infertility and its effect on a couple takes years of training and practice. With the hectic pace of medicine today, just keeping up with new developments is no small task. Condensing all of this information into explanations that patients can understand is an important but difficult challenge.

This book by Dr. Robert Franklin and Dorothy Kay Brockman, with a section on male infertility by Dr. Larry Lipshultz and a special chapter on Assisted Reproductive Technology (ART) by Dr. George Grunert, is designed to help meet that challenge. *In Pursuit of Fertility* presents detailed information, providing an extended consultation with doctors who have spent their lives studying the reproductive process. Although the written word can never substitute for your personal physician, this book should answer many of your questions. You will be given an in-depth look at the causes of infertility including the impact of stress. You will be able to make informed choices concerning the specialized medical care designed to improve your chances of having a baby. Those of you with younger sisters and teenage friends and daughters will want to pass on to them how some of the most important causes of infertility can be prevented.

Infertility is a unique and often complicated problem in that it involves two patients—a husband and wife. Usually neither is sick and both are relatively young. An extremely helpful approach in diagnosing infertility is to look at each partner individually and then to consider them as a couple. Frequently, there is more than one problem with one or both of them. The husband, obviously a key factor in the fertility equation, must not be neglected. Unless both of you are examined, your doctor might treat only one problem, stop with that, and lose valuable time out of your reproductive life. In some cases, by simply considering all the problems and treating them effectively, a potentially distressing period can be transformed into months of expectation—into a happy time leading to the birth of your long-awaited child.

While dealing with infertility is never easy, with this book in hand, you and your mate can work with your doctor as well-informed participants. You will find here authoritative information; you will learn what the latest technological breakthroughs can do for you. But such amazing medical advances are only part of the picture. Having worked with thousands of infertile couples, Dr. Franklin understands that triumphing over infertility involves much more than prescribing pills and expertly wielding the scalpel. Excellent therapy includes guidance and reassurance to help you through this difficult time. Filled with case studies that show how other couples have faced infertility, Dr. Franklin's book can serve as an invaluable "companion" as you work toward your goal. With the latest information at your fingertips, many of you will end the pursuit of fertility by realizing your dream—you will have the baby you've longed for.

Veasy C. Buttram, Jr., M.D.
Past President
American Society for Reproductive Medicine
(formerly the American Fertility Society)

Authors' Note

An important note to our readers. This book was written to educate and inform, and to enable you to understand the fundamental aspects of reproduction and the problems of infertility. The book is not designed to advise or instruct you on specifically what must be done in a particular case. Once you have informed yourself, you will be in a better position to work with your doctor in resolving infertility problems. But you must consult your doctor, and be under the care of your doctor, before following any procedure described in these pages. Similarly, solutions to infertility problems that involve persons other than the natural father and mother should be arranged only after consultation with lawyers or qualified social-service professionals.

Acknowledgments

First, we would like to thank contributing authors Larry I. Lipshultz, M.D., professor of urology, Baylor College of Medicine; George M. Grunert, M.D., director of the Assisted Reproductive Technology Program at the Woman's Hospital of Texas; and Sherry M. Wilson, M.S.W.

For their invaluable contributions to the chapter on assisted reproductive technology, Richard P. Marrs, M.D., director for the Center of Assisted Reproductive Medicine, Santa Monica Hospital Medical Center; and Eberhard C. Lotze, M.D., clinical associate professor, Baylor College of Medicine.

Without the help of Eleanor Tuck, former executive director of The Gladney Center; Michael McMahon, president of The Gladney Center; Ruby Lee Piester, vice-chairman, National Council For Adoption; Marilyn Anderson, former director of Adoptive Placements, The Gladney Center; Heidi Cox, general counsel, The Gladney Center; Kayte Steinert-Threlkeld, vice-president of Public Information, The Gladney Center; and William M. Schur, J.D., the chapter on adoption would have been impossible.

We would also like to thank the following experts for their helpful comments in reviewing our book: Veasy C. Buttram, Jr., M.D., professor emeritus and former director, Division of Endocrinology-Fertility, Department of Obstetrics and Gynecology, Baylor College of Medicine, and past president of the American Society for Reproductive Medicine; Russell L. Malinak, M.D., professor, Department of Obstetrics and

Gynecology, Baylor College of Medicine; N. A. Samaan, M.D., formerly
chief, Section of Endocrinology, M. D. Anderson Hospital and Tumor
Institute; Joseph R. Feste, M.D., clinical associate professor, Baylor
College of Medicine, and clinical associate professor, The University of
Texas Health Science Center at Houston, Department of Obstetrics and
Gynecology; William J. Schindler, M.D., Ph.D., Endocrinology, Ob-
stetrical and Gynecological Associates, Houston, Texas; Gail Schindler,
Ed.D.; Nina Kellogg, Ph.D.; Ruby Lee Piester, National Council for
Adoption; Emil Steinberger, M.D., president of the Texas Institute for
Reproductive Medicine and Endocrinology; Luigi Mastroianni, Jr.,
M.D., professor and chairman, Department of Obstetrics and Gyne-
cology, University of Pennsylvania; Charles E. Flowers, Jr., M.D., pro-
fessor emeritus of obstetrics and gynecology, University of Alabama;
Emery A. Wilson, M.D., professor of obstetrics and gynecology, Di-
vision of Reproductive Endocrinology, Kentucky Center for Reproduc-
tive Medicine; Roger D. Kempers, M.D., professor of obstetrics and
gynecology, Mayo Medical School, and past president of the American
Society for Reproductive Medicine; Sherwin A. Kaufman, M.D.; Mary
Lou Ballweg, executive director, the Endometriosis Association; and
Joe S. McIlhaney, Jr., M.D., author of *1,250 Health-Care Questions
Women Ask*. The opinions expressed in this book are the authors' and
are not necessarily those of the above individuals.

We are grateful for the enthusiastic efforts of our research assistants,
Melinda L. Smith, M.S., and Autumn Lowe Brown; our wonderful medical illustrator, Jan Redden; Lana Ama, R.N., who worked with us on
the chapter on AID; our editors at Henry Holt and Company, Channa
Taub and Jo Ann Haun; our literary agent, Heide Lange of Sanford J.
Greenburger Associates; and one of our copyeditors, Ted Stanton, professor and head of journalism, University of Houston.

Finally, we would like to express our appreciation to all the members
of Dr. Franklin's staff, especially his secretary, Debbie Perry, and all
the nurses.

In
Pursuit
of
Fertility

The Miracle of Fertilization

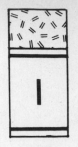

The instructions for life are written on a fragile thread of chemical memory to be passed silently from generation to generation, like a flame exchanged from burning wick to wick, the spark of life itself—first animating the living, then guarded by them, as they too reproduce so as not to let the sacred fires flicker out.

NATIONAL GEOGRAPHIC SOCIETY,
The Incredible Machine

The Reproductive Process

The woman's body is poised for pregnancy. On the surface of her left ovary a blisterlike bubble called a "follicle" bulges blood-red (see fig. 1.1). The follicle is about to burst and spew forth its life-giving fluid. Within this straw-colored brew sits the human egg—waiting to be set free. Smaller than the dot over an "i," the egg carries half of the instructions for life. The fragile egg's wait is short. The woman's brain is about to react to a powerful hormonal message emitting from the saclike follicle.

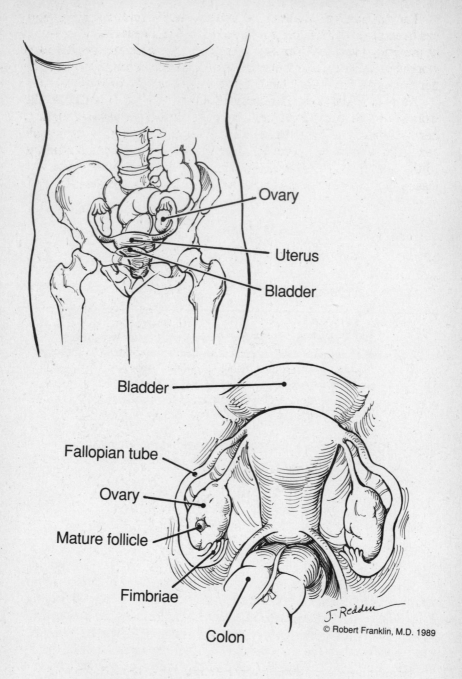

FIGURE 1.1. *The female reproductive organs, including the uterus, fallopian tubes, and ovaries.*

For the past two weeks, the woman's whole reproductive system has been preparing for this pivotal moment. Communicating via a series of precisely executed hormonal messages, her brain and ovaries have worked together in perfect synchronization to ripen a follicle and to make her uterus (womb) ready to accept the egg if fertilized (see fig. 1.2).

As with every creative effort, the spark of life is rekindled in the woman's head. Around the first day of her monthly menstrual period, her hypothalamus (lower brain), responding to low levels of the female sex hormone estrogen in the blood, sent an important chemical message to the pituitary gland (the master gland), at the base of her brain. Released approximately every ninety minutes, the hormonal message read:

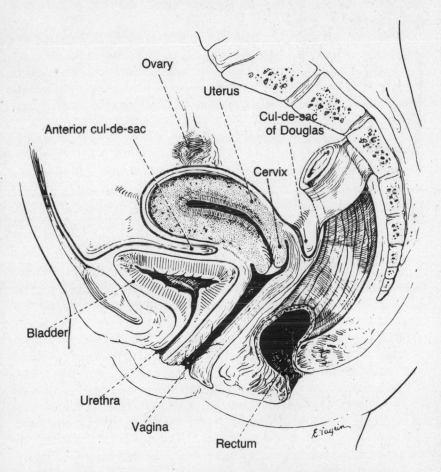

FIGURE 1.2. Sagittal or midline view of the normal female pelvis. (Reproduced with permission from R. W. Kistner, Gynecology: Principles and Practice, 4th ed., copyright © 1986 by Year Book Medical Publishers, Inc., Chicago.)

It is time to stimulate the ovaries to mature an egg! Secrete follicle-stimulating hormone (FSH).

Following orders, the pituitary released the sex hormone FSH into the bloodstream. Picked up by special FSH receptors on the ovaries, this hormonal message read: It is time to start maturing an egg! Tell the cells of the follicle surrounding the egg to start making the hormone estrogen.

Stimulated by FSH, eight to fifteen of the woman's lifetime supply of four to five hundred thousand eggs were recruited, although only one becomes dominant and fully matures during each menstrual cycle (see fig. 1.3). For some unknown reason probably related to the hormones, the rest of the eggs picked to ripen that month will stop growing and eventually die.

Now almost mature, the dominant follicle—called the "Graafian follicle"—signals that the egg along with its nutritive cells wants to be set free from the ovary. The message once again is hormonal. The cells in the ovarian follicles suddenly increase estrogen production to its highest monthly level. This burst of estrogen in the blood tells the pituitary that the egg is ripe.

Sensing the estrogen surge, the pituitary releases a large amount of another powerful sex hormone called "luteinizing hormone" (LH) into the bloodstream. This midcycle LH surge is picked up by LH receptors on the woman's ovary, which read the hormonal message as follows: Trigger the release of the egg! Within twenty-four to thirty-six hours, the follicle finishes maturing and the egg pops out into the abdominal cavity. This premier event is called "ovulation."

Once released, the precious egg is never left unattended. It is surrounded and picked up by the hormonally activated fimbriae (petallike fingers) on the end of one of the woman's two fallopian tubes or oviducts. Although these flowerlike tubal fingers sometimes miss, meaning that conception probably won't occur that cycle, this time they whisk the egg and its barely visible protective layers into the oviduct (see fig. 1.3). A muscular tube, the narrow oviduct acts as a conduit between its paired ovary and the hollow uterus.

Once inside the undulating fallopian tube, the egg surrounded by its "nurse" cells finds a friendly environment. The egg's tubal captor secretes a special fluid that nourishes the germ cell and helps convey it toward its goal—the uterus. Moved along by microscopic hairlike cilia that line the narrow tubal walls, the egg begins its eighty-hour journey through the approximately four-and-a-half-inch fallopian tube.

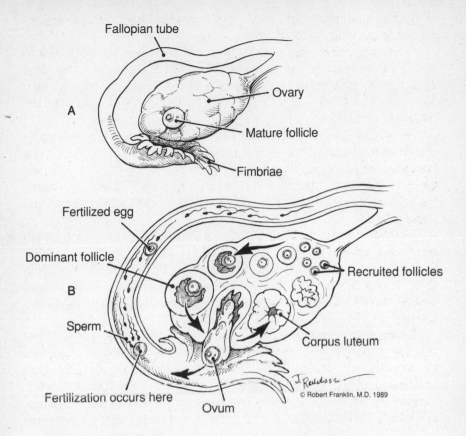

Fallopian tube

Ovary

Mature follicle

Fimbriae

A

Fertilized egg

Dominant follicle

Recruited follicles

B

Sperm

Corpus luteum

Fertilization occurs here

Ovum

© Robert Franklin, M.D. 1989

FIGURE 1.3. A. A nearly ripe egg-harboring follicle bulging from an ovary.
B. Cross-section of an ovary showing changes occurring during the menstrual
cycle. Each month, eight to fifteen eggs are recruited, but usually only one fully
matures. At ovulation, the petallike fimbriae whisk the egg into the oviduct.
Note how after the egg is released the follicle is transformed into the
progesterone-producing corpus luteum.

In about one to two hours, the egg arrives in a widened part of the tube called the "ampulla"—the place where fertilization usually occurs (see fig. 1.4). But at this point, the egg's descent through the oviduct suddenly stops. As if held by some mysterious force, the egg sits for hours in the ampulla waiting to be fertilized. Unless the sperm arrive in time—in less than twenty-four hours—the delicate egg will deteriorate and die.

Meanwhile, the initiators of fertilization, the sperm, are deposited by the father-to-be in the vagina near the cervix, which is the mouth of

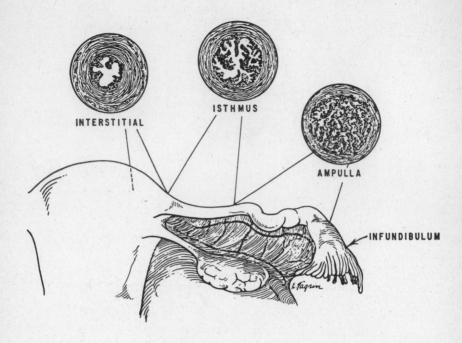

FIGURE 1.4. Sections of the fallopian tube or oviduct. The ampulla is where fertilization often occurs. (Reproduced with permission from R. W. Kistner, Gynecology: Principles and Practice, 4th ed., copyright © 1986 by Year Book Medical Publishers, Inc., Chicago.)

the uterus (see fig. 1.5). Before arriving in the hostile acidic environment of the vagina, the sperm have been carefully groomed for their difficult journey through the female reproductive tract. Their short, active life begins in the man's testicles, in the saclike scrotum (see fig. 1.6). Within each of the two testicles are tubes called "seminiferous tubules" that contain Sertoli cells and millions of sperm-cell generators known as "spermatogonia" or "mother cells." The Sertoli cells, which respond to the messenger hormone FSH from the pituitary, help the mother cells manufacture sperm. Lying between the tubules are the Leydig cells. When acted upon by pituitary LH, the Leydig cells produce the powerful hormone testosterone—the sex hormone that is responsible for a man's masculine appearance.

As the sperm develop within the testicles, they are protected and fed by the large Sertoli cells or "nurse" cells. When nearly mature but

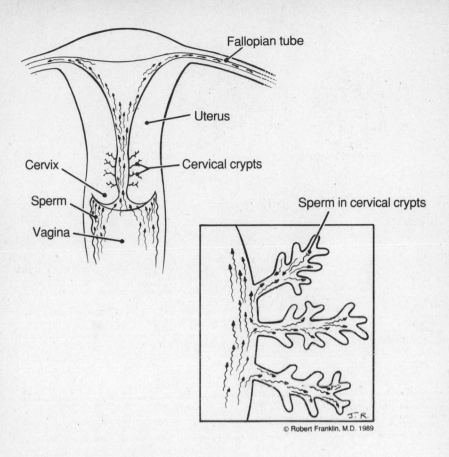

Fallopian tube

Uterus

Cervix

Cervical crypts

Sperm

Vagina

Sperm in cervical crypts

© Robert Franklin, M.D. 1989

FIGURE 1.5. After being deposited near the cervix, some sperm temporarily remain in the cervical crypts.

still unable to swim, the sperm are moved to the epididymis, located behind and attached to each paired testicle (see fig. 1.6). Once within the twelve-to-fifteen-foot coiled canal of the epididymis, the tadpolelike sperm attain their remarkable swimming ability.

When the sperm leave the epididymis during ejaculation, they move through the vasa deferentia (plural of vas deferens or ductus deferens), two long tubes each located within one of the two spermatic cords (see fig. 1.6). (The vasa deferentia are the pair of sperm ducts that are severed during a vasectomy to make a man sterile.) Before the sperm reach the urethra, they are mixed with other fluids to form the man's semen. In addition to the sperm, the semen is made up of the lu-

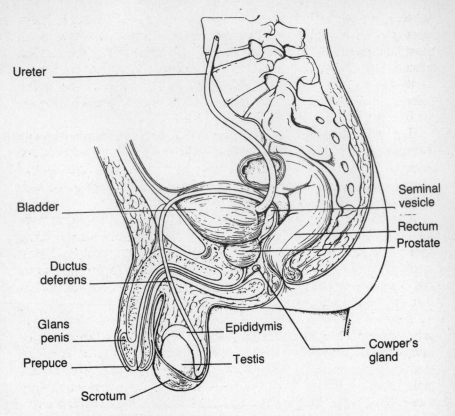

Ureter

Bladder

Ductus
deferens

Glans
penis

Prepuce

Scrotum

Seminal
vesicle

Rectum

Prostate

Epididymis

Testis

Cowper's
gland

FIGURE 1.6. A sperm's life begins in one of the testicles (testes), in the scrotum. Once nearly mature, the sperm is moved to the epididymis, behind and attached to the testicle. During ejaculation, the sperm moves through the ductus deferens, or sperm duct. In addition to the sperm, the semen also contains fluids from the Cowper's glands, the prostate gland, and the sugar-containing solution from the seminal vesicles. (E. E. Chaffee and E. M. Greisheimer, Basic Physiology & Anatomy, 3rd ed., Philadelphia: J. B. Lippincott, 1974.)

bricating fluid of the Cowper's glands, the alkaline fluid of the prostate gland, and a sugar-containing solution from the seminal vesicles (see fig. 1.6).

Once within the vagina, the sperm's tough journey has just begun. Not only is the vagina too acidic for the sperm, but even their own thick white seminal fluid is hostile and must be shed. If the sperm are unable to find their way into the more alkaline cervix within approximately one half-hour, they will perish.

Surrounded by more than two hundred million other hopeful competitors, one perfectly formed sperm is propelling itself toward its cherished goal—the waiting egg. To win a chance at immortality, this sperm must be a powerful, straight swimmer. It has to penetrate the cervical mucus, find the small entrance to the cervix, traverse the uterus—a cavity the size of an ocean in relation to its size—ascend one of the fallopian tubes, and be the first to penetrate the egg—no small challenge for one of the tiniest cells in the body (see fig. 1.7).

Determined to win the only race it will ever run, this vigorously swimming sperm sets forth on its long, difficult journey, its tail swishing behind it. Fueled by sugar-filled energy packets in its midpiece, the microscopic sperm swims upstream in the uterus through a specially prepared mucus coming from the cervix.

Capable of fertilization for at least forty-eight hours, the sperm finds the small passageway leading to the womb. The entrance is open. If the sperm had arrived at *any* other time except around ovulation, the cervix would have been shut tight. But under the influence of estrogen from the ovary, the cervix and the cervical mucus have been transformed so that the sperm can enter.

At *all* other times during the menstrual cycle, the cervical mucus acts as a remarkable filter that guards the upper reproductive tract against bacteria and sperm. But for a few days around ovulation, the number of sperm-killing white blood cells in the mucus drops, and the molecules line up in parallel rows that help direct the sperm as they ascend the cervix. At midcycle, the mucus changes from a thick pluglike barrier to a clear watery liquid with remarkable *Spinnbarkeit* or stretchability. Now copious and thin, the cervical mucus serves as a vehicle that allows the sperm to migrate toward the uterus.

As each sperm in the squadron travels through the cervix, it is washed by the cervical mucus. Molecular changes occur in the sperm's bulletlike head that prepare it to fertilize the egg. This process, whereby the enzyme inhibitor is removed from the sperm head, is called "capacitation." Unless capacitated, the sperm will be incapable of penetrating the relatively thick membrane enclosing the egg, called the "zona pellucida."

Once inside the cervix, the "chosen" sperm has outmaneuvered over 99 percent of its competitors. The misshapen ones especially are left behind. Although the race's formidable odds of two hundred million to one are now reduced to a "mere" million or more to one, the event is far from over.

In the race to perpetuate the human race, standard rules do not apply. The first sperm to ascend the upper female reproductive tract

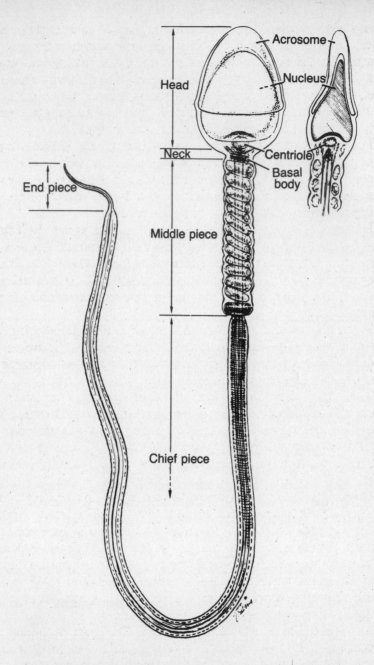

FIGURE 1.7. *Perfectly formed oval-shaped sperm fueled by energy packets in the midpiece. (Reproduced, with permission, from J. A. Pritchard, P. C. MacDonald, and N. F. Gant,* Williams Obstetrics, *17th ed., copyright © Appleton-Century-Crofts, 1985.)*

may *not* be the winner. Any of the following sets of unfortunate circumstances could mean certain death for the heroic sperm: if the egg has not arrived in the fallopian tube; if the egg is in one tube but the sperm picks the other; or if the egg is waiting but the sperm fails to penetrate the egg or misses its target completely. In some cases, the sperm might exit the tube near the ovary to find itself floating around the abdominal cavity, rather like a brave astronaut left to die in space.

The sperm that ultimately wins has perfect timing. Unlike many of its competitors, which temporarily remain in the cryptlike reservoirs of the cervix (see fig. 1.5), this sperm immediately ascends the woman's upper reproductive tract. With luck on its side, the sperm enters the left fallopian tube—the one that holds the prize.

Though a fierce competitor, the chosen sperm is not the first in line—it is the *twentieth!* Nonetheless, it valiantly pursues the leaders as they swim one inch per minute upstream through the tubal mucus. Within fifteen minutes, all top twenty rivals reach the ampulla, closely followed by fifty others. The cherished egg—the largest cell in the body—looms straight ahead.

As the first contenders approach the target, their movements spin the egg like a slow-moving top. By chance, or perhaps by destiny, every one of them either misses or fails to penetrate the egg—their opportunity to fertilize lost forever.

Now, at last, the chosen sperm's time has come. If it can penetrate the egg, no other sperm can enter. More by chance than by aim, it hits the egg straight on. Releasing enzymes from its oval-shaped head, the sperm tunnels through the egg's protective layers. The first to reach the egg's membrane, the penetrating sperm is pulled inside, stiffening its tail.

An electrical charge fires across the membrane, preventing further entry. Losing its midpiece and tail, the sperm head ruptures—spilling its life-giving contents within the egg. Forever losing their separate identities, the nuclei of the sperm and the egg fuse, their chromosomes uniting: a totally unique human is created; its future appearance and innate intelligence are now set. Determining the sex of its offspring, the winning sperm has carried its genetic code—the accumulation of ten thousand generations—to the egg. The race is won!

But the final outcome remains undecided. The future of the dividing fertilized egg is far from certain. To survive, it has only one week to traverse the fallopian tube and implant itself in the endometrium, the lining of the uterus. During most of this time, the "pre-embryo" (the dividing fertilized egg) will be nourished by its small amount of on-board yolk and by the tubal mucus.

After about six days, the fertilized egg passes from the oviduct into the uterus. Its lining is lush and at exactly the right stage of development. The female sex hormones estrogen and progesterone have prepared the uterine nest for its tiny guest. First, ovarian estrogen stimulated the growth of the endometrium. About two or three days after the woman's menstrual flow stopped, the uterine lining was only one to two millimeters thick (see fig. 1.8). Although still underdeveloped, by ovulation (day 11 to day 14 into the monthly cycle) the endometrium had increased to a thickness of six to seven millimeters.

Immediately following ovulation, an amazing transformation occurred in the ovary that indirectly affected the endometrium. When the egg was released from its sac, the abandoned follicle filled with blood and turned into an orange-yellow endocrine gland called the corpus luteum. Playing a vital role in the preparation of the uterine lining for pregnancy, the corpus luteum produces progesterone—the female sex hormone that makes the endometrium lush and calms down uterine contractions.

By day 20 to day 24—the time when implantation is most likely to occur—progesterone had made the lining of the uterus soft and velvety and seven to eight millimeters thick. If the corpus luteum had secreted progesterone either in too small an amount or for too short a time, the endometrium would have been "out of phase" when the embryo arrived. Unable to implant, the fertilized egg would have died and passed out of the uterus unnoticed.

But the woman's infinitely complex reproductive system has performed exquisitely. During this menstrual cycle, her hypothalamus, pituitary gland, ovaries, cervix, fallopian tubes, and uterus have worked together in perfect concert. When the sixteen-celled fertilized egg arrives in the uterus—exactly on schedule—all is in readiness.

Its cells dividing, the pre-embryo at first floats free in the womb (see fig. 1.9). But with its portable food supply dangerously low, the tiny organism hovers over a possible nesting place. Exchanging mysterious chemical messages with the lush uterine lining, the pre-embryo prepares to implant itself. It brushes against the wall of the uterus and quickly burrows its way into the nutrient-rich endometrium, tying into the maternal blood supply. The woman now is pregnant.

Carrying the sacred spark of life, the demanding human conceptus takes over its mother—body, spirit, and heart. Once again the fragile fire flickers on—passed through the centuries from flaming torch to torch, from sperm to egg, from parent to child, and from Genesis to Revelation.

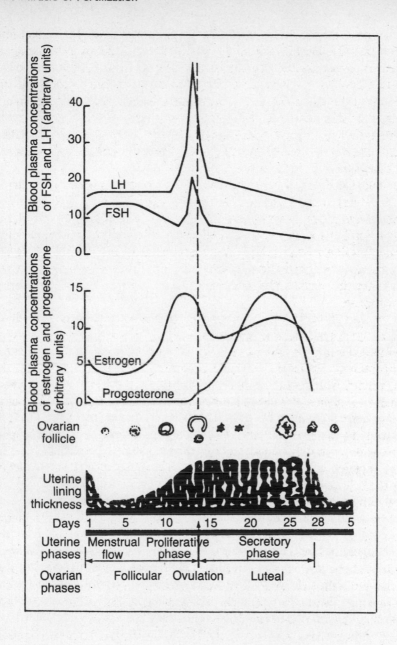

FIGURE 1.8. *Under hormonal influence, the lining of the uterus changes during the menstrual cycle. (Reproduced with permission from Arthur J. Vander, James H. Sherman, and Dorothy S. Luciano,* Human Physiology: The Mechanisms of Body Function, *3rd ed., New York: McGraw-Hill, 1980.)*

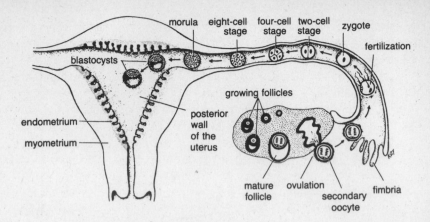

FIGURE 1.9. The ovarian cycle, fertilization, and human development during the first week. (From Keith L. Moore, The Developing Human, 4th ed., Philadelphia: W. B. Saunders Co., 1988.)

How Can You Help Make This Miracle Happen for You?

When a patient and her husband first come to see me, they want to know how they can help make the miracle of fertilization happen for them. Sometimes they have none of the reproductive problems covered throughout this book. Often all that may be necessary to shorten the time until pregnancy is some simple advice about the basics of conception. A patient may ask: "What can I do to increase my chances of having a baby?" "How can I tell if I am ovulating or releasing an egg?" "When is the most fertile time of my menstrual cycle?" "When and how often should we have intercourse?"

Sometimes, before I can answer, a patient will say: "Maybe the problem is that both of us are under a great deal of pressure. We work long hours to meet project deadlines. Often we are just too exhausted to have marital relations except on weekends." Some women tell me that, if they do have intercourse on a weeknight, they often are so tired that it is mechanical. In such cases they may use vaginal lubricants such as Vaseline or K-Y jelly.

Many patients say that the demands of keeping a job and running a household mean that they do everything "on the run," including eating. Said one woman: "I seldom sit down to a proper breakfast or lunch. And when I do, I worry that every bite will add to my weight."

I recommend that my infertility patients with hurried lifestyles set aside some time for themselves and for their mates. Most people know this is important, but they fail to do so for various reasons. Patients say: "I have to work overtime to pay the rent," "I'm saving for a VCR," or "I'm putting my husband through medical school." One woman said that she had to work weekdays, every evening, and weekends to buy a horse. Women under intense pressure often do become pregnant, but some patients who have difficulty coping with stress have problems conceiving. There are several reasons for this. As discussed in detail later in chapter 4, crash diets and severe stress can cause irregular ovulation and missed menstrual periods. In addition, if intercourse is mechanical and the woman isn't given time to become sexually aroused, she may not lubricate. This leads to the use of vaginal lubricants, many of which stop sperm dead in their tracks.

All of us have goals that are important to us. But if fertility is near the top of your list, you might consider temporarily setting aside some of those near the bottom, thus making more time for yourself and your mate. This doesn't mean that you need to quit your job, or that your additional time together necessarily should be spent trying to have a baby. You may just wish to enjoy each other's company and let nature take its course.

Sometimes you may want to wait until morning to make love. Because male hormone levels are highest at this time and most people are rested, mornings are an especially fertile time for some couples. If you are comfortable with this arrangement, you should wake up early enough to stay together for a while. I also recommend that a woman remain in bed for about one hour after intercourse.

Charting Ovulation

A woman's fertile time is around ovulation. Ideally, the sperm should be in the fallopian tubes when the egg is released. Normally, one of the two ovaries will ovulate at midcycle, meaning that the egg is released about fourteen days after the menstrual period starts. In other words, if a patient has a twenty-eight-day cycle, ovulation will occur on approximately the fourteenth day, plus or minus a day. If she has a longer cycle—for example, thirty-two days—the egg usually will be released on about the eighteenth day. For the patient with a short cycle, say twenty-three or twenty-four days, subtract fourteen days from the length of the cycle to try to predict the day of ovulation.

There are physical signs that suggest ovulation. Some women have pain in the lower part of the abdomen when they ovulate. Occasionally a patient will describe this as a "pinglike" pain on one side or the other, depending on which ovary has released an egg; some women describe the pain as lasting longer. Breast tenderness during the last part of the menstrual cycle may indicate that ovulation has occurred.

A fairly accurate way to track ovulation is to chart your basal body temperature (BBT). This can indicate whether and when you are ovulating. Following ovulation, the BBT goes up at least half a degree and remains elevated for approximately twelve to sixteen days. Since your temperature goes up *after* ovulation, you cannot use this to predict exactly when to have intercourse in order to achieve fertilization. But by charting your temperature over several months, you can get a good idea of when in your cycle you are likely to ovulate.

Your basal body temperature is your morning temperature before *any* activity, after sleeping for at least three hours. This means that the thermometer should be shaken down to 96.5 degrees Fahrenheit the previous night, and you should take your temperature immediately after you waken, before getting up or going to the bathroom, et cetera. To see if you ovulate, start taking your temperature the morning your menses begin (this is day 1) and continue taking it every morning until your next period. It is important to use a specially calibrated thermometer designed to detect temperature changes as small as 0.1 degree; a regular thermometer is not calibrated finely enough. (Fast electronic digital thermometers that are easy to read are available.) Record the results on a graph; this is called an "ovulation chart." Once you connect all the dots, you will see your ovulatory pattern for that menstrual cycle (see fig. 1.10). Menses are usually marked on the chart with an *M* or an *O*, and coitus with a *C* or an *X*.

If your temperature chart is higher during the last part of the cycle, this indicates that you probably released an egg. A flat chart indicates lack of ovulation. If you ovulate and become pregnant, your temperature will remain elevated; otherwise it will usually drop to its preovulatory temperature, and your menstrual period will begin (see the chart in fig. 1.11).

Why does the basal body temperature increase after the release of the egg? In a normally ovulating woman, the BBT shifts upward because of the thermogenic (heat-producing) effect of the sex hormone progesterone. You will recall that, after a mature ovum (egg) pops out of the ovary, the follicle (the now empty egg sac) is dramatically transformed: its cells, which nourished the egg before ovulation, turn into the semisolid corpus-luteum gland, sometimes called the "yellow body" (see fig. 1.12). This newly formed gland starts secreting progesterone—the hormone

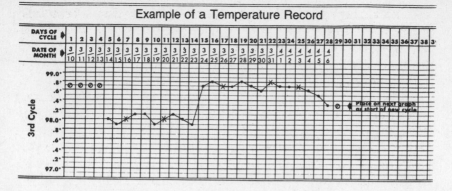

FIGURE 1.10. Ovulation chart, also called "basal-body-temperature chart" or "BBT chart." (Courtesy of Ob & Gyn Associates, Houston, Texas.)

that prepares the lining of the uterus for pregnancy. Since progesterone elevates BBT, the woman's temperature goes up during the last half of her cycle, indicating presumptive ovulation. (We say presumptive because sometimes an egg matures but is not released from its follicle, owing to a hormonal defect or an abnormal enzyme.)

Once you have taken your BBT for several months, you will have a clearer picture of your overall ovulatory pattern. If it is regular, it can be used to attempt to predict the fertile time of future cycles. The low point on the chart, just before the temperature shifts upward, is the most likely time for conception to occur (see figs. 1.10 and 1.11). You will have the best chance for pregnancy if you have intercourse every other day around ovulation. If you abstain until after the temperature shift, it might be too late. If your periods are irregular, predicting the release of the egg with the BBT is difficult, because the day of ovulation is unknown until *after* the upward temperature shift.

There is another method of predicting ovulation at home that can serve to indicate when a woman is about to ovulate, but it is more expensive and complicated than the one just described. A few women don't have the usual 0.5-degree upward temperature shift following ovulation. These patients, however, still can track ovulation with home ovulation kits that measure the pituitary sex hormone LH. Women make small amounts of LH during most of their menstrual cycle. But as you now know, just before ovulation a large amount of LH is secreted. This LH surge causes the amount of this hormone in the blood to increase five to ten times and usually occurs at the lowest point on the temperature chart. As mentioned earlier, this sudden increase in LH triggers ovulation about twenty-four to twenty-eight hours after LH starts to surge.

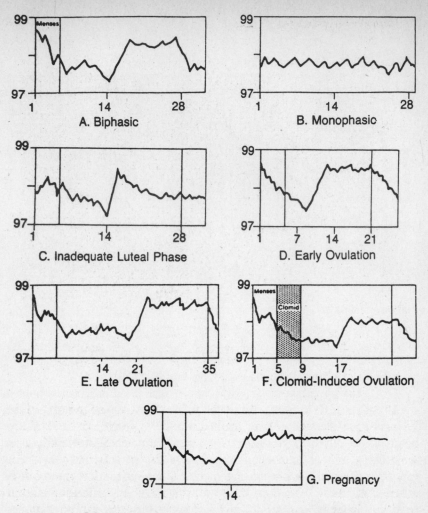

FIGURE 1.11. *Basal-body-temperature charts, including pregnancy. The low point is the most likely time for conception to occur. (From V. C. Buttram,* Surgical Treatment of the Infertile Female, *Baltimore: Williams & Wilkins Co., 1985.)*

Women can detect this LH surge by testing their urine with one of the self-test kits. These provide ovulation sticks that turn a specific color (usually blue) during the LH surge, indicating that the egg probably is about to be released. Since these home kits are expensive, we recommend them mainly for women with no thermal shift, for patients who need to predict the day of ovulation for artificial inseminations, or for women who don't want to take their temperature every day.

For most patients, simply taking the basal body temperature—if done carefully—remains a good method of documenting ovulation, because it is inexpensive, relatively accurate, and easy to do. (See chapter 4 for more information on ovulation.)

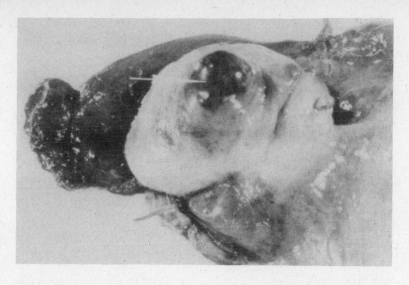

FIGURE 1.12. The corpus luteum (this one is of early pregnancy) secretes the sex
hormone progesterone. (Courtesy of Dr. R. Vogt, from J. A. Pritchard,
P. C. MacDonald, and N. F. Gant, Williams Obstetrics, 17th ed., copyright ©
Appleton-Century-Crofts, 1985.)

Although past ovulation charts can serve as a guide suggesting when
the egg might be available for fertilization in the future, don't let them
dictate your sex life. Knowing when ovulation probably will occur is
helpful, but a spontaneous approach to achieving pregnancy is more
important than a stack of ovulation charts indicating that intercourse
occurred at "baby" time. If you and your husband are exhausted around
ovulation, having "mechanical" sex just to have a baby can be counter-
productive in the long run. It is better to enjoy your time together.
Often this is the best way to make a baby.

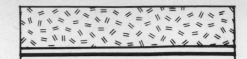

Part I

Female Infertility: Evaluation and Treatment

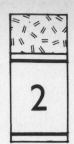

2

Endometriosis

I have waited far longer than nine months for the miracle of this moment—I have waited for six agonizing years.

For one second, my glance falls upon my husband. Standing beside me, he keeps his eyes riveted to the mirror at the end of the delivery table. His face is flushed with anticipation, but his warm, supportive hands have turned to ice.

As the strain of childbirth passes over me, my only thought is: Will our baby be OK?

Endometriosis has played havoc with my reproductive system—destroying all but a tiny part of each ovary. And yet, with the help of one of the best infertility teams in the world, we have beaten the heartbreaking odds stacked against us.

To me—at this moment—it seems unbelievable that the baby inside me could be perfectly healthy. But about one thing I have no doubt: I will love it forever, no matter what happens.

Our years of longing for a baby are rapidly coming to an end. In the mirror, I can see the top of a tiny rotating head being pushed into this unforgiving world. My spirit watches and marvels, almost as if detached, as my body births our child.

He has arrived! The healthiest, plumpest, and to us the most beautiful baby boy ever born, a tiny twin of my husband. The memory of his rosy-cheeked face is etched forever upon my heart.

As I look down at him, I feel as though the anguish of the past six years has made his birth seem still more of a miracle. The countless hours in my doctor's waiting room, the endless testing and retesting, even the pain of major surgery—all these memories fade before the glow of the tiny being in my arms.

"We prayed so hard for him, doctor," I whisper.

"We all did, Georgia, we all did," he says.

—Georgia

As I hurried across the street from the hospital to the office five years ago, my thoughts turned to my next patient, Georgia.* She and her husband, Paul, had been trying unsuccessfully to have a baby for four years. As I shook Paul's hand, I could tell by the way he glared at me from behind his black-rimmed glasses that he had been waiting in my office a little too long. His voice was friendly, but his restless manner indicated that he had many other things on his mind.

The couple had attended our Infertility Class, which explains the importance of getting the husband involved in the infertility workup right from the beginning. Nevertheless, I sensed that Paul, a busy tax attorney, felt that he was wasting his time by accompanying his wife to her first appointment with me.

My job as Georgia and Paul's infertility specialist was to find out why they had been unable to conceive. In time we would discover that Georgia's infertility was associated with a disease called endometriosis. But the challenge was more than making the diagnosis and treating the disease effectively. The couple needed help in dealing with the stress of infertility. Although cases involving endometriosis are similar, no two are exactly alike. The history of the progression of the disease—the pain and the patient's reaction to it—are described differently by every woman. Georgia and Paul's story was like no other. When our team succeeds in helping a couple have a baby, as we did with Georgia and Paul, our work is unbelievably rewarding.

When Georgia first walked into my office earlier that morning, my nurse of many years, Adele, introduced her to one of my fourth-year residents. He asked Georgia the routine medical questions necessary for a thorough gynecologic history. Since infertility is an extremely private subject, the questioning must be tactful. The medical workup delves into personal areas such as menstrual irregularities and the tension that a couple is experiencing in sexual activity. To Georgia, as is true of most patients, the inability to have a child was an overwhelming emotional problem. Our goal was to make her and Paul feel comfortable by treating

*The names and details have been changed throughout.

them in a warm yet efficient manner, with as much individual attention as possible. We wanted to eliminate any possibility that they might feel caught up in an uncaring medical machine.

Georgia said that she had stopped taking estrogen-dominant birth-control pills four years earlier. (As we will discuss later, this was the wrong type of oral contraceptive for her.) Planning for a large family, the couple had purchased a four-bedroom house across the street from an elementary school. After trying to have a baby for one year, Georgia had become worried and had visited her gynecologist of nine years. He had mentioned that her uterus was "tipped," but had reassured her that at twenty-four she just needed to relax and give herself a little time.

When another six months passed, however, and no baby was on the way, Georgia decided to visit another doctor. He suggested that she chart her basal body temperature (BBT) to see if she was ovulating (releasing an egg) each menstrual cycle. (For a review of charting ovulation, see chapter 1.)

As instructed, Georgia faithfully charted her BBT, starting on the first day of her menstrual flow (see fig. 1.10). Every morning, before any activity (she could not put one foot on the floor or even sip a cup of coffee in bed), Georgia took her temperature with a specially calibrated thermometer. She recorded the results on an "ovulation chart."

Around the fourteenth day of nearly every cycle, Georgia's temperature jumped at least 0.5 degrees Fahrenheit, indicating that she had ovulated. You will recall that the low point on the chart, just before the temperature shifts upward, is the most likely time for conception to take place (see fig. 1.11[A]). Georgia's doctor suggested that the couple have intercourse every other day around this time.

Although charting the BBT is the simplest way of tracking ovulation, the doctor must remember that the temperature chart can become an instrument that harms the marital relationship. As therapist Sherry Wilson discusses in chapter 10, the rigidity of taking the basal temperature every single morning, month after month, and having sex because the chart changes, can become stressful, especially for the male. If I sense this happening with one of my couples, I back off charting ovulation. In an infertility workup, any added tension is self-defeating—it is just what the doctor should *not* order for an already anxious patient. I want the temperature chart to help, not hurt, her chances of conceiving.

By the time Georgia came to see me, she was sick of sticking a thermometer in her mouth every morning. Exasperated, she handed me thirteen charts with "X"s marking every single time she and her husband had made love for over a year. In spite of all this effort, she had not conceived.

"Why do you think I haven't gotten pregnant?" Georgia asked me, her eyes glistening. "You can see that I ovulated every month last year." "That is exactly what we are going to find out," I answered.

What Is Endometriosis?

Many of the questions that we asked Georgia were directed toward finding out whether she had endometriosis. A "benign" invasive disease that affects between four and ten million women in the United States alone, endometriosis is one of the major causes of infertility. What is this mysterious-sounding condition that causes millions of women so much physical and emotional suffering? Simply put, it is a puzzling disease in which misplaced menstrual tissue identical to the endometrium (lining of the uterus or womb) grows *outside* the uterus—in the pelvis, for example (see fig. 2.1).

During menstruation, some of the menses can back up through the fallopian tubes (uterine tubes) into the pelvic cavity (see fig. 2.2). (Doctors call this backward flow "retrograde" or "reflux menstruation.") In some women this ectopic (out-of-place) tissue eventually implants itself on the pelvic organs, often on the ovaries. During each cycle, this tissue, now called "endometriosis," acts just like the uterine lining: Since it is usually hormonally responsive, it builds up, breaks down, and bleeds. But, unlike the endometrium inside the uterus, endometriosis in the pelvis has no way of leaving the body (see fig. 2.1). If it is left untreated, it is easy to imagine why this disease can become progressively worse with each monthly cycle, often causing pain and infertility.

What is the most common place in the pelvis for endometriosis to implant itself? Although some doctors will say it is on the ovaries, I find the disease most often on the left uterosacral ligament (one of several ligaments that support the uterus) (see fig. 2.2). Endometriosis also can grow on the outside of the uterus, around and inside the fallopian tubes, around the ureters (the tubes that carry urine from the kidneys to the bladder), on the bladder, on the rectum, and on the small intestines. Other common locations are in the pouchlike culs-de-sac in the front and the back of the uterus (see figs. 2.1 and 2.2).

Occasionally doctors find endometriosis in locations outside the pelvic cavity. These less common sites are the cervix (the neck of the womb, which sticks out into the vagina), the vagina, and the vulva. I have even seen patients with endometriosis in the lungs, nose, or eye. Fortunately, the disease rarely travels to these locations.

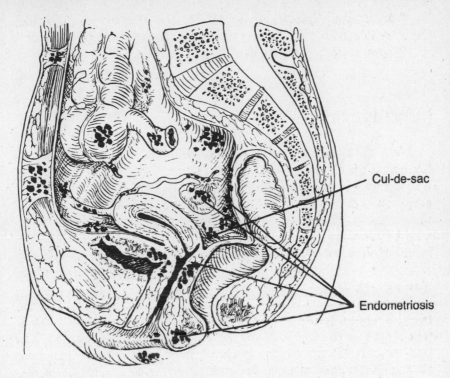

Cul-de-sac

Endometriosis

FIGURE 2.1. Endometriosis. The out-of-place endometrial tissue has no way of leaving the body. (Reproduced, with permission, from L. W. Way, Current Surgical Diagnosis & Treatment, 6th ed., copyright © Lange Medical Publications, 1983.)

Adhesions: Fertility Enemy!

Adhesions—the enemy of fertility—are one of the most common complications associated with endometriosis. These rubbery bands of scar tissue sometimes form between surfaces inside the body and tie down the pelvic organs (see fig. 2.3). Adhesions can be filmy and cobweblike or dense and fibrous. Some are almost as hard as concrete! Even the delicate weblike adhesions can cause infertility if they keep the fallopian tubes (oviducts) from picking up the egg. If the scar tissue covers the ovaries or the ends of the tubes, or pulls the entrance to each oviduct away from its ovary, the fimbriated ends of the tubes (the little tubal "fingers") will be unable to whisk the egg from the surface of the ovary into the tube (see fig. 2.4). The weblike adhesions can be removed during a minor surgical procedure, but major surgery is necessary to eliminate dense scar tissue.

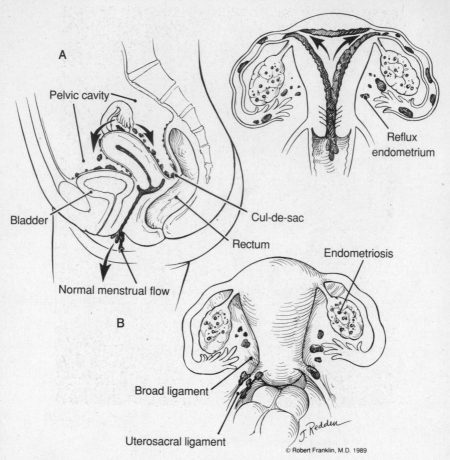

A

Pelvic cavity

Reflux endometrium

Bladder

Cul-de-sac

Rectum

Endometriosis

Normal menstrual flow

B

Broad ligament

Uterosacral ligament

© Robert Franklin, M.D. 1989

FIGURE 2.2. A. Reflux menstruation into the pelvic cavity. Note how the blood seeps backward through the tubes into the pelvis. B. Endometriosis is often found on the uterosacral ligaments.

Surgery can remove adhesions, but it also can cause them. For this reason, I always ask new infertility patients if they have had an abdominal operation. Even fertility surgery can lead to adhesion formation. I also see many young women with adhesions who had their appendixes removed during childhood. An infected or ruptured appendix, as well as the operation to remove it, can cause adhesions to form between organs, especially if microsurgical techniques are not used.

Exciting developments in surgical techniques have reduced but not eliminated postsurgical adhesion formation. The most extensively studied surgical aid to limit scar-tissue development is a satiny "cloth-like"

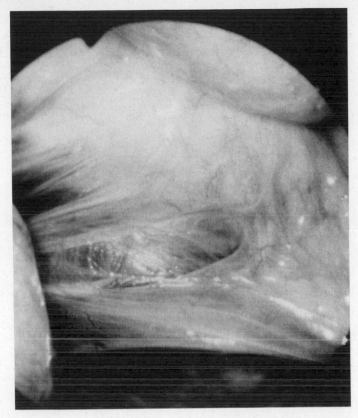

FIGURE 2.3. *Photograph of adhesions or scar tissue that can cause infertility.*
(Courtesy of Dr. E. Lotze.)

substance called Interceed. A specially prepared cellulose mesh, Interceed is applied to traumatized pelvic surfaces. Within an hour this operative aid turns to a Jell-O-like substance, adhering to raw tissues and keeping them from sticking together. Within a week—the critical time for preventing adhesions—Interceed is absorbed by the body. Two other barriers used to reduce adhesions, the GORE-TEX Surgical Membrane and the HAL-F Membrane have recently shown promise. In addition to these operative aids, microsurgery, gentle handling of the tissues, and judicious use of drugs that decrease inflammation and swelling are other key methods of lessening adhesion formation following surgery.

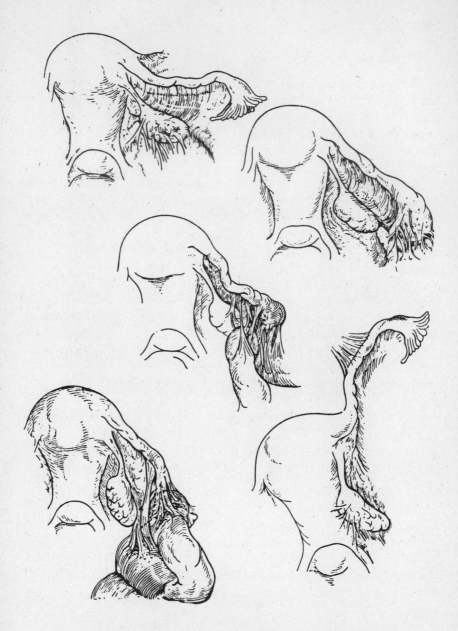

FIGURE 2.4. *Adhesions or scar tissue. The tubal fingers are unable to whisk the egg into the fallopian tube. (Reproduced with permission from R. W. Kistner and G. W. Patton, Atlas of Infertility Surgery. Boston: Little Brown & Co., 1975.)*

Symptoms

Menstrual Cramps

When an endometriosis patient first comes to see me, she usually has been trying to get pregnant for at least one year, sometimes for several years. She often complains of considerable cyclical pain related to menstruation, or what doctors call "dysmenorrhea." In fact, "worse than normal" cramping in an infertility patient often is an important clue pointing to endometriosis.

Not all endometriosis patients, however, have severe menstrual cramps—many women have no warning symptoms of any kind that they have the disease. The amount of pain does *not* necessarily correlate with the severity of the disease. I see some women who have few symptoms yet have extensive endometriosis, often in the ovaries, and others with minimal disease who have severe pain.

Georgia had said that her menstrual pain was "not too bad." However, after treating endometriosis patients for over twenty-six years, I have learned that women sometimes refuse to admit that their cramping is "worse than normal."

Why do some women feel ill at ease about discussing menstrual pain, even with their gynecologists? One reason is that they have had this kind of pain for so long that they have learned to discount it. Another reason is that in the past nobody (including doctors) thought that cramping was significant. In fact, even today severe pain with menses sometimes is brushed off with the comment "All women have cramps." The unfortunate inference drawn by the patient is: Since other women learn to live with this periodic discomfort, why can't I? So, even when their pain is severe, young women soon learn to stop complaining about it.

For these reasons, many patients with "worse than normal" cramping tend to downplay their pain, because they do not want their doctors to think that they are overstating it. Even though Georgia had severe cramping around the onset of her period every single month for over twelve years, she rated her pain at only about three on a scale from one to ten.

Often a clearer understanding of my patient's pain comes from talking with her husband. In front of Georgia and Paul, I said: "Is it really true that you have only slight pain with menstruation?"

By the time I asked this question, I had the advantage of having palpated (examined by touch) the endometriosis during Georgia's pelvic exam. From the tender beadlike endometrial nodules on the ligaments supporting her uterus, I knew that she should have considerable monthly backache and discomfort.

The husband frequently will say, as Paul did: "She hurts enough that she takes painkillers and goes to bed with a heating pad once a month. She certainly looks to me like she is hurting."

Georgia did mention that, when her periods first started, at age thirteen, she had such excruciating pain that she had to crawl across the room to the telephone to get help. I estimate that, like Georgia, if asked to describe their *first* periods at menarche, about 30 percent of endometriosis patients remember having had severe pain. In fact, this is when many infertility specialists feel that endometriosis usually gets started.

But, except for her first period at puberty, Georgia—as do many patients—avoided using the word "pain" when describing menstrual cramps. Instead she mentioned discomfort, aching, or pelvic pressure, when she really meant a dull, throbbing, deep-seated pain. She also had sacral backache during menstruation, as do many women, but she failed to label this "pain."

With endometriosis, sharp pain occurs when there is new growth, swelling, or rupture of a small implant of endometriosis or of an endo- metrioma. (An endometrioma, which we discuss in detail later, is a benign ovarian tumor filled with old chocolate-colored menstrual debris.) Oth- erwise the patient has a dull ache that waxes and wanes, getting worse before and during her period and also at ovulation.

Georgia's former doctor had suggested that she do pelvic tilts to relieve menstrual cramping. These exercises can significantly reduce this type of pain (see fig. 2.5). Doctors think that pelvic tilts make the uterus less tense or spastic by improving circulation to the area. This may decrease retrograde (backward) menstrual flow. Another plausible explanation of why exercise reduces cramping is that it changes the biofeedback from the uterine cramping to a different, more acceptable impulse. In biofeedback sessions, if the woman concentrates on her hand, for example, she sometimes does not receive the cramping im- pulses. Biofeedback techniques are also used to help relieve the pain of natural childbirth; the woman relaxes by concentrating on her breathing.

Today doctors treat dysmenorrhea with a series of drugs called the "antiprostaglandins," such as Anaprox, Motrin, and Naprosyn. The pros- taglandins—important chemicals now thought to be associated with in- fertility in endometriosis patients—are found in menstrual tissue. Some of these hormonelike fatty acids are known to cause smooth muscles such as the uterus to contract. Although at present the clinical effects of the prostaglandins are poorly understood, we think that the significant

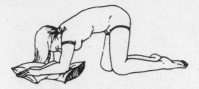

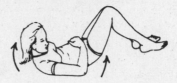

Rest on the elbows and knees, keeping the upper arms and legs perpendicular to the body. Hump the back upward. Contract the buttocks and draw the abdomen in vigorously. Relax, breathe deeply.

Lie flat on the back with the knees and hips flexed. Tilt the pelvis inward and contract the buttocks tightly. Lift the head while contracting the abdominal muscles.

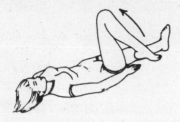

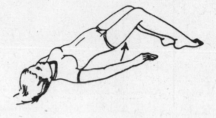

Slowly flex the knee and then the thigh on the abdomen. Lower the foot to the buttock. Straighten and lower the leg to the floor.

Lie flat on the back with the arms at the sides. Draw the knees up slightly. Arch the back.

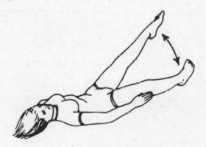

Raise first the right and then the left leg as high as possible. Keep the toes pointed and the knee straight. Lower the leg gradually, using the abdominal muscles but not the hands.

FIGURE 2.5. *Exercises to help relieve menstrual cramping. (Reproduced, with permission, from R. C. Benson,* Current Obstetric & Gynecologic Diagnosis & Treatment, *5th ed., copyright © Lange Medical Publications, 1984.)*

levels of some of these chemicals found in the pelvic fluid of endometriosis patients could be one of the reasons they have difficulty getting pregnant. Only since doctors have had the antiprostaglandin drugs, which reduce inflammation and pain, have we started to realize that the prostaglandins are related to uterine cramping and bladder and bowel dysfunction.

Pain with Intercourse

Another major complaint of at least 25 percent of endometriosis patients is painful intercourse. Doctors call this problem "dyspareunia." Many women with this disease have nodules of endometriosis on the uterine support ligaments or in the culs-de-sac. If endometriosis or scarring from it is hit during intercourse, the woman can have pain. If she is hurt enough times, she may become unable to "turn on." If she fails to reach a certain stage of sexual arousal, the vagina will not become moist, making intercourse even more uncomfortable.

Endometriosis also can cause vaginal dryness when the disease invades the nervous system to the cervical glands and the vagina. If the doctor has to remove extensive tissue in the treatment of deeply invasive endometriosis, the patient may have a problem lubricating, at least for a while.

Vaginal dryness can be related to other problems besides endometriosis. If a woman has a psychological block about sexuality, or if she is not going through all the stages of lovemaking leading to arousal, the cervical glands and vagina may fail to secrete enough mucus. Bothered by the dryness, many women use vaginal lubricants without realizing that they either kill sperm, reduce sperm motility (forward swimming power), or otherwise adversely affect sperm.

Painful intercourse obviously can cause severe marital tension, especially if the husband is a macho male who thinks that bells ought to ring for his wife every time he touches her. In fact, the loss of her sexual interest, added to the stress of infertility, can rip a marriage apart, particularly if the marriage is already unstable.

When Georgia bitterly told me that she had been unable to enjoy sex for several months because it hurt, I immediately thought of endometriosis. The pelvic examination would reveal that she had a knot of endometriosis on one of her uterine support ligaments. When hit during deep penetration, endometriosis hurts. It is like bumping a blister surrounded by scar tissue—when it tears, it hurts.

By the time I saw Georgia, her pain had become so intense that she had refused to have relations with her husband for over a month. Yet she loved him deeply and obviously wanted a child by him.

Like most husbands whose wives have pain with intercourse, Paul felt that Georgia was rejecting him. One of my challenges as their doctor would be to help Paul understand that his wife was unable to respond sexually because endometriosis was causing her pain. The more the husband understands that the disease is at fault, the less he feels personally rejected.

Pain with Exercise

Georgia told my resident that she had pelvic pain while jogging. Sometimes a blister forms where the body absorbs the misplaced endometrial tissue. Since this blister is weaker than normal tissue, not only intercourse but jarring exercise can tear a hole around the blister. This causes "windows" in the peritoneum (the smooth membrane lining the organs and walls of the pelvis and abdomen) (see fig. 2.6). Obviously this can cause pain.

Although I feel that exercise is of great benefit to women, I encourage my endometriosis patients to do smooth exercises, such as walking, bicycling, or swimming, rather than jarring activities, such as military sit-ups, aerobic jumps, or jogging. Yet I realize, as one leading gynecologist put it, that when joggers stop jogging they do get upset! For various reasons, some people seem to need strenuous exercise. Without doubt, jogging can elevate the runner's mood while decreasing the size of her hips and waist. Hence, for the patient with mild endometriosis, the benefits of jogging might be worth the small risk of injuring the pelvis. But for some patients, jogging can be a gynecologic disaster.

Jarring exercise can be harmful to patients with either mild or severe disease, but for different reasons. It is with mild endometriosis that I often see blisters on the ligaments that support the uterus. Jogging or any trauma (even the stretch of pregnancy or labor during childbirth) can cause these blisters to tear, resulting in large holes in the uterine support system. I have seen the ligaments that hold the uterus in place disappear, causing the womb to prolapse (drop down into the vagina) (see fig. 2.7).

Severe endometriosis, on the other hand, can actually strengthen the uterine support system because the disease causes heavy scarring that fixes the uterus in place. Nevertheless, these patients in particular should avoid jarring exercise. In the more advanced stages of the disease, the ovaries, which contain endometriosis, sometimes leak and form adhesions to the abdominal wall. Jogging can rip an ovary loose, spilling the endometriotic material into the pelvis. This obviously will make the disease worse.

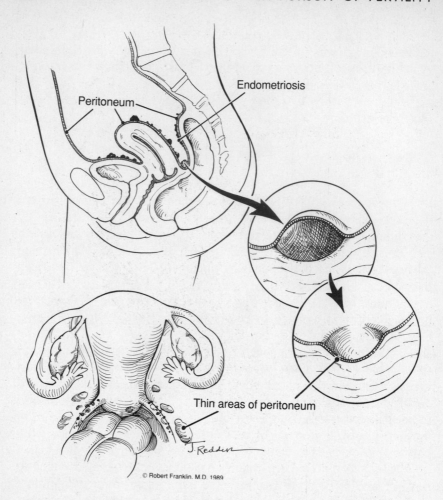

Peritoneum

Endometriosis

Thin areas of peritoneum

J. Redden

© Robert Franklin. M.D. 1989

FIGURE 2.6. The peritoneum is the smooth membrane that covers the organs and lines the walls of the pelvis and abdomen. Note the "windows" or thin areas in the peritoneum.

Premenstrual Syndrome

Patients with endometriosis, especially when it is in the ovaries, often have premenstrual syndrome (PMS). Georgia suffered from many of the symptoms of PMS, including headaches, bloating, acne, appetite changes, irritability, mood swings, and depression. These symptoms usually occurred one or two days before her period and were accompanied by menstrual cramps. PMS also afflicts many women who do not have endometriosis.

Doctors do not know what causes PMS. We think, however, that it

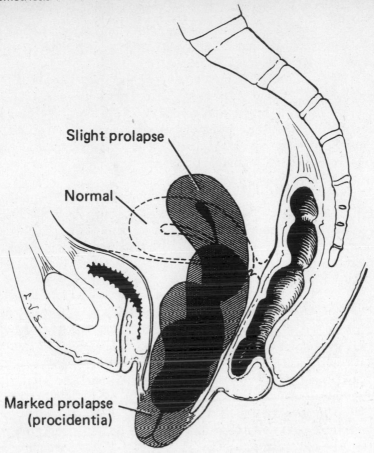

Slight prolapse

Normal

**Marked prolapse
(procidentia)**

FIGURE 2.7. *Prolapse of the uterus into the vagina. (Reproduced, with permission,
from R. C. Benson,* Current Obstetric & Gynecologic Diagnosis & Treatment,
5th ed., copyright © Lange Medical Publications, 1984).

may stem from more than one problem. One theory suggests that PMS
is associated with an abnormal estrogen-progesterone relationship. As
you know, these hormones are produced in the ovaries. When endometriosis invades and irritates an ovary, it can fail to function properly,
throwing its hormones out of balance. Although the theory remains
unproved, PMS may be caused when progesterone production is erratic
or inadequate in comparison with the amount of estrogen produced before
menstruation. A "high" level of estrogen, which is associated with fluid
retention and a bloated GI (gastrointestinal) tract, probably causes the
PMS symptoms.

If given in sufficient amounts, vaginal progesterone suppositories do
appear to relieve PMS symptoms in many patients. Some patients,

however, fail to respond to this therapy. Unfortunately, if a woman has ovarian endometriosis, her ovaries will continue to malfunction even when she is treated with progesterone.

One form of PMS may be associated with increased levels of prostaglandins. An injection of these chemicals can make the uterus contract and can cause headaches, bloating, and weird emotional feelings. Endometrial tissue secretes prostaglandins, which may be one of the reasons many endometriosis patients have more severe PMS than women without the disease. The antiprostaglandin medications help these patients.

Diet and exercise also play an important role in the treatment of premenstrual tension. PMS sufferers need to keep their blood-sugar level within a normal range. I recommend six small meals a day, as well as decreased caffeine and sugar intake. Such patients should also avoid social drinking, because the condition dramatically lowers their tolerance to alcohol. Although diuretics have been prescribed for years to treat PMS, only a few women are helped by them.

Like Paul, the husband of a woman with PMS may see his wife as a person who is fairly happy before she ovulates but who becomes suddenly irritable or depressed the last half of her cycle, especially a few days before and after menstruation begins. He may think to himself: What am I doing wrong? What am I going through here?

Many men have a tendency to take the burden of every problem directly on their shoulders. But if a husband is taking on the entire responsibility for his wife's responsiveness and her emotional problems, he may have too much to handle. He needs to take the emotional ups and downs of his wife less personally.

As his wife's doctor, I try to help him understand that stress accentuates PMS. If, for example, his wife is having pain with intercourse, this certainly can add to her stress. It is important for her to be able to be honest with her husband. If he can relieve some of the pressure on her to perform sexually, she may have less PMS. After the endometriosis is successfully treated, her PMS and pain should be reduced.

A Syndrome

Another clue in Georgia's history pointing to endometriosis was that she had the following problems that I often see associated with the disease: urinary-tract infections (often caused by various strains of E coli), yeast infections, and bowel irritability. In the preceding four years,

Georgia had had five urinary-tract infections including "honeymoon" cystitis (a urinary-tract infection during her honeymoon), many yeast infections, and alternating bouts of diarrhea and constipation.

During this time, she had suffered from bladder-related symptoms such as frequency, urgency, painful urination, and even blood in her urine. If a patient retains urine, the bacteria are not flushed out, and she can get a urinary-tract infection that may require treatment with antibiotics. Double voiding (standing up and sitting down again after voiding) may help a woman completely empty her bladder. Some patients occasionally require dilation of the bladder neck by a urologist. Women need to be aware, however, that overdilation can cause scar-tissue formation and even incontinence.

It is important for patients who are susceptible to urinary-tract infections to drink at least eight glasses of water a day. As one study showed, the old-fashioned treatment of drinking cranberry juice may prevent some urinary-tract infections by preventing bacteria such as *Escherichia coli* (*E. coli* normally dwell in the intestinal tract) from clinging to the bladder wall. Vitamin C tablets also may be helpful by creating a hostile, acidic environment for bacteria, thus discouraging their growth. Not all patients, however, can tolerate acidic drinks. Furthermore, if the woman already has an infection, the extra acid may increase her pain.

Although some patients have symptoms because of bacteria in their urine, many suffer from urinary-tract symptoms just before or during menstruation even though their urine cultures are negative. Like many endometriosis patients, Georgia sometimes had difficulty emptying her bladder because she had a relatively small or stenotic (abnormally narrowed) bladder neck. Nobody knows whether this tightening is caused by an anatomic problem or by bladder spasticity. I think that it could be either. The antiprostaglandins may help by reducing bladder spasm.

Georgia, unfortunately, not only had a small bladder neck, she also had endometriosis implanted on her bladder. This latter problem can cause bladder irritability. In fact, if it is extensive, the patient may have a very spastic bladder and may need to urinate frequently, especially during menstruation.

In addition to urinary-tract problems, Georgia also often had diarrhea during her period. When the menses back up into the pelvic cavity, a woman sometimes develops painful peritonitis—an inflammation of the peritoneum. You will recall that this membrane lines the abdominal wall and covers its organs (see fig. 2.6). GI-tract symptoms such as diarrhea may be caused by this peritoneal irritation. Doctors speculate that increased levels of prostaglandins in the pelvic fluid of endometriosis patients may lead to bowel irritability. The antiprostaglandins also seem to help relieve the diarrhea problem, especially if taken before the symptoms start.

Another reason that some endometriosis patients have GI-tract symptoms is that misplaced endometrial tissue on occasion implants itself on the bowel. This can cause alternating bouts of constipation and diarrhea. Fortunately, menstrual tissue usually does not stick to the bowel until very late in the progression of the disease. At that time, I often find the debris in an immobile area, such as caught in an adhesion (in scar tissue) or where the bowel enters the rectum.

Good dietary habits and exercise help patients with bowel irritability. The diet should include adequate fiber rather than refined products such as white bread. The colon's primary function is storage. If there is not enough volume, the patient can get a spastic colon and become constipated. As the colon contracts, it interferes with the blood supply. This sets the patient up for GI cramps—and they can be severe.

Over the years, I have observed that endometriosis patients often suffer from vaginitis (vaginal infections) because they sometimes produce copious amounts of cervical mucus. So although, as we discussed earlier, endometriosis sometimes causes vaginal dryness, the disease also can have the opposite effect. If the endometriosis irritates the nerve supply to the cervical glands and vagina or causes an abnormal hormone picture, the cervical glands can secrete excess mucus. This provides an abundant food supply for the various organisms in the vagina, allowing them to grow.

Vaginal infections can adversely affect fertility because they decrease the motility of the sperm. Even the common minor infections such as candidiasis (moniliasis), trichomoniasis, and gardnerella (also called "hemophilus vaginitis" or "HV") *sometimes* prevent conception. By increasing white-blood-cell count and acidity, vaginal infections create an unfriendly environment for sperm. In fact, the bacterial infection HV can immobilize sperm.

Many doctors think that emotions affect vaginal infections. Although this is impossible to prove, endometriosis patients often seem more tense to me than other infertility patients. One reason may be that the disease often is painful. Simple nervous tension can cause increased pelvic wetness or discharge because the cervical glands and vagina are affected by the autonomic (self-controlling) nerves, which also control the mechanism for wetness during sex. Although sexual excitation is related to the hormones, it is mainly the mental attitude that causes these autonomic nerves to work. The nervous system, however, cannot tell the difference between sexual excitation, hormonal excitation, and stress. Thus all three have the same effect on the vagina—they can cause increased wetness, sometimes leading to vaginitis.

Georgia had suffered considerable irritation, itching, and misery because of candidiasis, a common fungal infection. This kind of yeast infection is usually caused by the *Candida albicans* organism—a cousin of the familiar yeast that makes bread rise. Between 30 and 80 percent of all women harbor this fungus, although many women have few or no symptoms.

Yeasts love sugar and flourish partly because of the way women eat. Diabetics (patients with high blood sugar), for example, seem to have more yeast infections, because of the increased sugar content of the fluids in the vagina.

On several occasions, Georgia had been diagnosed as having hypoglycemia (low blood sugar) by her family physician. Since their blood sugar fluctuates widely—sometimes they have bouts of high blood sugar—patients with hypoglycemia have more yeast infections than other women. Some people with low blood sugar become diabetic when they are older, especially if they gain weight.

Both pregnancy and birth-control pills change a woman's blood sugars and cause increased mucus production, so that yeast infections grow more profusely. The increased hormonal stimulation of pregnancy causes the cervical glands to become much more active. Birth-control pills create a kind of pregnancylike state by raising levels of the ovarian hormones estrogen and progesterone in the blood. Since estrogen stimulates the cervical glands to make more mucus, birth-control pills—especially the estrogen-dominant ones—cause increased mucus production. There is a direct relationship between hormones, cervical mucus, and yeast infections.

Antibiotics in general and tetracyclines in particular also allow yeast to grow by killing off not only disease-causing germs but also the "good" germs that help keep the yeast population under control. Antibiotics kill the acidophilus bacilli that keep the vagina acidic and healthy. When these "good" germs are destroyed, the yeast can multiply.

Although doctors have an arsenal of powerful antifungal drugs to cure yeast infections, some patients still suffer from chronic vaginitis. I recommend that patients with this problem read *The Yeast Connection,* by William G. Crook, M.D. He advises avoiding sugars, refined carbohydrates (whole grains are recommended), alcoholic beverages, and foods containing yeast in order to help discourage growth of the microbe.

Is Endometriosis Hereditary?

Endometriosis probably occurs in the same family much of the time. I would estimate that up to 30 percent of patients with endometriosis, especially if the condition is severe, have relatives with the disease. For this reason, I asked Georgia if her mother or either of her two younger sisters had ever had it. Although Georgia had no knowledge of anyone in her family having the disease, I later would diagnose the problem in both of her sisters. As we will discuss in detail later, this disease often can be arrested in its milder stages if treated early.

Apparently, several factors other than heredity may influence whether a woman develops endometriosis. In my opinion, these include how long she delays childbirth, the position of her uterus, when she starts menstruating, and the way she handles stress. We will discuss each of these in detail later, but the point is that there probably are many factors besides familial predisposition influencing the way the disease develops.

Is Endometriosis Fatal?

The odds of dying from endometriosis are extremely low—perhaps roughly one in ten thousand. In fact, the risk is so small that I hesitate to mention it for fear of worrying you unnecessarily. Although cancer may arise from endometriosis, it rarely does.

Endometriosis can become fatal if it obstructs the ureters, the tubes that carry urine from the kidneys to the bladder. Fortunately, this also is rare. The disease is generally a surface condition that appears on the peritoneum and the internal organs. It takes a long time before it invades the ureters or the cavity of the bowel. The ureters are extremely tough little tubes made of thick muscle. Although endometriosis can grow all around them, the disease rarely gets inside and obstructs. Nevertheless, if the endometrial tissue is allowed to grow unchecked over a long period of time, endometriosis can eventually block renal outflow. Before a kidney is lost, however, tremendous pain usually warns the patient of this danger.

Diagnosis

A Special Kind of Pelvic Exam

Before performing Georgia's physical exam, I had carefully studied the medical history taken by my resident. I immediately noticed that she had many of the symptoms associated with endometriosis. Her complaints of severe cramping, deep pain with intercourse, PMS, heavy periods, yeast infections, bladder infections, and bowel irritability—especially when considered together—pointed to endometriosis.

The gynecologic examination is the second major part of the initial infertility workup. The doctor can learn a great deal about what is causing his patient's infertility from the pelvic exam. If the woman is slender, he can tell the size and position of both the ovaries and the uterus. If she has a large ovarian cyst or if she has BB-like nodules and scarring from endometriosis, the doctor can palpate these.

Making the diagnosis clinically depends not only on what the gynecologist palpates but also on how the patient reacts to the pelvic exam. If the patient shows evidence of discomfort when the doctor gently moves across an area, he often has hit endometriosis. Occasionally this will cause the patient literally to move off the table. A normal ovary will hurt when touched, but a diseased one will hurt more. Although the physician has to realize that every woman is different, the patient's response to her pelvic exam gives him important additional clues as to what is wrong.

The doctor must be extremely gentle if he hopes to establish rapport with a new patient, especially an endometriosis patient. If he does the pelvic exam like a boxer, he knows nothing and will learn nothing. The patient subconsciously will relate everything he does for her in the future—including surgery—to how gentle he is during the gynecologic exam.

The physical must be thorough enough to pick up the major problems without being uncomfortable for the patient. The woman with endometriosis has a very tense, tender pelvis. If the pelvic exam causes too much discomfort, I back off—I do not persist to the point of causing unpleasant feelings between us.

I have found that the best way to put a patient at ease is to listen to her. She will tell me the diagnosis. When she starts telling her story, I often not only understand her problem but can expand on it. If, when she says that she has premenstrual tension, I can anticipate some of her other feelings, we immediately will have rapport because she knows that I understand what she is going through.

Doctors must do everything possible to emphasize that they are going to hear out a patient's complaints. This takes varying amounts of time. Sometimes I am unable to do it during the initial visit. Often all I can do is survey the problems.

Years ago I worked with an old general practitioner who said: "Do not be in a hurry to make the diagnosis. Sometimes you will be unable to do it the first time you see the patient. If you talk with her enough times and carefully listen to what she says, you will make the diagnosis."

When talking with my patient, I try to pick the exact word that describes how she is feeling. Otherwise I may get a misleading answer. For example, when I asked Georgia if palpating each ovary *hurt,* she said, "No." But when I asked her if her ovaries felt *tender,* she said, "Yes." So the doctor has to pick the precise word that describes what the patient feels if he or she wants to get accurate information.

The beauty of pain is that it warns us that something is wrong. The ovaries, however, usually are silent. This is why some endometriosis patients present no history of pain or menstrual cramps. Since the ovaries seldom give any indication that they are under attack, endometriosis can destroy one or both of them—a lifetime supply of eggs—before the patient knows that her fertility is lost.

The Preliminary Diagnosis

Once Georgia's history and physical were completed, I met with her and Paul in my office. Although the diagnosis is often unknown at this time, in Georgia's case I felt that all the clues pointed to endometriosis, probably with ovarian involvement. My unhappy task was to explain to the couple that I strongly suspected that she had severe endometriosis, a condition often associated with infertility.

Most doctors feel that this disease causes 30 to 40 percent of infertility. In my infertility practice, which is primarily surgical, I find that the figures are closer to 40 or 50 percent. One reason I see more endometriosis patients than some other physicians is that I have a referral practice for infertility.

I told the couple that Georgia's history was compatible with the preliminary diagnosis of endometriosis in that she had debilitating pelvic pain with her periods, pain with intercourse, very heavy menstrual flow, and infertility. Her pelvic exam also pointed to endometriosis. I had palpated endometrial implants on the uterine support ligaments, in the

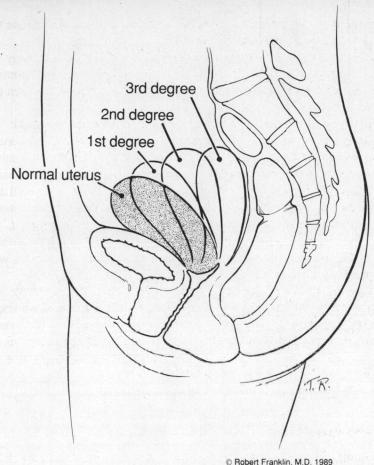

3rd degree

2nd degree

1st degree

Normal uterus

© Robert Franklin, M.D. 1989

FIGURE 2.8. Degrees of retroversion of the uterus.

cul-de-sac (see fig. 2.2), and on the surface of the uterine wall. Her ovaries were enlarged and tender.

Normally the uterus rests over the bladder, pointing to the front of the body, but in about one-third of women the womb is retroverted (tilted backward) (see fig. 2.8). It has been our experience that patients with a retroverted uterus have more problems with back pain, endometriosis, and infertility. Georgia's uterus was not only "tipped" but also scarred and fixed. Endometriosis can tip the uterus. If the disease implants itself in the ligaments and starts growing, the scar tissue can contract and pull the uterus backward. Some patients with a retroverted uterus, especially if it is fixed, have discomfort during sex because their ovaries are held in a position where they get hit during deep penetration.

After a couple has tried to have a baby for a year, the possibilities are at least 85 percent that there is a physical cause why they have not conceived. Since Georgia and Paul had been unable to get pregnant for almost four years, I felt that they needed a complete infertility workup. After considering Georgia's history, her pelvic exam, and her frustration level, I thought that we needed to set up a game plan designed to identify the factors causing infertility and attempt to eliminate all of them. This is how we get babies.

But before I did any invasive tests for Georgia, a semen analysis for Paul was necessary. If we restore the wife's fertility and fail to check the husband's sperm count, we might not see a pregnancy. Sometimes both partners are infertile. In addition, one patient can have several problems, although often in medicine these can be traced to a single cause. For example, the woman with endometriosis of the ovary may have irregular ovulation, a luteal-phase defect (abnormal progesterone production following ovulation), and cervical mucus problems. We think that endometriosis causes all of the above complications. (See chapter 5 for complete details of the semen analysis and of another study called the "Sims-Huhner postcoital test.")

Overcoming infertility is an extremely intense job. The ability to complete the medical workup and adequately treat the problems depends on how quickly we can find out what is wrong. Most patients can tolerate trying to have a baby for only a limited length of time: it may be six months; it may be a year. A doctor who takes too long to make the diagnosis will have a very short time to treat the patient before she gets discouraged. If what is wrong is discovered quickly, there is more time to help her.

The Definitive Diagnosis

LAPAROSCOPY

The only way to make a definitive diagnosis of endometriosis is to look directly at the internal reproductive organs. Doctors can see inside the pelvic cavity and abdomen with the aid of a miniature video camera attached to a lighted, pencil-sized telescope called a laparoscope (see fig. 2.9). A magnified flashlight-sized view of the inside of the body appears on the high-resolution video monitor. Inserted through a tiny hole in the lower edge of the navel, the laparoscope is our finest diagnostic tool. In fact, the ability to diagnose and treat with this instrument has revolutionized the science of infertility. A minor operation, diagnostic laparoscopy can require only a half-inch incision. Since it can be covered

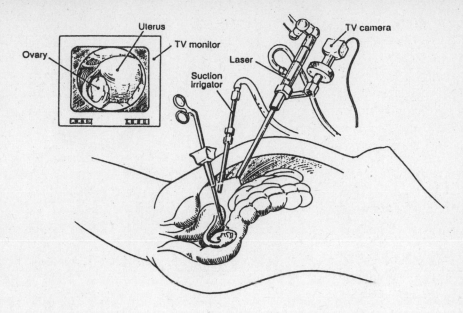

FIGURE 2.9. *Laparoscopy, a minor operation in which doctors use a pencil-sized telescope to diagnose and treat diseases of the pelvic organs. The laser can vaporize endometriosis and sever adhesions or scar tissue.*

with a large Band-Aid, nurses nicknamed laparoscopy "Band-Aid surgery."

Before I can offer medical or surgical treatment, I have to confirm the diagnosis of endometriosis with laparoscopy. When I palpate a thickening, a fixation, or an enlargement in a young woman, I think of endometriosis. But what I palpate could be an ovarian cyst or some other problem. I do not treat until I know what I am treating.

Laparoscopy helps me differentiate between endometriosis, cancer, and infection. When palpated they can feel the same—all three can cause a kind of scarring that is as hard as a rock. With the 'scope, I can tell whether an ovarian enlargement is a benign cyst, a functional cyst caused by ovarian malfunction, endometriosis, or a malignancy. Although it is extremely rare in a young patient, I have to make certain that I am not mistakenly treating a malignant tumor or some other disease. Anytime that I feel a mass, a thickening, or an enlargement, the thought of malignancy crosses my mind. Cancer is always a *remote* possibility, though certainly *not* a probability in a young patient.

To verify that Georgia had endometriosis and the associated adhesions, I suggested that she have a diagnostic laparoscopy. Right before

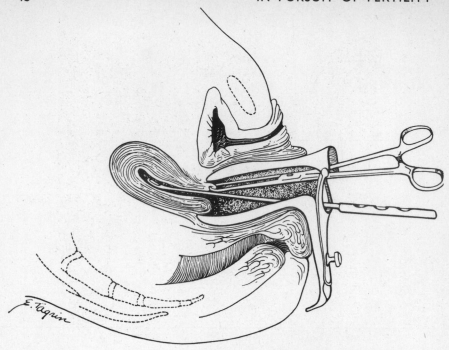

FIGURE 2.10. Endometrial biopsy to study a patient's hormones. (Reproduced, with permission, from R. W. Kistner, Gynecology: Principles and Practice, 4th ed., copyright © 1986 by Year Book Medical Publishers, Inc., Chicago.)

the 'scope, we do an X-ray to study the uterus and fallopian tubes. At the time of laparoscopy, we do an endometrial biopsy, whereby a sliver of the uterine lining is removed and studied to judge hormonal activity (see fig. 2.10). These tests are done on an outpatient basis. The laparoscopy should be set up for the third week of the cycle, when we can learn the most, not only about the endometriosis but also about the patient's hormones. The day before the 'scope, blood is drawn for tests including a serum pregnancy test to rule out a pregnancy from a previous cycle. The patient is instructed to use birth control during the cycle of her 'scope.

THE X-RAY (HSG) BEFORE THE 'SCOPE

The X-ray (hysterosalpingogram or HSG) is an important diagnostic test. It tells us if the fallopian tubes are patent (open). If the tubes are open, we can see the radio-opaque liquid iodine flow through the cervix into the uterus, in and out the tubes, and into the pelvic cavity (see fig. 2.11). If the dye runs up against a blockage, I can see on the X-ray

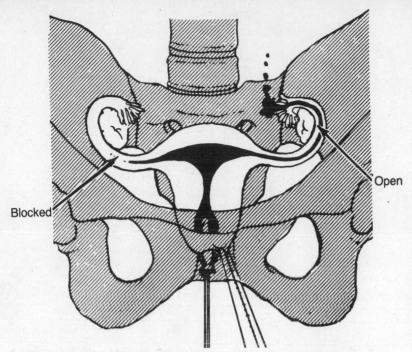

Blocked

Open

FIGURE 2.11. HSG X-ray of the fallopian tubes and uterus. (Reproduced, with permission, from R. C. Benson, Current Obstetric & Gynecologic Diagnosis & Treatment, 5th ed., copyright © Lange Medical Publications, 1984.)

exactly where the tube is occluded. Sometimes reflux menstrual flow or infection causes the inner walls of the tubes to stick together. (For detailed information on tubal blockage caused by infection, see chapter 3.)

I explained to the couple that the HSG also enables us to study the uterus. The normal uterus is pear-shaped and hollow, but a few patients have a womb that is heart-shaped or, as in fig. 2.12, partially or totally divided by a wall called a "septum." We diagnose those problems with the X-ray. It is important to discover uterine anomalies or malformations before pregnancy because patients with an imperfectly formed uterus often miscarry (see chapter 8).

Another advantage of the HSG is that it enables doctors to see scarring inside the uterus as well as abnormal growths such as polyps (small benign growths) and fibroids (leiomyomas, or benign muscular tumors). (See figs. 2.13 and 2.14.) Scarring inside the uterus, which may be the result of a previous abortion or a D&C (dilatation and curettage—dilatation of the cervix and scraping of the lining of the uterus), may prevent pregnancy by blocking the openings to the oviducts. If the

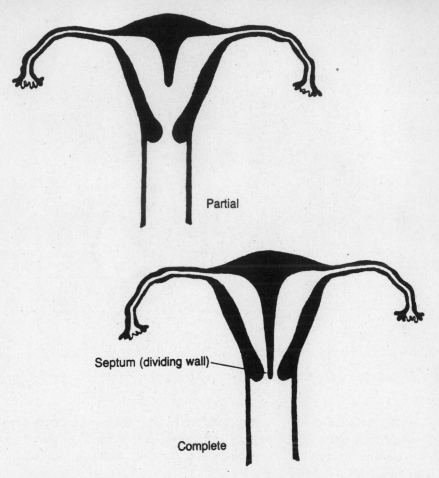

FIGURE 2.12. *Uterus with a septum or dividing wall. (From V. C. Buttram,* Surgical Treatment of the Infertile Female, *Baltimore: Williams & Wilkins Co., 1985.)*

sperm do manage to fertilize the egg but it implants itself on a scar, the woman may abort. It is like throwing a seed on a road or an unplowed field. In addition, scarring in the uterine cavity, if severe enough, can prevent expansion of the uterus and lead to abortion. And a fibroid or polyp may cause infertility if either obstructs the entrance to a fallopian tube.

For the convenience of the patient, we generally schedule the HSG right before laparoscopy, when the patient has been given a shot to relax her. There is, however, some controversy among physicians about doing the HSG during the third week of the cycle. Since the endometrium

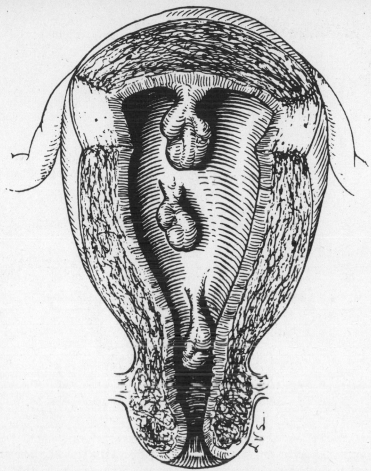

FIGURE 2.13. Polyps. (Reproduced, with permission, from R. C. Benson, Current Obstetric & Gynecologic Diagnosis & Treatment, 5th ed., copyright © Lange Medical Publications, 1984.)

is very lush then, it can plug the end of the tube that goes through the uterus, resulting in an abnormal X-ray. In other words, the fallopian tube can be blocked at this time but open around ovulation. Such temporary blockage rarely occurs, but when it does we recheck the diagnosis by running dye through the tubes during the laparoscopy.

DIAGNOSING LUTEAL-PHASE (HORMONAL) DEFECTS

One of the mechanisms of endometriosis that causes infertility that can be studied at the time of the 'scope is an abnormal hormone picture.

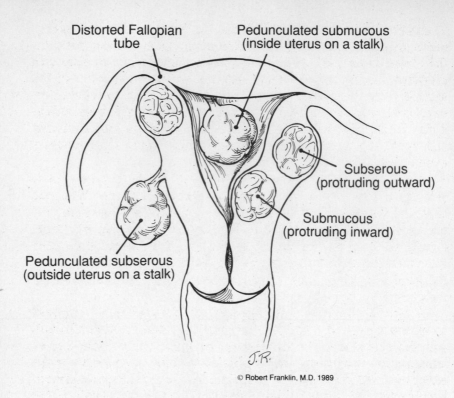

Distorted Fallopian tube

Pedunculated submucous (inside uterus on a stalk)

Subserous (protruding outward)

Submucous (protruding inward)

Pedunculated subserous (outside uterus on a stalk)

FIGURE 2.14. Fibroids (leiomyomas) are benign muscular tumors.

If the hormones aren't on target, the lining of the uterus won't be properly prepared to accept and support a pregnancy. You will recall that the corpus luteum (the orange-yellow gland that forms in the egg sac after ovulation) normally produces the ovarian hormone progesterone during the second half of the menstrual cycle. This hormone makes the uterine lining lush so that the embryo can "latch" on to it.

Sometimes endometriosis patients fail to have a clean biphasic (two-phase) cycle. The follicles appear to be growing and putting out progesterone too early. We can tell this by looking at the basal-body-temperature chart or by following the maturation of the follicle with ultrasound. A painless imaging process using high-frequency sound waves, ultrasound produces a picture of the internal organs on a TV-like screen. If the lining of the uterus is stimulated by progesterone before rather than after ovulation, the endometrium will be out of phase. When this happens, the fertilized egg will not implant itself, because by the time it arrives in the uterus the uterine lining is too old.

Endometriosis patients seem to have a higher incidence of spontaneous abortion (miscarriage) than normal. In some of these patients, the corpus luteum fails to secrete enough progesterone to support a pregnancy. If the corpus luteum secretes progesterone either in too small an amount or for too short a time, the uterine lining will be underdeveloped when the embryo arrives. Even if the embryo does attach, it may abort. Called a "luteal-phase defect," this may be one reason that endometriosis patients often lose babies early in pregnancy, sometimes even before they know they are expecting.

A luteal-phase defect shows up on the basal-body-temperature chart, although this method is too inexact to make the diagnosis. When we looked at Georgia's chart for March, we saw that her temperature remained elevated for too short a period of time, indicating that the corpus luteum quit secreting progesterone too early. If the temperature rises too slowly rather than abruptly, as hers did in May, this indicates that the gland failed to produce a large enough quantity of the hormone for the cycle.

A blood test called "serum-progesterone assay" helps diagnose an inadequate luteal phase. We compare the patient's hormone level with the normal level for that specific day of her cycle. If the corpus-luteum gland is abnormal that month, the progesterone level may be either too low or too high. For example, if the patient has a large corpus-luteum cyst, or if she has many progesterone-producing follicles (these don't release eggs), her progesterone level will be abnormal for that cycle.

We correlate the serum-progesterone level with the temperature charts and a biopsy of the endometrium taken on the twenty-first day of the menstrual cycle. At that time, the endometrium is supposed to be at a specific place in its development. If it is more than two days off, a luteal-phase defect exists—but perhaps only for that month. The following cycle, the patient may or may not have this problem.

To do an endometrial biopsy, we take a sliver of the uterine lining from the front and back of the uterus. We take the biopsy deep in the uterus (see fig. 2.10), because if the sample is taken too low (near the cervix, for instance) the test will always indicate a poor endometrium. Our specialized pathologist can tell if this tissue is properly developed for the twenty-first day of the cycle. If the uterine lining is out of phase for that day, the patient probably has a hormone deficiency that month.

Since the endometrial biopsy can be painful, we do it while the patient is asleep right before the laparoscopy. If the biopsy must be done at another time, an anesthetic called a "cervical block" is given. This is a fairly important diagnostic test, but it hurts. And not just a little—for some patients it hurts a lot. Obviously this is no way to develop rapport with a new patient.

Since a normal woman may occasionally have luteal-phase dysfunction, the doctor needs to prove that the corpus luteum malfunctions rather *regularly,* if not during every single cycle. But since I want to avoid subjecting my patient to repeated biopsies, I sometimes have to fudge on the diagnosis. By looking at several temperature charts, the endometrial biopsy, and the blood test of progesterone level, I usually can tell if the woman has a luteal-phase problem. If it is significant, I treat it with progesterone suppositories. I do not want my patient to start a pregnancy and lose it.

LOOKING THROUGH THE 'SCOPE

After the HSG is completed, the patient is moved to the operating room. At this time, I look directly at the reproductive organs through the laparoscope (see fig. 2.9). The patient feels nothing, because before the procedure the anesthesiologist gives her a light general anesthetic. Once she is asleep, we inflate the abdomen with carbon dioxide and insert the laparoscope through a half-inch incision at the lower edge of the navel. In order to manipulate the uterus, we place a blunt cannula (tube) into the uterus via the vagina. We also make a second, tiny incision in the pubic hairline to see underneath the ovaries.

Looking at a magnified picture of the inside of the body appearing on the TV monitor, I examine all the organs in a systemic, clockwise fashion with the 'scope. If I did not follow a pattern, I might miss something. I usually start on the left side and look at the left tube and ovary, underneath the left tube and ovary, at the back of the uterus and the cul-de-sac area, at the right tube and ovary, and at the bladder. I also look at the intestines, the appendix, the liver, and the gallbladder. I not only evaluate the location and severity of the endometriosis, but I also pinpoint other problems, such as kinks in the tubes, adhesions, and fibroids.

The laparoscope helps me diagnose ovarian malfunction and specific problems related to the ovarian hormones. A normal ovary is about one or two inches in length and is covered with little indentations or pits where an egg has popped out each month. If the patient has ovulated during the menstrual cycle of her 'scope, I see the yellow-orange corpus luteum where the egg was extruded (see fig. 1.12). If she has an ovarian cyst, I will see that. Occasionally the 'scope also reveals an LUF (luteinized unruptured follicle). This occurs when the corpus luteum forms, but there is no evidence that the egg has been released.

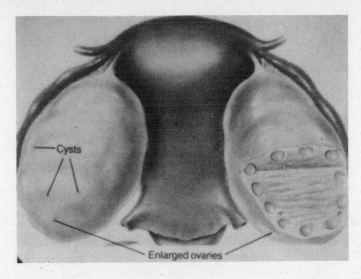

FIGURE 2.15. *Large polycystic ovaries. (Diagram courtesy of Parke-Davis, a division of Warner-Lambert Co.)*

Georgia's temperature charts showed evidence of ovulation, but some infertility patients seldom or never ovulate. The ovaries of the latter, or of the woman on birth-control pills, are very smooth and small; each ovary has a thin capsule with little or no evidence of pitting on it. This tells me either that the woman's hormonal axis between her brain and ovaries—the hypothalamic-pituitary-ovarian axis—is not functioning properly or that ovulation has been suppressed by the pill.

Not all ovaries that fail to ovulate are small. Occasionally doctors see large white cyst-filled ones called polycystic ovaries (PCO) (see fig. 2.15). Generally this type of ovary also fails to release eggs. (See section on "Polycystic Ovarian Disease" in chapter 4 for further information.) In addition to the small inactive ovaries and the large polycystic ones, we also see many ovaries where the distinction between types is not clear-cut.

Some patients have a kind of benign tumor that doctors call an "endometrioma" or "chocolate cyst." Filled with old blood that looks like chocolate-colored syrup, an endometrioma is the most common kind of ovarian tumor found during fertility surgery (see fig. 2.17 and fig. 2.18). During a pelvic examination, I noticed one of Georgia's ovaries was enlarged and fixed to the sidewall of the pelvis, making me wonder if she had an endometrioma.

A chocolate cyst starts as a little "blood blister" with misplaced endometrium in it. Stimulated by ovarian estrogen, the tumor grows larger every cycle. Each month, when estrogen is withdrawn, the endometrium bleeds inside the endometrioma, causing it to swell. If the tumor starts to rupture, the blood, which contains irritating free iron, seeps into the surrounding tissue. Sometimes the blood stays in the ovary, but usually it leaks out of the ovary, causing the organ to stick against the pelvic sidewall. Eventually very dense adhesions form between the ovary and the sidewall.

Often the patient with an endometrioma has a history of severe cramps as a teenager. She frequently remembers doubling up in pain during her first period, as Georgia did. But as she grows older, her cramps sometimes lessen, either because she starts taking oral contraceptives or because the endometriosis causes her ovaries to produce too much progesterone. Progesterone softens tissues and can reduce the pain. But the endometrioma does not get better. It continues to grow—giving little warning of its presence.

As I mentioned earlier, this is why a woman with severe endometriosis may complain very little, whereas a patient with mild disease sometimes complains bitterly. The woman with extensive disease in her ovaries (again, they have few pain fibers) often has no pain, whereas the patient with mild endometriosis may hurt in the early stages of the disease because she has endometriosis in the nerve supply to the pelvic area.

When the ovary does hurt, it is usually around ovulation or when it leaks or sticks to the pelvic wall. The patient may have a sharp, tearing pain at this time. Unfortunately, she usually forgets these brief knifelike stabs; she thinks that she has a virus or a GI upset. This is another reason a patient with a large endometrioma sometimes gives her doctor no history of pain until the tumor swells and ruptures. Then she starts hurting all the time.

Even though an endometrioma is rarely malignant, it can cause serious complications for the patient. If left untreated, the tumor can destroy an ovary. Worse yet, if the tumor ruptures, its chocolate-colored contents pour into the abdomen. Sometimes during this process a blood vessel can tear; it usually stops bleeding, but if it doesn't, the resulting hemorrhage can be life-threatening, although the woman should have warning symptoms.

Treatments

Lasering Through the 'Scope

Today, many of the infertility problems that we find during the diagnostic laparoscopy can be treated with videolaseroscopy. This is the newest way to eradicate endometriosis. By lasering through the operating channel of the 'scope, I can vaporize surface endometrial implants and cut filmy adhesions. This method of treatment reduces injury to the peritoneum (see chapter 9 for further information on the laser).

For many patients, the operating laparoscope eliminates the need for major abdominal surgery. Unfortunately, however, not all infertility problems can be handled with the 'scope. Some disease is too extensive to correct through a half-inch "belly-button" incision.

Patients need to be aware that, although complications during laparoscopy are rare, they have occurred. Bleeding, and perforation of blood vessels, the bowel, the stomach, and the uterus have been reported. The more experienced the surgeon, the less chance of complications. The mortality rate following this procedure is extremely low. Most of the deaths reported have been caused by complications from the general anesthesia. For a thin person, laparoscopy is a safe, minor operation if performed by an expert. Obese patients, however, are at higher risk than someone of normal weight.

Patients generally have minimal discomfort following the diagnostic 'scope. Although recovery after the operating 'scope is slower, it is much faster than following major abdominal surgery. After the diagnostic procedure, some patients say that the incision feels as if they had a mole removed. If a blood vessel is hit, causing a hematoma (a bruiselike accumulation of blood), there will be increased discomfort. Normally, however, recovery is fairly rapid. Most women go back to work in a day or two and resume exercise and intercourse after a week.

Immediately following laparoscopy, I tell the husband what we learned. After the patient is awake, I visit with her, but she doesn't have to worry about remembering everything. We go over our findings again one or two days after the 'scope and in detail three or four weeks later, when the results of all the tests are back. At that time, I sit down with the couple to discuss any problems and outline a game plan to help them.

This plan, however, is not set in concrete. A doctor has to be flexible enough to revise the workup about every two or three months. People do not always react to medication or surgery by the book. The secret of success in treating infertility is to be able to take another positive course of action if necessary.

How the Stage of Disease Affects Treatment

One of the big steps forward in the treatment of endometriosis is that we can gauge the severity of the disease with the diagnostic 'scope, using the point system of the American Society for Reproductive Medicine (ASRM) (see fig. 2.16). We can tell if the endometriosis is minimal, mild, moderate, or severe. The laparoscope gives us a good idea about the extent and location of the ectopic endometrium so that we can decide how to treat it.

Occasionally the endometriosis is so mild that no treatment is necessary. But since ovulation problems are associated with mild disease,

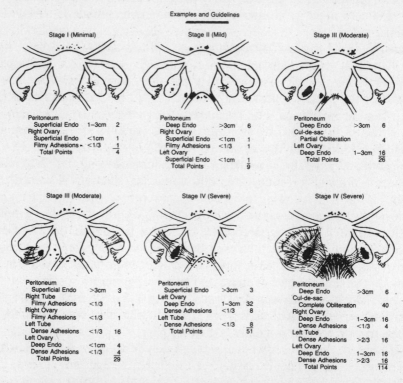

FIGURE 2.16. *Staging the severity of endometriosis and adhesions using the point system of the American Society for Reproductive Medicine. (Revised American Fertility Society Classification of Endometriosis, 1985, Fertility and Sterility, vol. 43, p. 351, 1985. Reproduced with the permission of the publisher, The American Fertility Society.)*

I continue to monitor the patient's temperature charts and cervical mucus. When necessary, I vaporize mild endometriosis with the operating laser through the laparoscope. If I am unsure whether I have destroyed all of the cells, I prescribe one of the drugs called "GnRH or LH-RH agonists" for three months to dry up any remaining disease. For patients who are unable or unwilling to take an agonist, I give a medication called "danazol" (marketed as Danocrine). Both of these medications are described in detail later.

In moderate endometriosis, we can take either of the following two therapeutic approaches: In the majority of cases, I do the diagnostic laparoscopy followed by the operating laser 'scope to remove as much of the endometriosis as possible. Following this procedure, I prescribe either an LH-RH agonist for three months or, in rare cases, danazol. After that, the patient allows a cycle for her hormones to readjust and then tries to conceive for about six months. During this period I carefully monitor her, checking her ovulatory process and cervical mucus, including sperm penetration. If she isn't ovulating, I prescribe fertility drugs. If she doesn't get pregnant, we re-evaluate her case.

An alternative therapy for moderate disease, especially if the patient is over thirty, is to follow the above treatment plan except that, immediately following the course of the agonist, I repeat the 'scope. If I am unable to remove the disease completely, I perform microsurgery to eliminate the endometriosis. This is major abdominal surgery (see fig. 2.17). In other words, if the second-look laparoscopy shows that the disease is deep or extensive, or if the adhesions are too thick to remove through the 'scope, this operation is our most effective treatment.

The purpose of this major procedure is to improve greatly the patient's chances of having a baby. With a "bikini" incision, I open up the abdomen (perform a laparotomy) and remove the endometriosis, using meticulous microsurgical techniques. Surgeons have nicknamed this surgery the "blue-plate special" because it involves a series of mini-operations. (Doctors refer to the operation as "conservative" surgery because the reproductive organs are "conserved" rather than removed, as during hysterectomy or radical surgery.)

With endometriosis, the doctor continually has to re-evaluate each case. Sometimes when I think that I have removed all the disease, I have not. Even with the magnification afforded by the operating microscope, we unfortunately are unable to see all of the endometriosis. Occasionally I miss some microscopic cells; other times, they reaccumulate. (See chapter 9 for further information on the operating microscope.)

Endometriosis

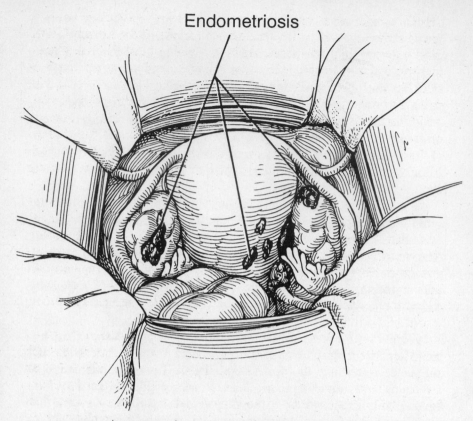

FIGURE 2.17. Laparotomy (surgery with the abdomen open) showing endometriosis in an ovary.

Dr. John A. Rock of The Johns Hopkins University School of Medicine says that, when doctors take random biopsies of areas that look clean, they occasionally find microscopic endometriosis where the specimens have little white blebs (blisters containing fluid) or changes in them. These need to be eradicated because they can grow. We try to eliminate enough of the endometriosis so that the body's defense system can destroy the rest.

The problem is that surgeons must balance their desire to destroy the endometriosis with the goal of preventing postsurgical adhesions. For this reason, we follow the advice of the late T. S. Cullen of Johns Hopkins, who said: "Remove as much as necessary but as little as possible."

For the patient with severe disease, the treatment plan generally is as follows: After the diagnostic 'scope, I prescribe three months of a

LH-RH agonist or, in rare cases, danazol. These medications not only dry up some of the endometriosis but reduce swelling and inflammation, making surgery much easier. Usually at this time I perform reconstructive microsurgery, because in cases of severe endometriosis this provides the best hope for restoring fertility. I seldom treat severe disease solely with the 'scope, unless the patient chooses this therapy. Finally, if the ovaries are involved, I prescribe an additional month of an agonist, or rarely danazol, following the laparotomy. This reduces the number of remaining microscopic cells and gives the ovaries a chance to heal. If the ovaries start working too soon after surgery, they can become cystic.

One of the problems in treating endometriosis is that, when I first look at it, I am unable to tell exactly how deep the disease is. A small spot of endometriosis on an ovary, for example, may be a little surface disease, or it may be the tip of an iceberg—like a big endometrioma affecting most of the organ (see fig. 2.18). Until I actually open an endometrioma, I cannot tell how extensive the disease is. If I am lucky and the endometriosis is superficial, I will simply vaporize it with the laser.

If I find a large (over three centimeters) blood-filled endometrioma—and I have seen some as large as a grapefruit I will not treat it through the 'scope. Instead I remove the tumor through a bikini incision following two or three months of agonist or danazol therapy. Unfortunately, sometimes I also discover many small endometriotic cysts spread throughout the ovary. They look as though someone squeezed a blood blister inside the ovary and the endometriotic fragments scattered in all directions. We treat this diffused type of ovarian endometriosis by performing a wedge resection: with the abdomen open, we carefully cut the diseased area from the ovary.

How does the endometriosis get inside the ovary? One of the most respected authorities on endometriosis, Dr. Robert W. Kistner of Harvard Medical School, says that when the disease gets implanted on the surface of the ovary, the normal cells surround the ectopic endometrium and try to bury it. This theory explains how endometriosis becomes internalized and why the surface sometimes looks normal at first glance. Often when I laser a pinpoint spot on the ovary, the endometriosis will seep to the surface like an oil well.

Patients frequently ask if they can get pregnant when a piece of each ovary is missing. Since the ovary is filled with eggs, a woman usually can conceive with only a part of an ovary. I have patients with only a tenth of an ovary who have good ovarian function. They can conceive as long as the tube can pick up the egg. These patients, however, may not ovulate as long as normal and may have their final menstrual period sooner.

Expert laparoscopists sometimes treat severe ovarian endometriosis with videolaseroscopy and report good results following this therapy. Nowadays surgeons are removing large endometriomas through the 'scope. But this is long surgery performed under the worst possible operating conditions. The risk of missing endometrial cells is high.

One of the secrets of success with laparoscopic surgery is to know its limitations. Imagine yourself looking at a TV monitor at a magnified flashlight-sized section of the internal organs of the pelvis (see fig. 2.9). When you first take the surface off the endometrioma, a brown syruplike liquid comes out. If some of the endometrial cells spill into the pelvic cavity, the endometriosis can spread. Each time you laser, a layer of carbonized material forms—a chocolate-colored coagulum that immediately insulates the endometriosis below it. This prevents you from removing all the endometrial cells through the 'scope, because the layer of carbon blocks the carbon-dioxide laser.

Although the recovery time is much longer for the patient, in some cases the surgeon can do a better job during a major procedure. With the abdomen open, I often can remove ovarian endometriosis more thoroughly. Incomplete removal may mean that the disease is back in six months.

After the 'Scope

After listening to the preliminary diagnosis, Georgia and Paul decided to go home and think about my recommendations. Three days later, Georgia called and scheduled a laparoscopy for her next menstrual cycle.

The following month, after Georgia's laparoscopy, as I walked down the long hall from the operating room to the surgery waiting area, I thought of how I would break the news of her condition to Paul.

I said: "Georgia is doing fine. The laparoscopy confirmed my preliminary diagnosis that she has severe endometriosis. I lasered as much of the surface disease as possible, but I was unable to get it all. Some of the implants are deep, and both ovaries are involved. I suspect that one has an endometrioma deep inside it and that the other has endometriosis scattered throughout the whole organ. There are two pea-sized fibroids within the muscle wall of the uterus, but I don't think that they are positioned to interfere with conception. On the positive side, both of Georgia's fallopian tubes are open, and she ovulated this cycle."

"Do you think that we will be able to have a baby?" Paul asked.

"With proper treatment, many of my patients with severe endometriosis do get pregnant. I would like you and Georgia to come in and talk with me in a couple of days, so that we can sit down and discuss the laparoscopy in detail and how we can help her."

A few days later, the couple returned to my office for discussion. I had already told Paul that his semen analysis was normal. His sperm count was sixty-five million per milliliter, with greater than 55-percent motility. This simply meant that there were plenty of sperm and that they were good swimmers.

Although endometriosis sometimes makes the cervical mucus abnormal, Georgia's mucus was abundant and of good ovulatory quality. This helped reinforce the findings of the laparoscopy that the problem was in the upper genital tract.

With controlled optimism, I told the couple how we could attempt to treat the endometriosis. Since Georgia had severe disease I felt that I eventually would have to operate. My goal was to guide them by presenting as much information as possible. I wanted to help Georgia and Paul choose the approach that was right for them, but they had to make the major decisions.

Although I presented the facts in a positive way, I was realistic about Georgia's chances for pregnancy. If I had been overly optimistic, she would have expected to get pregnant immediately. I wanted her to be prepared to carry on with her life even if she failed to conceive right away; I did not want her to become profoundly depressed every time she got her period. So I pointed to a reasonable time in the future, like six months to a year after surgery, when she might conceive. This approach causes less stress than if the patient expects pregnancy each cycle.

Medical Treatments: Helpful and Harmful

POWERFUL NEW DRUGS: THE AGONISTS

I recommended that Georgia take one of the synthetic GnRH agonists for two or three months before her major surgery. These drugs, which cause pseudomenopause, can dry up some of the endometriosis, reduce adhesion formation, possibly lessen pain, and improve surgical results. But before giving this medication, I wanted her to know more about it.

I explained: "These powerful new man-made drugs called 'gonado-tropin-releasing hormone (GnRH) agonists' or 'LH-RH agonists' can cause endometriosis to regress and fibroid tumors to shrink. When given in continuous therapeutic doses, by monthly injection, GnRH agonists—which cannot be taken orally—suppress ovarian production of estrogen and progesterone. When the drug is stopped, hormone levels return to normal in about four to six weeks. Most patients get their menstrual period back within eight to ten weeks."

I explained that in nature, a woman's hypothalamus sends bursts of GnRH to the pituitary (the master gland) approximately every ninety minutes. As you now know, this pulsatile release of GnRH signals the master gland to secrete FSH and LH to stimulate the ovaries into production. When GnRH is sent to the pituitary in sustained levels—rather than in intermittent pulsing bursts, as found in nature—the ovulatory process is halted. After an initial elevation in FSH and LH—which can be partially avoided by starting therapy during the second half of the menstrual cycle—levels of these pituitary hormones drop. This obviously decreases ovarian estrogen production. Since endometriosis typically is estrogen-dependent, the disease gets better. In some women, the condition is suppressed enough to permit laparoscopic surgery. Unfortunately, however, although endometriomas sometimes shrink, their disease stage rarely improves. Regrettably, once the drug is stopped and estrogen production resumes, the endometrial implants eventually return. For this reason, the medication usually gives the patient only a "window" of time to attempt pregnancy, or if the disease is severe, to have conservative surgery for endometriosis.

"So what you are saying," said Georgia, "is that an agonist probably will *not* cure my disease, especially since some of it is in the ovaries. These medications, however, should significantly suppress my endometriosis, at least temporarily. This should improve the outcome of my surgery."

"That's right," I said. "Following agonist therapy, not only is the pelvis drier, but the blood vessels are smaller and easier for me to laser. Ovarian surgical results are improved, because the drug changes the ovary from an active, soft organ, which is easy to traumatize and to make bleed, to a quiet, dry organ.

"Sometimes we just do not know how endometriosis causes infertility. We have observed, however, that some women get pregnant more easily when their ovaries resume ovulation after resting on GnRH therapy. As I mentioned before, endometriosis can cause the ovary to malfunction. Sometimes it becomes luteinized (predominantly progesterone-producing) too early so that when ovulation occurs the endometrium is out of phase (at the wrong stage of development). Following GnRH therapy, this problem sometimes improves."

By shrinking endometriosis, an agonist also may prevent some cases of miscarriage. Endometriosis patients frequently have a history of losing babies. During the first three months of pregnancy, the endometriosis gets worse. Apparently the extra estrogen on board speeds up the progression of the disease. I have followed pregnant patients with a nodule of endometriosis in the cul-de-sac (see fig. 2.2). As the pregnancy progresses, the nodule also grows, sometimes from the size of a pea to that of a marble. The woman gets more and more cramps, backache, and uterine irritability. Eventually the uterus starts contracting, which may cause the patient to lose the baby. A difficult experience for any woman, miscarriage can be emotionally devastating for the infertility patient who has been trying to have a baby for years!

I try to prevent this by pretreating with an agonist, before conception. By shrinking the endometriotic implants before pregnancy, a GnRH agonist sometimes helps the patient carry her baby to term.

While a patient is taking an agonist, I see her monthly to determine if the endometrial nodules mapped out at laparoscopy are shrinking and if they are still tender. If the agonist is working, the nodules get very soft—eventually I cannot feel them anymore. Unfortunately, in the small group of patients in whom I still detect active endometriosis following agonist therapy, the pregnancy rate is low.

GnRH agonists, which lack the androgenic side effects of danazol such as weight gain, are more effective in reducing estrogen levels. Although estrogen deficiency usually causes endometriosis to regress, lack of this hormone unfortunately can cause menopauselike symptoms, including hot flashes, insomnia, vaginal dryness, mood swings, and increased levels of cholesterol in the blood. Following ovarian surgery for endometriosis, I often continue GnRH therapy for one or two months. If the ovary starts ovulating too soon after surgery and swells, the suture line might tear, causing more adhesions.

Although GnRH agonists are available as nasal sprays, we rarely use this delivery method because absorption through the nose is unreliable, especially if the patient has a sinus infection or head cold.

DANAZOL: THE DRUG THAT CAUSES PSEUDOMENOPAUSE

Some doctors prescribe danazol for a few months before major surgery to suppress endometriosis. I seldom use this expensive drug anymore because the GnRH agonists are more effective, have fewer side effects, and require a shorter treatment period. For the rare patient who cannot or will not take an agonist, danazol still offers some relief. For a woman with mild disease, we sometimes get away with using danazol without surgery, but for the patient with more advanced disease, we use the drug as a pre- and/or postoperative adjunctive therapy.

By suppressing a woman's hormone levels, danazol puts her reproductive system into a rest state, causing the endometrial implants to regress. Superficial peritoneal implants seem to respond the best; these often disappear in two or three months.

The drug acts on multiple sites: it works centrally on the brain, indirectly suppressing the ovaries; and secondarily on the endometrium, causing the endometriosis to shrink. By working on the brain control center, danazol suppresses the midcycle surge of the pituitary sex hormones FSH and LH. (Since doctors call these hormones "gonadotropins," they refer to danazol as an "*anti*gonadotropin.") Without stimulation from FSH and LH, the ovaries will not ripen and release an egg. Once the ovaries are quiet, the circulating levels of estrogen and progesterone drop, menstruation ceases, and the endometriosis shrinks. Edema (swelling), inflammation, and pain are reduced. (Remember, usually neither the endometrium inside the uterus nor the endometriosis outside the uterus can grow without hormonal stimulation.)

Although danazol suppresses endometriosis and improves surgical results, it does *not* make the disease disappear completely—the drug is not a permanent cure. It simply suppresses the endometrium to where we cannot see it; it gets down to a one-cell layer. But over time it usually comes back. If the patient is to get pregnant, the lining of the uterus has to regenerate. The same hormones that rebuild the endometrium in the uterus cause the cells of endometriosis to grow. What this means is that, following danazol therapy, there is usually only a short period of time when the patient can get pregnant before the disease recurs.

During the first cycle following danazol therapy, the patient must not get pregnant. Her reproductive system will need a menstrual cycle to readjust after it has been suppressed. It takes time for the pituitary and the ovaries to recover and the endometrium to rebuild. If a woman gets pregnant immediately after stopping the medication, she might miscarry, because she will be fighting a poor hormonal situation.

During the next cycle, however, the patient should try to conceive. If she waits too long, the endometriosis might recur. With short-term danazol therapy, the second cycle is usually normal. In other words, patients on three months of preoperative therapy are back to a normal endocrine system within two months. The endometrial biopsies are usually normal, and the basal body temperature usually indicates ovulation.

Before taking danazol, every patient needs to be informed that, since it is a very weak androgen (male hormone), the medication has significant side effects. The most common problems that I see are weight gain, irritability, temporary decreased breast size, oily skin, acne, and muscle cramping. Some patients also experience menopauselike hot flashes and a change in libido (sex drive). On short-term therapy, only a small percentage of patients have deepening of the voice or increased hair growth. I have heard of cases of increased hair growth and a lowered voice—one woman was an opera singer—but I have never seen a patient with these side effects.

The most common problem by far is weight gain. But if the patient increases her physical activity by doing aerobic exercises like walking, bicycling, or swimming—any smooth activity—she should not gain weight. Exercise helps mobilize body fluids to reduce excess water retention. And increased physical activity helps alleviate the jittery, irritable feeling that causes danazol patients to eat.

Patients on danazol appear to act like people who have hypoglycemia. While they are taking this drug, they must follow a special complex-carbohydrate diet that is relatively low in sugars and fats. The purpose of this diet is to keep the blood sugar from fluctuating widely. My patients who have followed this advice, eating six small meals a day and exercising, have gained little weight on danazol.

There is a wide variation in the doses of danazol that doctors prescribe. Even though the larger dosage costs more, I primarily give eight hundred milligrams rather than four hundred because on the smaller amount a patient will occasionally ovulate and get pregnant. The patient on eight hundred milligrams does not ovulate, nor does she suffer from significantly worse side effects than on the lower dosage. Pregnancy on danazol is a disaster—it is a real worry because the drug is a teratogen, an agent that can cause a defect in the embryo. The medication can masculinize a female fetus, causing the baby to have a large clitoris and fusion of the labia. So, as a double precaution, I insist that all of my danazol patients use a local contraceptive. A patient on this medication must be followed monthly to determine not only how she is feeling, but also if the disease is regressing.

FERTILITY DRUGS: FERTILIZER FOR ENDOMETRIOSIS?

The fertility drug clomiphene citrate (marketed as Clomid and Serophene) has been used for years to induce ovulation in women who have irregular periods. This drug, however, can make endometriosis worse! By stimulating the ovaries and thus increasing the amount of estrogen produced, clomiphene can make endometriosis grow. In fact, I have known patients with ovarian endometriosis who have taken clomiphene and subsequently had a large ovarian cyst rupture. For this reason, it is important to treat the endometriosis *before* giving clomiphene (see chapter 4 for details on clomiphene).

Conservative Surgery for Endometriosis

One month after Georgia's laparoscopy, the couple were back in my office to learn the final results of all the tests.

"Dr. Franklin," said Georgia, "do you think that I am going to get a baby?"

"We will do our best," I answered. "Although your endometriosis is severe, I think that we can increase your chances to between thirty and fifty percent or better. Here is what I feel would be the most effective plan to help you get pregnant: First, since you had endometriosis in your ovaries, I want you to continue taking the agonist. In two or three months, I will do a second-look laparoscopy. At this time, we should be prepared to follow the 'scope with conservative microsurgery—the operation that gynecologists call the 'blue-plate special.' (See fig. 2.17.)

"This major operation should greatly improve your chances of having a baby. Using microsurgical techniques, we will attempt to eliminate the rest of the endometriosis, sever the remaining adhesions, and remove the endometrioma and smaller endometriotic cysts from your ovaries. To relieve your menstrual cramps and pain with intercourse, I will sever the presacral nerve during a procedure called a 'presacral neurectomy.' This may reduce uterine and tubal contractility. In fact, many doctors think that this procedure enhances fertility, although we cannot prove it.

"In my opinion, the presacral neurectomy also helps prevent recurrence of the endometriosis. Since we remove some of the nerve supply to the cervix, it relaxes. This reduces the harmful syndrome of reflux menstruation. If necessary, we also will suspend the uterus so that it is no longer retroverted. This should further decrease the amount of retrograde flow.

"When the patient does not cramp, it usually means that the menstrual flow is going forward more easily. In the majority of women, cramping is greatly reduced after childbirth. During delivery, there is a certain amount of crushing of the nerve ganglia that end up in the cervix. This is one reason why having a baby breaks the cycle of the progression of endometriosis."

"I have heard that cutting this nerve makes childbirth less painful," said Georgia. "Is that true?"

"Yes, it can help, especially during the first stage of labor."

"Can you promise me that surgery will enable me to get pregnant?" asked Georgia.

"We will certainly do everything humanly possible to restore your fertility and cure this disease that has caused you pain for years. But, as much as I would like to be able to promise you a baby, I can't guarantee anything—if I did, it would be false. Unfortunately, I don't have a warranty on your parts, Georgia.

"There are other approaches to starting a family, such as adoption, that you may wish to explore. We have an effective treatment for the majority of our patients—for about two-thirds of them. These will get pregnant, but the rest may not. I feel that it is the doctor's responsibility to tell patients that, since it can take several years to adopt, they may run into a time problem if they wait too long to apply. How do you feel about adoption?"

"I don't want to think about that yet," said Georgia.

"I understand," I said, "but you might wish to join one of the infertility support groups such as Resolve, Inc.,* or the Endometriosis Association,† where you can talk with people for whom adoption has been a terrific success. Adoption gives a couple an alternative way to end the struggle to have a family. You are young, but for a patient in her late twenties or early thirties I suggest at least applying with an adoption agency. Many agencies have a cut-off age of forty-five. Knowing that the option of adoption exists relieves some of the pressure of infertility."

"Is conservative surgery for endometriosis painful?" asked Georgia.

"Patients are concerned that they will have severe pain following the laparotomy. Although any surgery is painful, the major procedure is much less painful than it used to be. This operation and the way we manage postoperative pain have improved in the last fifteen years. With

*Address: 1310 Broadway, Somerville, Massachusetts 02144-1731; telephone: (617) 643–2424.
†Address: 8585 N. 76th Place, Milwaukee, Wisconsin 53223; telephone: (800) 992–3636; in Canada, (800) 426–2END.

the advent of the laser and the newer medications, it is unbelievable how well most patients do."

I explained to the couple that nowadays we manage pain by delivering an analgesic either through an epidural in the lumbar spine *or* intravenously using Patient Control Analgesia (PCA). If the patient has an epidural, which can be left in place for about two days after surgery, she can walk earlier because sensation is blocked below the insertion point. If the woman has PCA, when she hurts, she gets the analgesic instantly by pushing a button on a computer-controlled machine that has been preset using the doctor's pain-medication orders. The patient no longer has to wait for a nurse to give her a shot for pain. To avoid overdosage, PCA will give no more medication during a four-hour period than the doctor has ordered, and no more than a preset number of milligrams in ten minutes. PCA is monitored by a nurse who checks the machine every four hours to see if the doctor needs to increase the dosage. In addition, we put little electrodes on both sides of the incision to block the pain impulses.

It is extremely important for the patient to receive pain medication immediately when she starts to hurt. We have found that, with intravenous PCA, the patient needs less pain medication than when it was given by injection because she gets relief sooner. When a patient has to wait for a shot, five minutes can become twenty minutes, and twenty minutes can seem like a hundred years.

Generally the laparotomy patient now needs one or two pain shots after surgery. When we did the surgery by the old method, the patient asked for a pain shot every two or three hours. In addition to pain medication, I give cortisone, because it reduces swelling and increases the patient's sense of well-being. Surprisingly, some women say that the operating-laser laparoscopy (not the diagnostic laparoscopy) is more painful than the laparotomy.

Of course, every individual perceives pain differently. The doctor may say a patient doesn't have pain, but the patient may say, decidedly, that she does. What is important is that to the patient the pain is real.

Recovery after major surgery is rather lengthy. The patient is hospitalized for three days and receives only intravenous fluids for the first twenty-four hours and clear liquids for the next twenty-four hours before resuming a regular diet. Some patients are constipated for a while, especially if they have had a presacral neurectomy. They require a mild laxative, a diet with adequate bulk, and a stool softener. Intercourse should not be resumed until five or six weeks after surgery.

The morning of Georgia's microsurgery, my faithful internal alarm clock goes off at 5:00 A.M. Not wanting to go back to sleep, I slip out of bed and head for my study. I have a speech on tubal surgery to write, but my mind keeps coming back to the day's work before me.

Georgia's surgery is scheduled for 7:00 A.M. For a second, I see her slender fingers tightly grasping Paul's hand when she asked me: "Dr. Franklin, can you promise me that surgery will enable me to get pregnant?" I had wanted to answer, "Yes," but instead I had told her the truth: "As much as I would like to be able to promise you a baby, I can't guarantee anything."

Women such as Georgia, who are used to solving problems with analytical thinking, sometimes go to pieces when confronted with infertility—a problem to a large extent beyond their control. But, regardless of their background, I doubt that most of my young patients really understand their own maternal drives and needs. To an infertility patient, the desire for a baby often becomes an all-consuming passion. Georgia desperately longed for a tiny infant to cuddle and to love. Why should any woman have to live through agony to realize this dream? After all, is not parenthood a "right" that most of us take totally for granted?

At 7:30, I am in Operating Room 3 of the hospital, looking down at my deeply sedated patient. She is being closely monitored by the anesthesiologist. Surrounded by my two residents, a nurse, and scrub tech, we begin the series of organ-specific mini-operations that constitute reconstructive microsurgery for infertility.

I start by making the horizontal bikini incision in Georgia's abdomen in the pubic hairline. As I look directly into her pelvis, I see that the agonist has dried up some of the endometriosis and reduced the inflammation. While my assistant surgeon continually irrigates the area with a special warm solution to help prevent adhesions, I confirm the operative plan mapped out during the laparoscopy.

Georgia's reproductive organs are fixed by dense adhesions connecting one organ to another. I want to free up her pelvis and do everything possible to prevent additional scar tissue from forming following surgery. Along with the endometriosis, adhesions are the enemy. To help prevent their formation, I handle the tissues extremely gently—this is crucial to excellent fertility surgery. We use every surgical technique and medical therapy available to prevent adhesions, but even with the most exquisite handling the patient sometimes forms additional adhesions following surgery.

Alternating between the magnification provided by the microscope and my wide-angle operating loupes, I begin removing adhesions, systematically lasering the surface endometriosis and excising the deeper lesions. Each vessel is cauterized, and the operating field kept free of blood. As we noted during the laparoscopy, the bowel is disease-free. And since the appendix has no endometriosis on it, I do not remove it. Appendectomy is necessary only if the appendix is diseased.

As I carefully examine both ovaries, I see a discoloration on the capsule of the left ovary, indicating that the endometrioma still lurks beneath the surface. The right ovary, which has adhered to the pelvic wall, is enveloped in tentlike adhesions and appears enlarged. I strongly suspect that it has tiny spots of endometriosis scattered through part of the organ.

I always operate on the best ovary first—the one with the least disease. The GnRH agonist has reduced ovarian endometriosis and inflammation, making it easier to remove the disease without hurting the normal tissue. Using meticulous microsurgical techniques to save as much of the ovary as possible, I peel a large tumor out of Georgia's left ovary (see fig. 2.18). I am extremely careful to avoid injuring the ovarian blood supply. If anything interferes with this life-giving fluid, the ovary will malfunction because it cannot communicate hormonally with the pituitary.

Next I operate on the right ovary. After removing the adhesions, I dissect the tiny endometriotic cysts scattered through about two-thirds of the organ. The only treatment is to perform an ovarian-wedge resection. I literally cut the disease out of the ovary. After I am finished, about one-third of the right ovary remains intact. Georgia's ovaries are now free of endometriosis, and she appears to have sufficient ovarian tissue left to have children.

After examining every area with the microscope, I feel that I have removed all of the endometriosis. Although it is sometimes unnecessary, in Georgia's case I suspend the uterus so that it is no longer retroverted. If the uterus and ovaries are allowed to fall back into place where they were adherent, the two raw surfaces might readhere. When the uterus is pulled forward so that there is no contact between the two surfaces, fewer postsurgical adhesions form. Finally, since Georgia suffers from severe menstrual cramping, I perform the presacral neurectomy to reduce pain if the disease should recur.

As I walk out of the operating room, I am encouraged. I immediately tell Paul that Georgia is doing fine and that I am more optimistic about her chances of having a baby.

I say: "I want Georgia to take the agonist for one more month. After

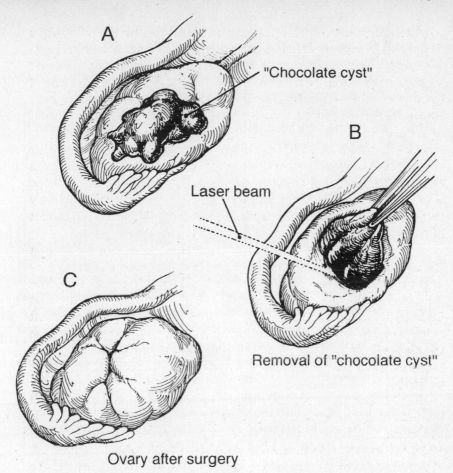

A

"Chocolate cyst"

Laser beam

B

Removal of "chocolate cyst"

C

Ovary after surgery

FIGURE 2.18. An operation to remove a large endometrioma or "chocolate cyst" from an ovary.

discontinuing the medication, you must keep using effective birth control for another month. But after that I want Georgia to get pregnant."

The day Georgia leaves the hospital, she smiles and says to me: "Dr. Franklin, one year from today I will be back in this hospital, only I will not be on this floor—I will be in labor and delivery."

Ten months later, Georgia and Paul decided to apply for adoption. At last the constant push for pregnancy was over. The following month, Georgia became pregnant.

What Causes Endometriosis?

The Theories

There are several theories about the causes of endometriosis. The most widely accepted is that the menses regurgitate backward through the fallopian tubes into the pelvic cavity. I know that this happens because I have seen it through the 'scope many times. Many doctors think that almost all menstruating females have some backup. In one study, red cells were found in the culs-de-sac of ninety out of one hundred women. The question is: Why do only 5 to 15 percent of premenopausal women develop endometriosis? In other words, why do the endometrial fragments adhere in some women but not in others?

One theory holds that the development of endometriosis depends not only on the amount of menstrual flow running into the pelvic cavity but also on how intact and powerful the woman's immune mechanism is. If her immune system is weakened—by chronic stress, for example— her body may be unable to destroy the misplaced cells. Think how some people almost never get colds, because their immune mechanism is intact, whereas others pick up every sniffle of the season.

A good working theory is that the woman who develops endometriosis keeps throwing menstrual blood back into the pelvis until the debris alters the peritoneum. At first, the endometriosis does not grow. But over time, the menstrual debris breaks down the immune system, and the body allows the misplaced endometrium to implant itself and grow. Endometriosis causes a very peculiar kind of scarring. When blood is injected continually into tissue, it gets hard and thick and remains irritated.

Every patient's immune system handles endometriosis differently. Some women contain the disease *too* well, whereas others have little resistance to it. Some black women, for example, lay down very heavy, thick scars. These patients often wall off the disease, putting a large scar around it. These are the same women who are likely to form keloids (excessive scar tissue). When we operate, we find a thick, invasive type of endometriosis. Oriental women have a different reaction to this disease. They seem to have less resistance to endometriosis because of the softness of their tissues. Once the out-of-place endometrium starts to grow, the disease often penetrates into the tissues and invades the ovary.

Dr. W. Paul Dmowski created endometriosis in monkeys and studied their immune system. The researchers diverted each monkey's uterus directly into the abdominal cavity. The animals' immune systems protected them for a while, but eventually they lost their ability to resist the implantation of the disease. But even with the menses spilling directly into the pelvis, the monkeys generally took one or two years to develop the disease.

Scientists think, however, that lower animals have a better immune system than humans. In women, just one gross contamination is sometimes sufficient for endometriosis to implant itself. This is especially true of the lush endometrium of pregnancy. For example, some women develop endometriosis in their incision following a cesarean section.

We had a tragic case at Baylor College of Medicine that graphically illustrates the amazing ability of the endometrium to transplant and grow outside the uterus. One of our pregnant patients developed endometriosis in her leg after she was shot by a jealous boyfriend. The bullet struck the uterus, killed her baby, and lodged in her thigh. A surgeon carefully removed the bullet, but several months later the woman developed thigh pain during her menstrual cycles. Eventually the pain became so severe that she required exploratory surgery. When the doctors reopened the wound, they found active endometriosis in the bullet's path. The endometrial cells spread by the bullet had bled and grown during each menstrual cycle, causing her thigh to hurt.

Now let's go back and support the reflux-flow theory further. In a young woman with an imperforate (abnormally closed) hymen, the menstrual blood cannot flow out of the vagina (see fig. 2.19). With each period, more debris builds up in the vaginal cavity. At first, her cervix is closed and keeps blood from backing up from the vagina into the womb. Eventually, however, the menses start refluxing through the cervix and accumulate in the uterus. Before long, the blood seeps backward through the fallopian tubes into the pelvis.

When I see a woman with an imperforate hymen or even a poorly developed hymen, I worry that she might have endometriosis. The incidence of the disease is higher among women with any anomaly (malformation) of the genital tract, especially if the abnormality causes in-

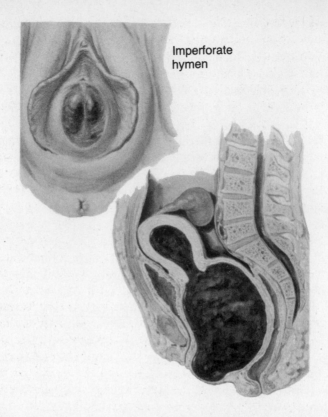

Imperforate
hymen

FIGURE 2.19. Imperforate hymen causing buildup of menstrual blood. (Copyright © 1954, CIBA-GEIGY Corporation. Reproduced with permission from the CIBA Collection of Medical Illustrations by Frank Netter, M.D. All rights reserved.)

creased reflux flow. If a woman's genital tract is narrow or small, she is more likely to develop endometriosis.

I think that reflux menstruation leading to endometriosis accounts for several complications that occur with the disease. For instance, doctors see a condition associated with reflux menstrual flow called "agglutination of the fallopian tubes" whereby endometriosis (or any irritant, such as an infection) causes the fimbriated ends (the little fingers that pick up the egg) of the tubes to stick together.

This could lead to another complication of endometriosis: a higher incidence of ectopic pregnancies. Many doctors think that not all tubal pregnancies have an anatomic cause. They feel that the estrogen-progesterone imbalance sometimes associated with endometriosis may cause some of these ectopic pregnancies. Since estrogen increases tubal activity and progesterone decreases it, excess progesterone may lead to a tubal pregnancy. In addition, the hormones not only affect the nerve supply and muscle activity but also influence the secretory activity inside the tubes. Thus hormones might cause the fertilized egg to move more slowly through the tube, leading to a dangerous misplaced pregnancy.

Another theory about the way in which endometrial cells are transported to sites outside the uterus is that the cells are disseminated through the lymphatic and vascular systems. A large duct called the "thoracic duct" drains all of the abdominal cavity. It is certainly possible that cells from the uterine lining could break off, fall into this duct, and be carried to distant locations, especially if the patient has a rupturing endometrioma.

If there is a break in the circulatory system, the contraction of the uterus or a trauma such as a D&C can cause cells to be released into the blood vessels. Anytime a doctor does a D&C on a patient with cancer of the endometrium, some of the cancer cells are released into the vascular system. I think the same thing happens with endometriosis.

This theory is supported by the presence of endometriosis in distant locations such as the eye, lung, or thigh. The physician can actually see the endometriosis in the eye in the form of a blood blister or scar tissue. Since it is usually hormonally responsive, it cycles with the woman's periods and hemorrhages. I have seen patients cough up blood during their periods when they have the disease in their lungs.

Another hypothesis about the origin of endometriosis is that the continuous irritation caused by the free iron in the menstrual blood stimulates a change in the cells of, for example, the surface of the ovary. Doctors call this transformation of cells "metaplasia." Probably *both* retrograde flow and changes in the cells are important factors in the development of this disease.

Doctors also theorize that endometriosis could develop during the formation of the genital system. It is possible that the endometrial cells might end up in the wrong place—somewhere outside the uterus. What happens to the fetus in the womb is that the cells start up on the urogenital ridge (a ridge of tissue that forms the urinary tract and female genital tract) and migrate down until they finally form the endometrial cavity. Along the way, some of the endometrial cells might be left behind in the pelvis. These cells are totipotential (have the ability to develop in any direction—to become any part of the body). Under the hormonal stimulation occurring at puberty, the misplaced cells might proliferate, causing the symptoms of endometriosis.

Is There a Link Between Environmental Toxins and Endometriosis?

Some doctors have worried for years that some environmental toxins might disrupt the immune system indirectly leading to endometriosis. In 1977, the EPA funded research on the effects of varying doses of dioxin exposure on a small colony of rhesus monkeys. Twelve years into the study one exposed animal died. Severe widespread endometriosis was the cause of death.

When EPA funding ran out, the Endometriosis Association provided emergency financing for laparoscopic study of these monkeys. Their research linked dioxin to endometriosis in the animals. Says president Mary Lou Ballweg: "Seventy-nine percent of the animals exposed to dioxin in the study developed endometriosis versus thirty-three percent of the unexposed animals. The presence of the disease was directly correlated with dioxin exposure, and the severity of the disease was dependent upon the dose administered." The National Institute of Environmental Health Sciences is currently testing the blood of women with endometriosis for chemicals related to dioxins.

Career Woman's Disease: A Misnomer

Endometriosis is sometimes called the "career woman's disease" because infertility specialists see many professional women who have this condition. Although this disease is not confined only to women who work outside the home, it most commonly affects women who have postponed having children. Postponing pregnancy gives the disease more time to progress. Remember that having babies breaks the cycle of the progression of endometriosis. Women who have frequent, early pregnancies seldom develop this condition. Rather, they have fewer periods, and, because pregnancy softens and stretches the cervix, menses flow normally from their bodies.

I do see a few patients, however, who have symptoms of endometriosis as teenagers, have one or two children, and then remain symptom-free—for a while. When they reach their forties, the symptoms return. One might speculate that the early pregnancies bought them time.

My picture of the "typical" young woman with endometriosis is the patient with a high estrogen-to-progesterone ratio. Although studies suggest that endometriosis is unrelated to body weight, I have noticed that these patients are often tall and thin—rarely are they overweight, at least not in the early stages of the disease. Over the years I have seen thousands of patients who fit this "classic" description, but it obviously doesn't apply to everyone.

The earlier a girl starts menstruating, the more likely she is to develop endometriosis. Not only does she have more periods during which menstrual flow can back up onto her ovaries, but, theoretically, her cervix is not softened by progesterone (this is the hormone that further softens the cervix during pregnancy).

During a girl's first menstrual cycle, her ovaries may not ovulate, so they produce only estrogen, no progesterone. This means the lining of her uterus has been built up by estrogen, but until she starts ovulating her cervix will not be softened by progesterone. Since at this time her cervix is not only firm but also often relatively small in relation to the size of the uterus, the menstrual flow—which may be heavy and filled with clots—may not exit the body easily. This is when reflux menstruation may start, and why so many girls suffer from painful first periods.

Some young women who start menstruating rather late also develop endometriosis. They may be tall, theoretically because a large amount of estrogen has not sealed the epiphyses (the little plates of cartilage at the ends of the long bones). Typically, when this girl's periods finally begin, her ovaries appear to produce a preponderance of estrogen. I think that her "high" estrogen/progesterone ratio causes her cervix to be harder than the progesterone-dominant woman's. Her small, hard cervix restricts the outward flow of menstrual blood into the vagina, so that she also may have increased backward flow through the fallopian tubes into the pelvis.

Many infertility specialists think that there is a syndrome that goes with "high" estrogen. I put "high" in quotation marks because the theory is difficult to prove. These doctors believe that the estrogen-dominant woman is more likely to develop endometriosis, fibroid tumors in the uterus, and fibrocystic breasts (breasts in which there are little knots).

How Does Endometriosis Cause Infertility?

We have already discussed how endometriosis causes adhesions and is associated with luteal-phase inadequacy, both of which can cause infertility. In the past, doctors assumed that endometriosis caused spasm of the uterus and tubes because the disease irritates the nerve supply to the uterus. Today we think another reason for spasm is that the endometrial implants produce increased levels of prostaglandins (the hormonelike fatty acids) in the pelvic fluid. These chemicals probably also lead to the erratic corpus-luteum formation mentioned earlier.

If the tube is in spasm, the sperm may not meet the egg. The time when uterotubal spasm (sudden involuntary contraction of the tubes and uterus) is important is right at ovulation, when the tubes need to be wide open. Since prostaglandin production from endometrial cells is governed in part by estrogen, and since estrogen levels are the highest around ovulation, the prostaglandin level is probably also the highest at this point. The narrowest portion of the tube (the cornual end), near the uterus, is the most sensitive to these chemicals. If this part of the tube is in spasm, the sperm might not reach the egg.

Women with endometriosis frequently miscarry, often before they even know they are pregnant. There are probably three main reasons for this: the disease has a toxic effect on the early embryo; the condition causes uterine spasticity, so that the embryo is expelled, often before the pregnancy is detected; and the corpus luteum fails, so progesterone production stops.

Researchers at Baylor are trying to learn whether such miscarriages are related to the prostaglandins, to some other toxic substance released from the endometriosis, or to the immune system. Scientists think that there is a relationship between prostaglandin levels and this disease, but the big problem is proving it. The *in-vitro* fertilization laboratory is helping us do just that. Scientists add some of the pelvic fluid removed during laparoscopy to a rat system that parallels the human system. This fluid keeps the rat system from reproducing. In other words, the fertilized egg stops developing (the cells stop dividing after a certain cleavage). Doctors know that this happens in animals, but we lack proof that it occurs in humans.

Nobody doubts that extensive endometriosis causes infertility, as, for example, when adhesions tie down the fallopian tubes. But although infertility specialists believe that even mild and moderate endometriosis causes infertility, researchers have difficulty *proving* this.

In the 1960s, when the Baylor group started concentrating on infertility, we had difficulty convincing some doctors that mild endometriosis keeps women from conceiving. Since that time, we have done at least three series of studies in my practice. Our findings are that infertility is associated with even the milder forms of endometriosis. Some patients with mild or moderate disease do get pregnant—but it often takes longer. Instead of achieving pregnancy in six months or a year, which is normal for a woman, these patients may take three or four years to conceive.

Once pregnant, some of them, unfortunately, miscarry and have to start all over again.

We continue to investigate all the ways that endometriosis might cause infertility. Although it is difficult to prove, I know in my own mind that the disease keeps women from getting pregnant. If all other factors are normal, these patients get pregnant when we clear up the endometrial implants.

A Related Condition: Adenomyosis

Some women have trouble having babies because they have adenomyosis—a disease associated with abnormal ovulation and frequent miscarriage. Many of these patients have pelvic pain, backache, extremely heavy menses, bleeding between periods, clotting, and pain with intercourse. In adenomyosis, some of the glands and cells of the endometrium are found *within* the myometrium (the muscle *wall* of the uterus). (See fig. 2.20.) For this reason, doctors used to call this condition "internal endometriosis," but now it is classified as a separate disease. At some time in their lives, 20 to 30 percent of women with proven endometriosis also develop adenomyosis. The majority of cases get worse just before menopause.

Adenomyosis responds rapidly to a GnRH agonist or to danazol; both reduce symptoms and allow some patients to carry a baby. These drugs help control uterine swelling, reducing the size of the womb so that the section of each fallopian tube near the uterus opens wider. This may allow the sperm to reach the egg.

Since both medications are expensive and have side effects, I don't give either long term. Unfortunately, when adenomyosis patients stop these medications, the symptoms can eventually come back. Nevertheless, these drugs often give patients a "window" of time in which to have a baby. Sometimes it helps them reach menopause without requiring a hysterectomy.

Adenomyosis often goes untreated because it is difficult to diagnose. In fact, misplaced endometrium hidden within the uterine wall frequently remains undetected until after the patient, usually in her forties, has had a hysterectomy and the pathologist has dissected the uterus.

I think that adenomyosis can be diagnosed, at least presumptively, at a younger age. The patient with this condition often has a relatively large, tender, knotty uterus with the symptoms already mentioned. A physician looking at the X-ray of the uterus and tubes of this patient

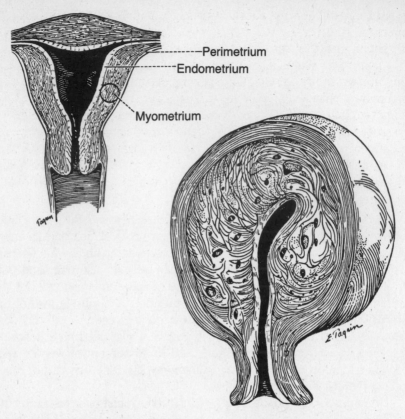

Perimetrium
Endometrium

Myometrium

FIGURE 2.20. Adenomyosis. Misplaced cells of the lining of the uterus are found in its muscle wall. (Reproduced with permission from R. W. Kistner, Gynecology: Principles and Practice, 4th ed., copyright © 1986 by Year Book Medical Publishers, Inc., Chicago.)

often sees a halo effect. In addition, since adenomyosis causes the uterus to be spastic, the patient with this problem usually complains of more discomfort than normal during her X-ray. A final diagnostic clue is that, unlike the endometriosis patient, the woman with adenomyosis usually continues to hurt when given birth-control pills.

Although adenomyosis is diagnosed with the laparoscope, the disease often remains undetected even when the doctor is looking directly at the uterus. Sometimes he sees no sign of disease—not even any endometriosis. If he is inexperienced in recognizing adenomyosis, he may forget that misplaced endometrium could be hidden within the uterine wall and may miss the diagnosis. More often, however, the uterus of an adenomyosis patient is granular and larger than normal. It is boggy (like a sponge full of water) and has little areas that appear to be in spasm even under anesthesia. But since fibroids (benign muscular tumors) also can make the uterus look knotty, it is often difficult to differentiate between fibroids and adenomyosis.

You may wonder how the endometrium gets *inside* the muscle of the uterus. In my opinion, the condition occurs because the patient has a narrow cervix and a relatively tight cornual end of each fallopian tube. (The cornual section of the oviduct goes through the muscle of the uterus; see fig. 2.21.) In some women, this part of the tube takes a relatively straight route; in others, it has a kink; and in still others, it takes a circuitous route. As the uterus contracts to empty itself during menstruation, the cornual end of the tube can close, forcing the cells of the uterine lining into the muscle wall.

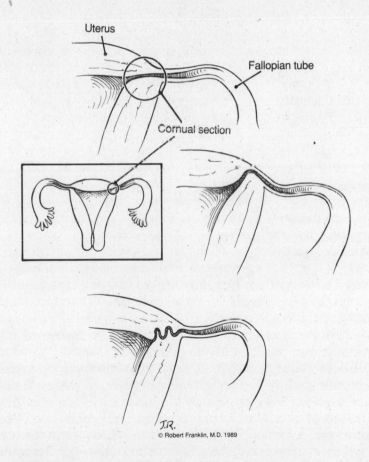

FIGURE 2.21. *The cornual section of the oviduct goes through the muscle of the uterus.*

Some doctors think that rapid, hard labor with twins or a relatively large baby can also cause adenomyosis. There is a higher incidence of adenomyosis in women who have had a prolonged or difficult labor that ends in cesarean section because the cervix never completely dilates.

Conversely, rapid, hard labor may be the *result* of adenomyosis. In other words, the disease could be present before the labor started. If the condition is mild, a pregnant patient may carry her baby to term, even though she has uterine irritability and contractions. But if the disease gets worse, as often happens following childbirth, this same patient may abort a subsequent pregnancy.

Prevention: Younger Sisters

Since Georgia had severe endometriosis, I felt that it behooved me to ask about her sisters because the aggressiveness of this condition tends to run in families. After examining the two younger women, I found that the middle sister, Laura, had moderate disease, and that the youngest, Dawn, was starting to develop the condition.

At only sixteen years of age, Dawn was suffering from severe menstrual cramping. She often spent the first two days of her period in bed. When I did a pelvic exam for her, I discovered that she had a large uterus and a relatively hard, narrow cervix that did not allow the blood to pass easily into the vagina. Furthermore, her uterus was spastic, tender, and markedly retroverted ("tipped"). Considering her family history, I felt that she was set up for endometriosis.

Since mild endometriosis often gets worse unless pregnancy breaks the cycle, it is extremely important to diagnose and treat it as early as possible. For this reason, I carefully started following Dawn as a teenager. I wanted her to be able to avoid developing an infertility problem like her older sisters.

My first line of treatment for Dawn was to prescribe one of the antiprostaglandins, such as Motrin, Ponstel, or Anaprox. Sometimes treating severe cramps early with these drugs will break the cycle and prevent retrograde flow. Unfortunately, however, in Dawn's case this therapy failed to relieve her cramping.

The second medical treatment to prevent the progression of endometriosis was to convert Dawn's firm, estrogen-dominant cervix to a soft, progesterone-dominant one. In order to do this, I prescribed four to six months of low-dose progesterone (ten milligrams of Provera per day for the last ten to fourteen days of each cycle). This medication does three things: First, the pituitary hormones FSH and LH are suppressed so that ovarian estrogen and progesterone production is reduced. Second, the cervix is softened, allowing the menses to escape easier. Third, less endometrium is formed; hence the patient has lighter periods.

Unfortunately, Dawn continued to have cramps on Provera. This suggested that the treatment was inadequate, probably because progestins (progesteronelike hormones) are a poor suppressor of pituitary and ovarian function. The cramping indicated that she was still having considerable uterine spasm, retrograde menstrual flow, or both. The endometrial lining needed to be reduced further.

Since Dawn had failed to get relief on progesterone, my next treatment was to prescribe a low-dose progesterone-dominant oral contraceptive (OC) such as Desogen or Ortho-cept. Each contains both estrogen and progestin and is a better suppressor of pituitary function than progestin alone. When a woman takes one of these birth-control pills, the buildup of the endometrium is further suppressed and the menstrual flow is reduced.

Patients hear that the pill makes endometriosis better. But if the patient with this condition is put on an *estrogen-dominant* pill, as Dawn's sister Georgia was, rather than one such as Desogen or Ortho-cept, the disease will get *worse*. As we mentioned earlier, estrogen stimulates growth of the out-of-place endometrium and makes the cervix harder.

Although the hormonally low-dose contraceptives are less likely to cause side effects than those containing higher hormonal dosages, Dawn's mother was concerned about the pill's long-term effects. I explained to her that OCs, which have been studied extensively since the 1950s, are thought to be one of the safer drugs on the market. In fact, most doctors still think that the pill protects against breast, ovarian, and endometrial cancer.

Some patients experience mood changes on oral contraceptives. Sometimes simply thinking that the pill may cause problems makes patients feel uncomfortable. They may worry that OCs will make them gain weight. Teenagers may be afraid that some people will disapprove of them taking oral contraceptives.

A few patients develop postpill amenorrhea (lack of menstrual cycles)—a condition that is treatable. The pill also slightly increases the chances of liver disease, but the risk is extremely low.

Occasionally a patient on a progesterone-dominant OC such as Desogen or Ortho-cept has more premenstrual tension than if she were taking an estrogen-dominant pill. Furthermore, a progesterone-dominant OC can make acne worse because most of the progestins are actually weak androgens, which can exacerbate acne. This is enough of a problem so that if my patient has acne and needs contraception—but does *not* have endometriosis—I do prescribe an estrogen-dominant pill because estrogen has a beneficial effect on the skin.

Since Dawn had seen both of her older sisters suffer from infertility, she was motivated to stay on oral contraceptives for a while. Exactly how long each individual needs to take the pill varies. As we mentioned earlier, a girl in her early teens has a firm cervix, which will tend to grow and become softer as she matures. When she gets older, she may not need the pill to protect her from endometriosis.

I told Dawn to take one low-dose OC every day for twenty-one days and then to stop for seven days. Although she menstruated at this time, her periods were light, because the endometrium was scant. She had no nausea or weight gain, as some patients do on the pill. With this treatment, her menstrual cramping almost stopped. Since the amount of blood pouring back into the abdominal cavity was reduced, the progression of the disease was halted.

Unfortunately, even Desogen or Ortho-cept sometimes fails to stop menstrual cramps. Depending on the circumstances, the doctor can increase the dosage of the pill or try to make a definitive diagnosis with the laparoscope. Progesterone-dominant OCs can be given continually, allowing the patient to have only three periods a year. In many cases, however, I recommend a diagnostic laparoscopy, because over the years I have noticed that about 50 to 75 percent of patients who have cramps on a low-dose progesterone-dominant OC also have endometriosis. But sometimes the severe cramping is from an entirely different problem, such as a pelvic infection. Quite clearly, accurate diagnosis is extremely important; if a woman has either one of these conditions, it can affect the rest of her life.

It is almost never necessary to do a major surgical procedure on a teenager, although I frequently vaporize endometriosis through the 'scope. The exception to this is if the patient has a large ovarian endometrioma. In such a case, I know that I have to operate because unless the chocolate cyst is removed the patient could lose her ovary. Although it is rare, I have seen fifteen-year-old girls with endometriomas as large as grapefruits. In fact, some of the worst tumors are found in teenagers. Endometriosis probably often gets started while women are in their teens.

When Dawn turned twenty, she got married and continued taking OCs. Like many endometriosis patients on the pill, she had few symptoms from the disease. Two months after she had discontinued the drug, I performed a pelvic exam for her. If the disease still exists several months postpill, I generally can feel the endometriotic nodules. In Dawn's case, however, the therapy had worked—I noticed no palpable endometriosis at this time.

Dawn's case had a happy ending. Unlike her older sisters, Dawn was able to have a baby as soon as she wanted one. I cannot prove that preventive medicine deserves the credit. Perhaps her disease would have stopped progressing without treatment—but her older sisters certainly got worse.

As an infertility specialist, I am often asked the question: "What should I do about having children? Should I have a child right now?" My absolute feeling is that, since children require a great deal of effort, a couple should have them only when both the husband and wife really want them—not because they fear infertility.

If a couple elects to delay having a baby, or decides not to have one at all, that is their right. But if the wife has endometriosis, I feel it is my responsibility to tell them that the disease might get worse. Although theoretically the condition should steadily progress to ever-worsening stages, what generally happens is that endometriosis has a long latent phase. As a rule, the disease seems to accelerate and become severe in the late twenties and early thirties, although this sometimes happens in patients as young as fifteen.

I think that it is my job as a physician to help my patient keep her fertility intact. This means not only treating moderate and severe endometriosis but also preventing mild cases from becoming worse. I want to try to prevent patients from having to face the physical and emotional pain of infertility that Georgia experienced. If I can do that for my young patients, when they want a baby they can have one.

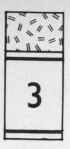

3

Diseases of the
Fallopian Tubes

*Every time I look at my childhood doll collection in my
mother's house I get furious. I want to throw them all
out the window.*

GINGER

Sexually Transmitted Diseases

When I looked at the video monitor showing a flashlight-sized view of Ginger's reproductive organs, I instantly knew why she had failed to conceive. The fiber-optically lighted laparoscope showed that a previous inflammation of the reproductive tract had severely damaged and blocked both fallopian tubes (oviducts). Thin bands of scar tissue called "adhesions" had formed around the outside of her right tube and ovary. Although I couldn't see inside her oviducts, I thought that at least the right one might be lined with adhesions.

After the laparoscopy, I had to tell my patient and her husband, Don, the unhappy news: the 'scope had confirmed my earlier tentative diagnosis; Ginger had pelvic inflammatory disease (PID), an inflammation of the upper reproductive tract involving the uterus, the fallopian tubes, and the ovaries, generally caused by sexually transmitted diseases or other infections. Carried into a woman's fallopian tubes by vigorously swimming sperm, infectious organisms that cause gonorrhea and chlamydia can scar and block the oviducts so that sperm no longer can reach the egg. Although sexually transmitted diseases such as gonorrhea and chlamydia are the most common cause of PID, it can also occur after an abortion or after childbirth.

Even the string of an IUD (intrauterine device) may act as a disease-carrying "wick" between the vagina and the uterus. Furthermore, some doctors think that the trichomonad microorganism, which causes the common vaginal infection trichomoniasis, can swim into the upper genital tract, carrying other, more serious infections to the tubes. Unless treated in time, the inflammatory process can lead to pelvic adhesive disease (PAD). As you now know, adhesions can form inside the body where one surface sticks to another. Without major surgery to unblock Ginger's oviducts and to remove the adhesions, she had almost no chance of having a baby by conventional means.

Chlamydia

As is true of about half of my patients with damaged tubes, Ginger's medical history gave no clues of a previous infection. But even though she had never been diagnosed as having gonorrhea or chlamydia, I strongly believed after looking at her pelvic organs through the 'scope that she probably had suffered from a "silent" chlamydial infection in the past.

Caused by the *Chlamydia trachomatis* bacterium and spread during sexual intercourse, chlamydia is a major cause of PID or disease of the upper genital tract. Without early and adequate treatment with the appropriate antibiotics, chlamydia can set up an acute or chronic infection that can scar the fallopian tubes, making the woman infertile.

Although chlamydia is the most common sexually transmitted disease, many people have never heard of it. According to the Centers for Disease Control, an estimated 12 million persons, two-thirds of whom are under twenty-five years old, acquire a sexually transmitted disease each year in the United States. Of these new cases, approximately 4 million are caused by chlamydia infections. Although nobody knows the exact incidence of chlamydia (many cases aren't reported), the number of infections seemed to increase after the Vietnam War. Until the 1980s, good diagnostic tests were unavailable. Only during that decade did chlamydia become a reportable disease.

When one kind of destructive bacterium such as chlamydia or gonorrhea infects and weakens a patient, other, secondary bacteria, which usually cause no harm in a well person, can set up an opportunistic infection. For example, the common *E. coli* bacteria from the intestinal tract, which generally are benign, can become invasive following tissue damage by another primary bacterium. One might compare gonorrhea to a shark that cuts up its prey, chlamydia to a piranha that nibbles away at its victim, and the secondary infections to the little fish that feed on the remains. Unfortunately, some of the secondary infections take a long time to cure.

Besides causing infertility, chlamydia can lead to other serious consequences for the patient and, if she does conceive, her baby. PID greatly increases its victim's chances of a tubal ectopic pregnancy (a misplaced pregnancy in the fallopian tubes). In addition, if the woman has the disease during childbirth, her baby is at higher risk of prematurity, stillbirth, eye infection (conjunctivitis or "pinkeye"), and pneumonia.

One positive aspect of pain is that it warns us something is wrong. Although chlamydia can be cured with antibiotics, 70 percent of women with the disease—like Ginger—have few or no symptoms. When patients do have symptoms, they may experience only mild lower-abdominal discomfort, a low-grade fever, and a light-yellow mucopurulent (composed of mucus filled with pus) vaginal discharge. Used to menstrual cramping, women often ignore pelvic pain. Some patients have irregular bleeding, itching, and burning, but attribute such symptoms to something else. Occasionally women mistakenly think they have a bladder infection. Even on physical examination, many infected women do not show the usual signs of the disease: they do not have a mucopurulent discharge or a red-looking cervix.

In males, chlamydia causes an inflammation of the urethra called "nongonococcal urethritis" (NGU). Although the disease is usually less serious in men than in women, the infection, if left untreated, can reach the epididymis (the long, coiled canal over each testis where sperm finish maturing). Once within the epididymis, chlamydia takes a long time to cure and can cause sterility.

Ninety percent of men with chlamydia have symptoms, such as a watery discharge or painful urination, that are sufficiently alarming to cause them to see a doctor. Unfortunately, however, some patients stop taking the medication after the symptoms disappear but before they are cured. With no indication that they are infected, these men can become silent carriers, transmitting the disease to their sexual partners.

It was a tragedy that Ginger's chlamydial infection had never been diagnosed. Even today the disease is sometimes missed by physicians. One reason for this is that the routine gram stain (a kind of Pap smear), which detects the well-known venereal disease gonorrhea, doesn't pick up a chlamydial infection. To complicate matters, gonorrhea and chlamydia—which often coexist within the same patient—share some common symptoms; both cause a yellow vaginal discharge and fever. In the 25 to 60 percent of gonorrhea patients who also have chlamydia, gonorrhea masks the chlamydial infection. Unless the doctor performs a special test for chlamydia, he or she may treat the gonorrhea with penicillin but fail to diagnose and treat the chlamydial infection. Since the latter is unresponsive to penicillin therapy, the disease grows unchecked—often making its victim sterile.

One important diagnostic clue for chlamydia: although the infection seldom elevates the patient's white-blood-cell count, as bacteria do, the disease does raise the patient's sedimentation or "sed" rate. This blood test, which shows how fast red cells settle, can indicate a silent underlying disease.

In the past, doctors lacked a practical test for chlamydia. Test results took from three to four weeks. By that time, the disease had done most of its damage. Nowadays, however, we are able to diagnose chlamydia quickly, using the newer enzyme immunoassay (EIA) techniques. If a woman visits her doctor immediately at the onset of the infection, the current four-hour-turnaround Chlamydiazyme test results enable us to diagnose and treat the disease while it is still in the cervix—before the bacteria have time to spread to the uterus and oviducts. If I suspect this infection, I immediately prescribe the antibiotic doxycycline, or erythromycin if the patient is pregnant. A follow-up examination is essential to make certain that the patient is cured.

Gonorrhea

Although many people are aware that untreated gonorrhea can eventually spread through the entire body, causing skin lesions and arthritis, some patients don't realize that the disease can cause infertility. At first concealed within the cervix, gonorrhea can travel up the endometrium and invade the fallopian tubes. Filled with toxins, the bacteria rupture and destroy the delicate tubal lining, causing the walls to stick together.

Acute PID occurs within forty-eight hours of the onset of symptoms. In severe cases, the inflamed and reddened oviducts ooze pus-filled mucus from the fimbriated tubal ends (flowerlike ends near the ovaries). In the next stage, the disease spreads from the inside of the oviducts to the outside. When this happens, adhesions form around the outside of the tubes. The woman now, unfortunately, has chronic PID and PAD.

Although approximately 80 percent of women with gonorrhea have few early symptoms, by the time I see patients with this disease they usually are in tremendous pain. Their symptoms are high fever and greenish-yellow, pus-containing vaginal discharge. Of infected males, 20 to 30 percent are asymptomatic. Some patients also have an oral or anal infection.

We have had good tests for diagnosing gonorrhea for years. Once detected, the disease usually can be cured with antibiotics such as penicillin or tetracycline, although special antibiotics are needed for penicillin- and tetracycline-resistant gonorrhea. These drugs kill bacteria, but sometimes the disease is merely suppressed rather than cured. As with chlamydia, patients with gonorrhea—thinking that they are well—often give the infection to their sexual partners.

A study by L. Westrom found that 12.8 percent of women had tubal blockage after one episode of PID, 35.5 percent after two infections, and 75 percent after three or more infections. Some of these patients may have had one chronic episode that was suppressed rather than cured, instead of several consecutive infections. Since antibiotics reach diseased fallopian tubes slowly, patients require prolonged, aggressive treatment. When a patient is in danger of losing her fertility from an infection, she should be hospitalized.

Mycoplasma?

Doctors are still trying to pinpoint the role of mycoplasma infections in infertility. These microorganisms, which are bacteria with viruslike qualities, are found in different species in humans and are difficult to culture and eradicate. The two most commonly cultured in the female genital tract are *Mycoplasma hominis* and *Ureaplasma urealyticum*. They are sexually transmitted. Although the mycoplasmas may be associated with infertility and habitual abortion, researchers have been unable to prove that these infections cause reproductive problems. Reports are conflicting. One well-known study indicated that mycoplasma patients have a higher conception rate following antibiotic therapy, whereas another suggested that treatment didn't improve fertility.

I have noticed that patients with mycoplasma often do seem to take longer to become pregnant than uninfected women. Patients with this disease are also more apt to miscarry. Even though doctors can't prove that it causes infertility, I think that a mycoplasma infection should be treated with the antibiotic doxycycline. Not only are microorganisms not supposed to be present in cervical mucus; they also make it more toxic and hostile to sperm. As we will discuss in chapter 5, mycoplasma can cause a decrease in sperm motility or swimming ability.

Ectopic Pregnancy: A Dangerous Complication of PID

A serious complication of PID is that it can lead to a dangerous ectopic pregnancy if the fertilized egg implants in a fallopian tube that is scarred and narrowed. Unless the embryo is medically treated or sur-

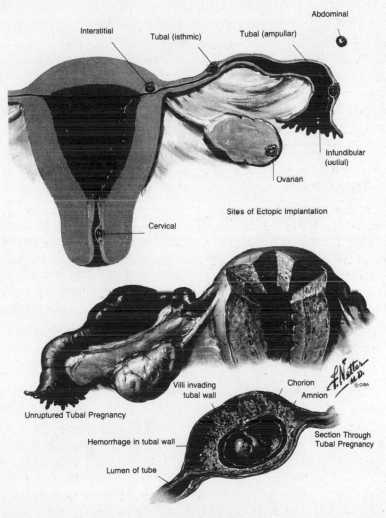

FIGURE 3.1. Some sites of ectopic or misplaced pregnancies. (Copyright © 1954, CIBA-GEIGY Corporation. Reproduced with permission from the CIBA Collection of Medical Illustrations by Frank Netter, M.D. All rights reserved.)

gically removed it will grow and eventually cause the tube to rupture. This is life-threatening (see fig. 3.1).

Westrom's study found that women who have had one tubal infection have six times more misplaced pregnancies than uninfected women. Unfortunately, an ectopic pregnancy can impair a woman's fertility by increasing the chances of a second tubal pregnancy and by causing adhesions.

The earlier the diagnosis of ectopic pregnancy is made, the less tissue damage, the less blood loss, the less adhesion formation, and the less danger to the patient. Patients at high risk for ectopic pregnancies must watch for missed or irregular periods and contact their doctors before the onset of symptoms. Such warnings of a misplaced gestation can vary from intermittent cramping as the affected side swells, to shoulder pain, fainting, and shock. The colicky pain is so distinctive that, once a woman has felt it, she instantly recognizes it if she has a second tubal pregnancy.

The group of women who are at greatest risk are those who have had a sexually transmitted disease, an IUD, a previous ectopic pregnancy, or tubal surgery. Any tubal disease puts a patient in this category. In addition, patients requiring one of the Assisted Reproductive Technologies (ART) such as *in-vitro* fertilization (IVF) or "test-tube" fertilization and "gamete intrafallopian transfer" (GIFT) must be carefully monitored for ectopic gestation. During the IVF process, eggs are removed from the ovaries, fertilized in a petri or laboratory dish, and transferred to the woman's uterus—often exposing the woman to more than one pre-embryo. During GIFT, eggs are removed through the laparoscope and, together with the sperm, immediately placed directly into the oviducts (see chapter 9 for detailed information about these ART procedures).

Doctors also must be on the alert for misplaced pregnancies, especially in high-risk patients. Unfortunately, it is common for women to see their physicians a few times before the doctors think of this diagnosis. Once the doctor is suspicious, he or she can do a blood test for the hormone beta-hCG (human chorionic gonadotropin), a hormone of pregnancy secreted by the placenta. Since the blood supply is less in tubal pregnancies than uterine pregnancies, beta-hCG levels are usually lower in ectopic gestations. Besides carefully monitoring beta-hCG titers, I follow the patient with judicious use of ultrasound imaging of the uterus. In fact, since ectopic pregnancies are the leading cause of maternal death in this country, I think that *all* high-risk pregnancies should be followed with ultrasound imaging. If no gestational sac is observed when specific levels of serial beta-hCG titers are reached, I perform a diagnostic

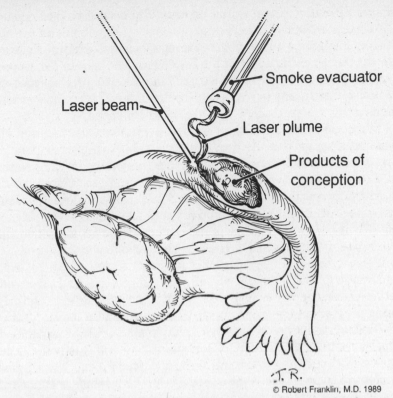

Laser beam

Smoke evacuator

Laser plume

Products of conception

J. R.
© Robert Franklin, M.D. 1989

FIGURE 3.2. Removal of an ectopic (misplaced) pregnancy from a fallopian tube during laparoscopy. After the ectopic pregnancy is carefully "teased" out of the tube, the products of conception are removed through the operating channel of the laparoscope.

laparoscopy. Physicians also must always keep in mind that a woman can have both a uterine and an ectopic pregnancy at the same time, especially if she has taken fertility drugs.

If the doctor diagnoses a patient with a misplaced pregnancy early enough, it sometimes can be treated medically with methotrexate (MTX). Obviously, this patient must be carefully selected and closely monitored using sensitive beta-hCG assays and sonograms. If the pregnancy is too advanced, if the woman has medical problems that preclude the use of MTX, or if the ectopic is leaking or about to rupture, it must be treated immediately with surgery.

Often an ectopic pregnancy is removed with the 'scope and the patient can go home the same day (see fig. 3.2). Sometimes, however, if the gestation is in the isthmic portion of the oviduct (see fig. 1.4), where the tubal muscle is very firm, a laparotomy (major surgery with the abdomen open) is required to resect (surgically remove) the misplaced pregnancy.

Although removal of the ectopic pregnancy sometimes is possible with the laparoscope, repair of the tube may require major microsurgery. Keeping the patient's desire for future pregnancies in mind, the surgeon has to consider on a case-by-case basis if the patient's tubal function can best be restored using the 'scope or major surgery. Often I have better results using the microscope with the abdomen open.

There are times when the damaged oviduct can be repaired with tubal plastic surgery at the same time the misplaced pregnancy is removed. For this to be possible, the ectopic pregnancy must be unruptured (or at least not leaking into the pelvis) and relatively small (no larger than two or three centimeters in diameter). But unless the doctor is an experienced microsurgeon and the hospital is equipped for twenty-four-hour microsurgery, repair of the oviduct should be postponed until a later date. This unfortunately means another operation.

Without the aid of magnification, tubalplasty (repair of the oviducts) immediately following emergency surgery can result in a low chance of uterine pregnancy and a high probability of another tubal pregnancy. During pregnancy, the blood supply increases, and the tissues, which are swollen and edematous, are easily traumatized. Blood loss, bloody surgery, or trauma can cause adhesions. Although this is still a factor with microsurgery, microsurgical techniques reduce the risk of post-surgical adhesions to the point where it is to the patient's advantage to remove the ectopic pregnancy and repair the tubes during the same operation. This can keep the woman from having to go through two major surgeries.

To keep the patient's fertility intact, it is important to do everything possible to preserve the other oviduct—the one without the pregnancy—including postsurgical testing to see whether this tube is open. Unfortunately, when PID leads to ectopic pregnancy both tubes are often involved. In fact, sometimes the tube with the ectopic pregnancy is the best oviduct, because the other one is clubbed at the fimbriated end (the tubal end near the ovary is filled with fluid). Often the little tubal fingers are inverted and may even be destroyed. When this is the case, I wait three to six months to repair the tube without the pregnancy. By this time, the uterine blood supply is back to normal. I feel that this is the best way to preserve the patient's fertility.

Prevention of PID

Obviously the best way to prevent pelvic inflammatory disease is to avoid getting an infection in the first place. Since the more sexual partners a woman has the more she is at risk of getting PID, sexual monogamy is the best prevention against tubal disease. Nevertheless, women with multiple partners can reduce their risk of infection by using barrier methods of contraception. Although there is no risk-free sex, the latex condom offers the best protection. Even condoms can break or leak, however, and the disease can be transferred with the hands during foreplay. The diaphragm, which has sperm- and bacteria-killing jelly on it, may help keep the bacteria out of the cervix. In addition, the contraceptive sponge and spermicidal foams and ointments containing nonoxynol 9 can provide a little protection. Finally, even a woman's own cervical mucus has some antibacterial qualities.

Birth-control pills, which provide less protection against VD than barrier methods, are nonetheless more effective than using no contraceptive. By preventing ovulation, the pill keeps the cervical mucus thick during the woman's entire menstrual cycle. Although unreliable, this pluglike mucus helps keep the infection out of the upper reproductive tract.

One form of contraception, the IUD, may increase the risk of infection. As mentioned earlier, the string used for removal may allow bacteria to travel to the upper reproductive tract. Not all IUDs are implicated, but many have been taken off the market; the price of the few still available has escalated. Although I don't recommend an IUD for a young woman, it sometimes is an ideal method of birth control for women who have already had children.

A woman who has the slightest suspicion that she has chlamydia or gonorrhea must immediately seek diagnosis and treatment. Even though she has no symptoms, a woman at high risk of infection should be tested routinely. The tendency in this country is to treat infections with oral antibiotics, partly because doctors and patients alike worry about the escalating cost of health care. The problem is that sometimes oral medication merely suppresses the disease. If the doctor thinks that the fallopian tubes are involved, more aggressive treatment could save his patient's fertility. If she has an acute episode of PID, there is a strong case for culturing her, putting her directly in the hospital, treating her with intravenous antibiotics, and looking at her reproductive organs with the 'scope. If we give antibiotics intravenously first, higher doses enter the system faster than with oral medication. Although this is expensive,

IV therapy is worth the cost if it saves a young woman's fertility. The patients in Westrom's study who had a 75-percent chance of tubal blockage after three infections had been treated primarily as outpatients. After release from the hospital, the woman should take oral antibiotics, because it takes much longer to get drugs into diseased and scarred fallopian tubes than into healthy oviducts.

Tubal Damage from Other Factors

Appendicitis

Childhood appendicitis can lead to infertility later in life by causing adhesions that tie down the fallopian tubes. The pus from an appendicitis infection can irritate the tissue around the tubes, causing the body to form scar tissue that can prevent the end of an oviduct from picking up the egg. It is like trying to pick up a grain of sand with your hand tied behind your back. Although appendicitis primarily affects the right side, where the inflamed appendix is located, often both tubes are involved. Fortunately, these adhesions usually can be severed with the laser laparoscope or by other methods.

Beta-Hemolytic Streptococci and Other Infections

Beta-hemolytic streptococci bacteria—which are on the skin most of the time and usually aren't sexually transmitted—can become invasive and can cause infection under certain conditions. Acute or chronic streptococcal infections of the genital tract, as well as many other bacteria, sometimes travel through the lymphatic or blood vessels, causing adhesions around the outside of the fallopian tubes.

Some women appear to be colonizers of strep. In other words, in these patients the bacteria are always in the vagina. In most cases, the source is probably the rectum. After an induced abortion, a D&C (dilatation and curettage) following a miscarriage, delivery of a baby, or a biopsy, strep can multiply and spread, because the bacteria feed on blood. Releasing tissue-dissolving chemicals, strep produce symptoms of reddening of the vaginal walls and a thick discharge, but the inside of the tubes usually aren't destroyed. Instead these patients often form adhesions around the outside of the tubes. If left untreated, however, the infection can penetrate the tubal walls and eventually destroy the inside of the oviducts. The woman with adhesions on the outside of her tubes has a better prognosis than the patient with the type of intratubal scarring caused by chlamydia or gonorrhea. Surgeons can remove adhesions on the outside of the tubes with the 'scope, whereas scarring within the tubes requires complicated microsurgery with the abdomen open.

To prevent strep infections secondary to a D&C following miscarriage or delivery, I immediately prescribe antibiotics for a short time. Although this use of antibiotics is empiric (treatment based on past experience instead of exact scientific evidence), I think it is justified to prevent infection and pelvic adhesions.

Endometriosis and Salpingitis Isthmica Nodosa (SIN)

Doctors suspect that endometriosis may alter the way the egg, sperm, and fertilized egg move through the fallopian tubes. We think that the disease increases the levels of some of the prostaglandins in the fluid surrounding the oviducts. Although a change in tubal function has been demonstrated in monkeys, this theory has yet to be proved in humans. To complicate matters, endometriosis may reduce sperm motility by altering hormonal relationships—by increasing progesterone and decreasing estrogen.

Another condition that can adversely affect the fallopian tubes is salpingitis isthmica nodosa (SIN), a disease in which the end of the tube near the uterine conjunction is thickened with irregularly shaped nodules (see fig. 3.3). Although the disease isn't malignant, nodules from several millimeters to 2.5 centimeters in diameter can block the oviducts, causing infertility.

SIN is diagnosed with an X-ray of the tubes and uterus, followed by a laparoscopy. Once the condition is detected, fertility sometimes can be restored with reconstructive tubal microsurgery during a procedure called "cornual resection" (surgically cutting or removing) and "reanastomosis" (putting back together). This simply means that the diseased section of the tube near the uterus is removed, and the remaining, healthy segments are meticulously realigned and sewn back together. Since this requires major abdominal surgery, which we will discuss in detail later, some of these patients may wish to consider IVF first.

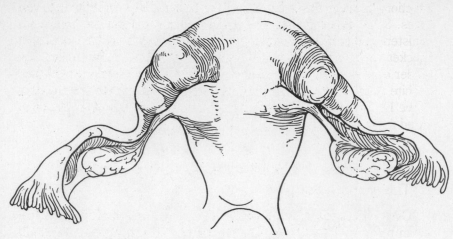

FIGURE 3.3. *Salpingitis isthmica nodosa, a mysterious disease in which the end of each fallopian tube near the uterine junction is thickened with irregularly shaped benign nodules. (Reproduced with permission from R. W. Kistner,* Gynecology: Principles and Practice, *4th ed., copyright © 1986 by Year Book Medical Publishers, Inc., Chicago.)*

Diagnosis of Tubal Obstructions

X-ray (HSG): Pinpointing the Blockage

When I first performed Ginger's pelvic examination, I noticed a cystic mass or thickening around her right tube and ovary. It was not tender. At that time, the thought crossed my mind that she might have a clubbed tubal end called a "hydrosalpinx." This medical term becomes easy to understand when broken down: "hydro" simply means "water," and "salpinx" means "tube." As you now know, infection can cause the fimbriated end of the tube, near the ovary, to close, to fill with fluid, and to swell. In the process, the delicate little tubal fingers that pick up the egg often are inverted and sometimes may be destroyed.

An X-ray (hysterosalpingogram or HSG) of Ginger's fallopian tubes and uterus indicated that both of her oviducts were blocked: the right one near the fimbriated end, the other near the uterus or cornual end (see fig. 3.4). When radio-opaque iodine was injected through the cervix, the liquid didn't flow out of either oviduct. Although in about 30 to 40 percent of patients this is caused by temporary tubal spasm, both of Ginger's tubes were actually closed because of the previous infection.

Before the doctor does the HSG X-ray, it is extremely important for him or her to make certain that the patient doesn't have an active infection, because the iodine can carry bacteria into the uterus to the tubes. Some gynecologists give antibiotics to every patient before administering the HSG. Even if the disease appears to be inactive, a "pocket" of infection might be opened by the dye. If the patient has tender ovaries or tubes or other signs of an active infection, a culture, a white count, and a sed rate are indicated. If test results are positive, I give her antibiotics. I do the X-ray only after the infection has been cured for three to six months.

Laparoscopy: Assessing the Condition of the Tubes and Uterus

Ginger's laparoscopy had confirmed a hydrosalpinx of the right fallopian tube. As I suspected, the fimbriated end was closed, enlarged, and filled with fluid. Furthermore, dense adhesions connected the hydrosalpinx to the right ovary (see fig. 3.4).

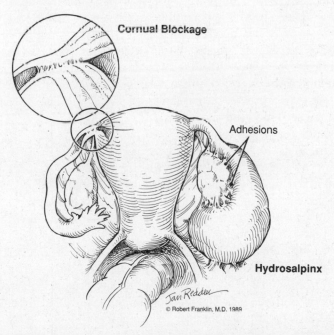

FIGURE 3.4. Both fallopian tubes are blocked: the right one near the fimbriated end and the left one near the uterus. The insert shows the inside of the left tube. Note the adhesions (scar tissue) connecting the hydrosalpinx (clubbed tube) to the right ovary.

Chromotubation (injecting dye into the tubes via the uterus during the 'scope) confirmed the results of the HSG X-ray. Both tubes were occluded (blocked). Ginger's left oviduct appeared surgically repairable, with little evidence of adhesions. Her left ovary looked good; I could see tiny pits all over it where an egg had popped out each month. This confirmed that she was ovulating, as indicated by her temperature charts. In some cases, expert laparoscopists now can repair the tubes through the 'scope. In fact, I'd estimate that 70 percent of the tubal operations that I perform are done this way. Unfortunately, since Ginger had a cornual blockage, I believed that tubal microsurgery, the major procedure, or IVF offered the best chance of getting her a baby.

Treatments

Medical Therapy—GnRH Agonists

After the laparoscope, I met with Ginger and her husband to discuss the medical and surgical options to help her get pregnant. I felt that she should take a GnRH agonist for at least three months because this medication occasionally opens the fallopian tubes. Although an agonist won't unblock a clubbed tube, the drug does open some cases of cornual blockage near the uterus. If tubal surgery is necessary, an agonist reduces the capillary bed, cutting down on bleeding. (The agonist is discussed in detail in chapter 2.)

Doctors really don't know why an agonist opens this kind of tubal occlusion. In cases where the drug helps, we assume that the blockage is caused by endometriosis rather than by infection. A second reason the end of the tube near the uterus opens with an agonist could be that the drug, which keeps the ovaries from making estrogen, causes the endometrium to shrink. In fact, without estrogen stimulation the entire uterus tends to become smaller.

Following agonist therapy, I repeat the X-ray to determine if the drug has opened the tubes. If the tube blocked near the uterus has opened, I often push ovulation with the fertility drug clomiphene citrate (Clomid or Serophene). The goal is to increase the number of eggs released each month. Doctors have learned that the more eggs available to the sperm the higher the pregnancy rate. By using clomiphene, we also often make both ovaries ovulate every month. Normally the left one produces an egg one month and the right the next, although this can vary. If the patient has one abnormal tube, Clomid or Serophene can help make an egg available to the good oviduct every month. This increases the chances of pregnancy each cycle.

In Ginger's case, the agonist failed to unblock the left cornual occlusion. Although not unexpected, this was disappointing.

Tubal Microsurgery

The advent of the operating microscope in the 1970s made tubal microsurgery (tuboplasty) a treatment option for patients, like Ginger, whose oviducts are blocked. Through the use of microsurgical techniques with the abdomen open, the diseased portion sometimes can be removed and the healthy segments carefully realigned and sewn back together. This is delicate surgery, and the outcome is heavily dependent on the skill of the surgeon. Under the microscope, every movement is exaggerated. Although the technique of operating with a microscope can be learned in days, it takes many years of experience to gain the judgment necessary to be a good microsurgeon. When the operation is successful, the sperm once again can reach the egg, and the fertilized egg can retrace the path of the sperm to the uterus.

Patients considering tuboplasty need to be aware not only of the factors that influence the potential pregnancy rates following this operation, but also of the possible complications, the recurrence rate, and the long-term risks.

I wanted Ginger and Don to understand that the probability of success with surgery—which must be stated in terms of live births following a particular kind of procedure—depends on many factors, some of which are beyond the doctor's control. Of primary importance is the presurgical condition of the tubes, the ovaries, and the adjacent peritoneal surfaces (the smooth membrane lining the organs and walls of the pelvis and abdomen). The chances of pregnancy after repairing an occlusion at the cornual end of the tube generally are higher than after reconstruction of the flowerlike fimbriated end. Keep in mind that if the tubal fingers are involved the entire length of the tube is often damaged, although this depends to some extent on what blocked it. When the tube is damaged in several places, the prognosis following surgery is poor. If only the tubal end near the uterus is closed, the section of the tube beyond the blockage usually is healthy, although occasionally the oviduct is closed all the way out to the fimbriated end. As might be expected, a patient with a small hydrosalpinx usually has a better chance of pregnancy than a woman with a large one or with no fimbriae. Furthermore, the more damage to the hairlike cilia and the mucosal folds within the tube, the worse the prognosis.

The length and section of the tube remaining after surgery are critical! Unless at least two or three centimeters of tubal length and one centimeter of the ampulla can be salvaged, the patient will probably never conceive, at least not by ordinary means (see fig. 1.4). I have had patients get pregnant with very short tubes, but the ampullary portion was adequate, and the fimbriated end of the tube that picks up the egg was movable.

Since fertility prospects are poor following surgery when the oviducts have multiple occlusions, patients with this problem may benefit from *in-vitro* fertilization because this procedure totally bypasses the fallopian tubes. In fact many doctors believe that, if the oviducts can't be repaired through the 'scope, IVF should be considered rather than major surgery.

A few patients have a healthy ovary but a poor tube on one side, and no ovary but a good tube on the other side. There is an operation that may enhance fertility in these women. Maintaining the ovarian blood supply, the surgeon simply moves the healthy ovary over partway toward the good oviduct and attaches the ovary to the uterus. The doctor then brings the open tube as close as possible to the good ovary and places the tube so that it can reach the egg. Several of my patients have conceived following this procedure. Some of the new reproductive technologies (ART), specifically IVF and GIFT, offer alternative methods of helping these women. With GIFT, eggs can be transferred from the healthy ovary to the opposite, good tube.

Before offering tubal surgery or some other treatment, I try to determine whether the rest of my patient's reproductive system is working. It is important to know if she ovulates and if her husband's sperm are capable of initiating a pregnancy. Furthermore, the patient's age and health are important factors influencing the success rate following tubal surgery. Few pregnancies have occurred after repair of the oviducts in women over forty.

As with any major surgery, the possibility of complications exists. Anytime we perform a laparotomy with the patient asleep, there is always a slight chance of infection, as well as the risk of complications from the general anesthesia.

Following tubal surgery, the patient has an increased long-term risk of ectopic pregnancy. Although our incidence of misplaced pregnancy is significantly less, the rate of tubal gestations can run as high as 15 to 20 percent, depending on the cause of the problem. After tubal surgery, there is also the possibility that the tubes will kink or that they will reblock because of adhesions. As stated earlier, they can be filmy without blood vessels, thick with many heavy vessels, or stuck together. With the new surgical techniques that help reduce the amount of scar-tissue formation, adhesions are becoming less of a problem after surgery.

The doctor has to consider all these factors when trying to determine the best treatment for his patient with tubal disease. The choice between major surgery and IVF can be a difficult one, especially if the couple can afford the latter. As discussed in detail in chapter 9, success rates following IVF vary, depending on many factors. In general, however, pregnancy rates are higher following microsurgery, if it is performed by an expert. Nevertheless, for tubal problems with a postsurgical pregnancy rate that is the same as the success rate with IVF, *in-vitro* fertilization certainly is an important option. In Ginger's case, if both her tubes had had a large hydrosalpinx (the larger the hydrosalpinx, the more pressure within the tube and the lower the postsurgical pregnancy rate), I would have recommended "test-tube" fertilization over tubal surgery.

Although IVF is a relatively minor procedure compared to tubal microsurgery, *in-vitro* fertilization must be repeated if the fertilized egg fails to implant. When the tubes remain blocked, each time the couple wants another child they must go through the expensive IVF process. In Ginger's case, her health insurance covered tubal surgery but not test-tube fertilization.

As much as physicians would like to be able to predict the chances for success following tubal repair, we often cannot. The prognosis depends on the amount of internal tubal damage caused by the original infections. Until the oviducts are actually opened, this is unknown. Every case is different; hence treatment must be highly individualized. Keep in mind that the location and extent of the damage to the oviduct have a major impact on the potential pregnancy rate following surgery. But even if there is severe damage around the outside of the oviduct, the prognosis is often good if the inside is healthy.

In my opinion, Ginger's chances for pregnancy after surgical removal of the left cornual occlusion were approximately 30 to 40 percent. Considering the size of the hydrosalpinx on Ginger's right tube and the extent of the increased pressure inside it, I roughly estimated that her potential pregnancy rate from her right ovary after surgery would be about 30 percent. The success rate partially depends on whether the oviducts are completely clubbed and the tubal fingers are missing or whether the little fimbriae come floating out and are healthy.

In one study of 868 cases, the pregnancy rate following repair of a hydrosalpinx was 18 percent after one year. Since the tubes may take as long as two years to heal—with possible regeneration of the cilia taking even longer—a more realistic pregnancy rate probably should cover two years after surgery. Although I suggest that my patients start attempting pregnancy two months after surgery, I tell them not to "start counting" until after one year. I think that this takes some of the pressure off them.

After carefully considering all the factors, Ginger decided to have tubal surgery. To repair Ginger's left tube, blocked near the uterus, I did a procedure called a "cornual anastomosis" (see fig. 3.5). During this operation, all of the diseased portion was removed from the left

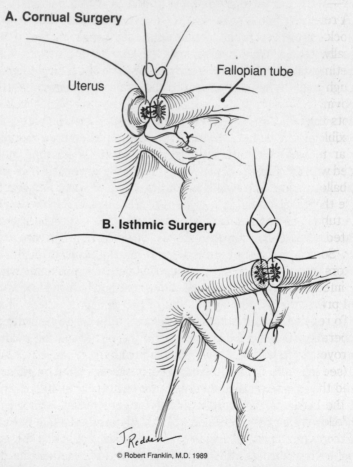

A. Cornual Surgery

Uterus

Fallopian tube

B. Isthmic Surgery

J. Redden

© Robert Franklin, M.D. 1989

FIGURE 3.5. A. Cornual surgery. A blockage at the junction of the uterus and fallopian tube has been removed. The tube has been carefully realigned with its passageway through the uterus. The two sections are rejoined so that the sperm can reach the egg. B. Isthmic surgery. A blockage has been removed from the isthmic portion of the tube, and the two sections are stitched back together.

tube. I used the laser to cut through the tubal muscle and microsurgical techniques to sever the section surrounding the tiny lumen (opening) of the tube. The openings of the two remaining, healthy portions were meticulously realigned so that the sperm could reach the egg and the fertilized egg could travel to the uterus. In the cornual portion of the oviduct, the opening is only about the size of the period at the end of this sentence. After the openings were matched, the three layers of muscles—a central circular, an inner longitudinal, and an outer spiraling layer—were carefully sewn back together.

A relatively new two-'scope procedure sometimes allows doctors to unblock cornual occlusions without major surgery. With the aid of a fiber-optically lighted hysteroscope inserted through the cervix, a surgeon sometimes can reopen a blocked fallopian tube by passing a small dilator through the 'scope into the obstructed part of the oviduct. Rather than removing the blocked portion during abdominal surgery, the doctor attempts to open the tube by running a tiny modified Novy catheter with a flexible guide-wire probe into the oviduct. This procedure is rather similar to balloon angioplasty, in which constricted blood vessels are dilated with an inflated balloon. During fertility surgery, a catheter instead of a balloon sometimes can widen a narrowed oviduct. The doctor looks inside the pelvic cavity with a laparoscope, constantly checking for possible tubal perforations. If the operation is successful, contrast medium injected through the catheter should spill out the fimbriated end of the tube. Some pregnancies have been reported following this procedure. Doctors worry about possible complications such as perforations, bleeding, infection and reblockage of the oviduct, damage to its lining, and tubal pregnancies.

To repair Ginger's right, clubbed tube, or hydrosalpinx, I performed an operation called "salpingoplasty." Although the tubal fingers had been destroyed by infection, I was able to design new ones to pick up the egg (see fig. 3.6). Once the scar was removed with the high-beam laser, I used the low-beam laser to shrink the outer surface of the oviduct so that the inside of the tube fanned out into a flowerlike shape.

Following surgery, we X-rayed the fallopian tubes to make certain that they were open. The radio-opaque dyelike substance flowed in and out of each oviduct easily. Four weeks later, I performed a second-look laparoscopy. Since I noticed that a few adhesions were just beginning to form, I immediately severed them with the laser.

Two years passed, but Ginger didn't become pregnant. By this time, she and her husband had managed to save enough money to try *in-vitro* fertilization. During the IVF process, five of her eggs were removed from her ovaries via a hollow needle. Her husband's sperm were placed

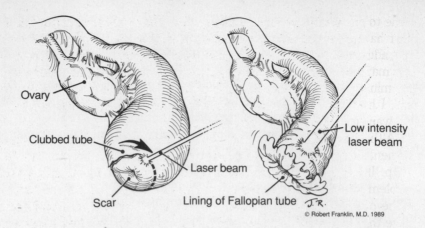

Ovary

Clubbed tube

Laser beam

Scar

Low intensity
laser beam

Lining of Fallopian tube

© Robert Franklin, M.D. 1989

FIGURE 3.6. The tubal fingers have been destroyed by disease, but a new, fun-nellike structure is created to pick up the egg.

right next to each egg in a laboratory dish. Four fertilized! But our hopes were short-lived. Ginger and Don were to be disappointed one final time. When the resulting embryos were transferred to her uterus, none implanted. The couple now had no more medical options, because they couldn't afford to try IVF a second time.

Two months passed. Then one day Ginger came to see me because her period was two weeks late. I could tell by the expression on her face that she knew she was pregnant. Nine months later, Ginger delivered a healthy six-pound baby girl.

Reversing Tubal Sterilization

Every year over eight hundred thousand women in the United States are sterilized by tubal ligation (by having the fallopian tubes "tied"). Of these, approximately 1 percent will request reversal surgery, the operation doctors call "reanastomosis" of the fallopian tubes. Why do so many women ask for reversal surgery? The reasons include an increase in divorce, a younger age at sterilization, the fewer babies available for adoption, and the relative ease of laparoscopic sterilization.

Considering the large number of requests for reversals each year, I feel that women under thirty-five should have counseling before becoming sterilized. I have had patients as young as twenty years of age come to me wanting reversal surgery. They have had their tubes "tied" after having several children—usually one right after another. Worried that additional pregnancies will ruin their daughter's health, Mom and Dad may encourage their offspring to become sterilized. But sometimes, the minute a young woman has the tubal ligation, she is unhappy. In fact, I have had several patients ask for reversal even though they did not want any more children for a while.

Although tubal ligation is a satisfactory birth-control method for some women, the patient needs to be told in advance that problems can develop. It has been sold as an invasive procedure with an extremely low problem rate, but some women have pain afterward. If the blood supply to the ovaries is disturbed during the ligation, they will swell and hurt. Since the blood vessels to each tube and ovary are very close together, the surgeon must be exceedingly careful not to damage the ovarian blood supply. The doctor also must avoid damaging the ovarian support system, because, if the ovaries twist, the pain can be excruciating.

Before performing reversal surgery, I try to determine whether the rest of my patient's reproductive system is working. Here again, it is important to know if she ovulates and if her husband's sperm are capable of initiating a pregnancy. Often her previous fertility history indicates whether there might be a problem.

Sometimes it is necessary to do a complete infertility workup on the couple before performing reversal surgery. This generally includes charting ovulation, a semen analysis, and a postcoital test. The day of the reversal, I do an HSG X-ray and laparoscopy before beginning the reanastomosis, to see how much of the tube has been destroyed and how many adhesions have formed.

The pregnancy rate following reanastomosis of the fallopian tubes depends on the condition and the length of the remaining tubal segments, how well the ovaries are functioning, the age and health of the patient, the quality of the husband's sperm, and the skill of the tubal microsurgeon.

To a great extent, the condition of the oviducts after tubal ligation depends on which sterilization method was used, where the tubes were damaged, and the length of time since ligation. Of the different tubal sterilization methods, which include cautery, surgical resection of part of each tube, the falope ring, the clip, and fimbriectomy (removal of the fimbriae), the falope ring and the clip afford the best reversal rates, fimbriectomy the worst. Although the overall pregnancy rate is approximately 58 percent, patients having isthmic-isthmic reanastomosis, in which two isthmic portions of the tube are rejoined, have a 75-to-80-percent pregnancy rate, whereas those requiring ampulla-ampulla surgery have only a 42-percent rate. Although repair of the ampullary portion is technically easier, the pregnancy rate is lower because the ciliated and secretory activities are more important in this segment than in the isthmus.

In general, the longer the time interval since ligation, the more damage. As many as 71 percent of patients requesting reversal surgery have disease between the point of tubal ligation and the uterus. The farther each tube is tied from the uterus, the more likely that it will have endometriosis, scarring, fistulas (abnormal openings), and tubal polyps (little growths that often develop where there is chronic irritation).

If a sterilized woman decides that she wants reversal surgery, she needs to be aware that she will be at increased risk of tubal pregnancies. To some extent, the ectopic-pregnancy rate following reversal depends on the sterilization method used. Fewer than 1 percent of my patients have tubal pregnancies after this surgery, although much higher rates have been reported.

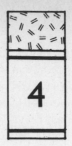

Hormonal Imbalances

Irregular Ovulation

When I first met Annie, eleven years ago, she was a twenty six year-old bride of nine months. Friendly and self-confident, Annie had an open personality that seemed to say: "Here I am. I am wonderful, and I know you are going to like me."

Annie told me that she and her husband wanted a large family and that they had never used any form of birth control. She was worried because she had not conceived and wondered if it was because her menstrual periods had become increasingly irregular.

During a normal menstrual cycle, a woman's reproductive system ripens the follicle surrounding an egg and releases it. This is called "ovulation." In Annie's case, I suspected that this process was not working exactly right, causing the shedding and regeneration of the lining of the uterus to be unpredictable. After carefully listening to her problems and performing a thorough pelvic examination, I felt that, once Annie started ovulating properly, she would have a good chance of having a baby.

Irregular ovulation is the most common cause of infertility; approximately 40 percent of my patients have erratic periods, including ovulatory disturbances. Why do so many women have irregular ovulation and menstrual cycles? To answer this question, one must begin by examining the sequence of events surrounding ovulation. A woman's ovulatory mechanism might be compared to the inner workings of a fine timepiece. If any part of the clock's delicate movement is off, it will be unreliable, gaining or losing time and causing the alarm to be unpredictable. Similarly, if the process by which a woman ripens a follicle is out of sync, she may not conceive, because her hormones also will be out of balance. An egg may not be released on schedule, or even if it is, the lining of the uterus may be inadequately prepared to support a pregnancy.

Since the ovulatory process involves an extremely complicated and exquisitely timed interplay of chemicals, there are many reasons ovulation can become irregular. Before an egg can pop out of an ovary, all the parts of the hormonal axis—the hypothalamus (lower brain), the pituitary gland (the master gland), and at least one ovary—must work together in perfect synchronization. If the blood-borne hormones that feed back and forth between the governing center in a woman's head and her ovaries are not released on schedule at relatively precise levels, ovulation may be erratic or fail to occur at all. In addition, blood levels of thyroid and adrenal hormones also must be on target. Although the body's system of checks and balances generally can compensate for slight hormonal irregularities, if one part fails to function correctly the woman will not conceive.

A woman can have menstrual periods and not be releasing an egg. In menstruating patients who fail to ovulate, the endometrium (the lining of the uterus) is stimulated by the ovarian sex hormone estrogen but not by the hormone progesterone. Without ovulation, the corpus luteum, which produces progesterone, never forms. (You will recall that the corpus luteum develops out of the egg sac following ovulation and produces progesterone to prepare the uterine lining for a possible pregnancy; see chapters 1 and 2 for review of the function of the corpus luteum.) If the endometrium has been built up by estrogen and the estrogen level drops, bleeding occurs. It can be profuse or slight, depending on the amount of estrogen available to promote the growth of the endometrium that cycle.

To determine whether Annie was ovulating, I asked her to take her basal body temperature (BBT) before rising each morning. After Annie had taken her BBT for three months, I examined her temperature charts. They indicated that her ovulatory pattern was erratic. As mentioned previously, normally a woman ovulates around the thirteenth or fourteenth day from the beginning of menstruation, and her period occurs approximately every twenty-eight days, with a range of twenty-six to thirty-four days. Over a three-month period, however, Annie had ovulated on the ninth day, the twelfth day, and the fourth day (during her period) of her menstrual cycle.

Even so, Annie's ovulatory problem was mild in that, although her periods were irregular, she did appear to ovulate. Her "picture tube" basically was working, but her hormonal axis just needed a little fine tuning. If she had not ovulated at all, it might have meant that she had a more severe problem.

Ovulatory disorders can be easy or difficult to treat, depending on what is causing them. When I see a new patient such as Annie, I always look for clues pointing to reasons her cycling mechanism is off. Is there an organic cause? Is her diet adequate? Does she have more stress than she can handle at home or at work? Did she experience a major psychological or physical trauma during puberty, such as a divorce in the family, sexual molestation, a severe burn, or a fracture, that could have triggered the problem?

Annie's history gave few clues as to the cause of her irregular ovulation. Her teenage years had been relatively uneventful. She had no family history of endometriosis, diabetes, or genetic problems, any of which could have caused her irregular periods. Furthermore, her physical and pelvic examination revealed no endometriosis or pelvic inflammatory disease. All of her other tests, including her "Pap" (Papanicolaou) smear, were normal, and her husband's semen appeared adequate to initiate a pregnancy.

Since Annie was over twenty-five years old, had never had a previous infertility workup, and had only mild ovulatory dysfunction, I decided to give her the fertility drug clomiphene citrate, marketed as Clomid or Serophene. Often referred to by the press as Clomid, this well-known drug, which we discuss in detail later, has helped many women conceive. I felt that clomiphene might synchronize Annie's hormonal system, making a more drastic type of investigation unnecessary.

This turned out to be the right game plan for Annie. The first month that she took clomiphene, Annie became pregnant. Although some women's periods become regular after having a baby, Annie's did not. Each time she and her husband wanted another child, she took clomiphene. Today, with the help of this amazing fertility drug, Annie has four healthy children and another on the way. Since her hormonal axis needed only a little help to start cycling properly, clomiphene caused her to ovulate on schedule. During her first or second cycle on the medication, she would conceive. If clomiphene hadn't worked after three to six months, I would have discontinued it and proceeded with further diagnostic tests, including hormonal studies and a laparoscopy.

Types of Mild Ovulatory Disorders

There are several main types of mild ovulatory abnormalities, although they are difficult to categorize in the early stages. The first group includes irregular ovulation, in which women release an egg at the "wrong" time in the menstrual cycle. These patients may have persistently early or late ovulation and thus have irregular periods. Not all such women, however, have difficulty getting pregnant. Sometimes they have unpredictable menstruation at one time in their lives but become regular later.

Some patients ovulate late and have a menstrual period every thirty-six or thirty-seven days. The proliferative phase (the first half of the cycle, before ovulation—days 1 through 12 or 14) is too long, meaning that ovulation occurs around day 21 or 22 rather than on day 13 or 14. These patients not only have more difficulty getting pregnant than normal, but they also seem to have more miscarriages and ectopic pregnancies than the general population.

One theory suggests this occurs because during long cycles the follicle has more time to age before ovulation. Another hypothesis is that these patients have defects in the enzymes (protein catalysts) that prepare the uterine lining each cycle for a possible pregnancy. This might cause the endometrium to be at the wrong stage of development when the fertilized egg arrives.

There is a second category of ovulatory disorder, one that's extremely difficult to define. It occurs in patients who often begin having problems as teenagers. They develop large fluid-filled corpus-luteum cysts and have grossly irregular periods (see fig. 4.1). The hormonal cycling mechanism in these patients appears to get out of balance. The problem may originate with a defect in the corpus luteum or in the governing center in the woman's brain. Sometimes the hormonal feedback from the ovary to the pituitary fails to shut off, so that too much LH (luteinizing hormone) is produced. When this happens, the corpus luteum enlarges and may continue functioning, resulting in a prolonged luteal phase, after ovulation. The egg probably isn't always extruded from its follicle. If it should be released and fertilized, it may not implant because the uterine lining has been improperly prepared by progesterone. When the corpus luteum becomes cystic, it either produces too much or too little progesterone to support a pregnancy.

A third group of patients appear clinically to be ovulating and menstruating regularly, but they have either poor or intermittent progesterone production. This can occur if the progesterone-producing corpus luteum malfunctions or dies. A patient with this problem sometimes gets

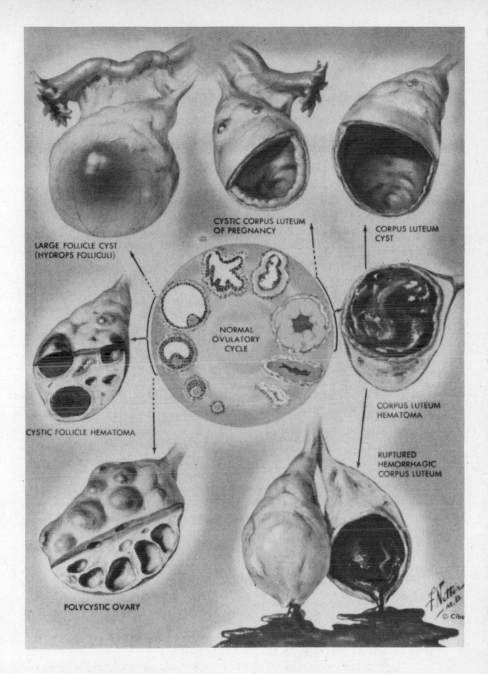

LARGE FOLLICLE CYST
(HYDROPS FOLLICULI)

CYSTIC CORPUS LUTEUM
OF PREGNANCY

CORPUS LUTEUM
CYST

CYSTIC FOLLICLE HEMATOMA

NORMAL
OVULATORY
CYCLE

CORPUS LUTEUM
HEMATOMA

RUPTURED
HEMORRHAGIC
CORPUS LUTEUM

POLYCYSTIC OVARY

FIGURE 4.1. Corpus luteum cyst and other cysts. (Copyright © 1954, CIBA-GEIGY Corporation. Reproduced with permission from the CIBA Collection of Medical Illustrations by Frank Netter, M.D. All rights reserved.)

pregnant and at first appears to be doing fine. Then suddenly she has a severe pain in her side. If the doctor is monitoring her progesterone level during early pregnancy, he will notice it drop, indicating that the corpus luteum has hemorrhaged and died. Without progesterone to support the pregnancy, the woman will abort in one or two days. If the doctor can anticipate this, he sometimes can save the pregnancy by giving progesterone.

Not every early pregnancy, however, can be saved with progesterone. Sometimes the reason the hormonal level suddenly drops is that the baby has died—often because it is not forming properly. Sensing that progesterone is no longer needed to support the pregnancy, the woman's amazing body halts corpus-luteum function. Shortly thereafter, the pregnancy is usually expelled.

Pregnancy can have a positive or an adverse effect on a woman's cycling mechanism. Some patients have irregular periods before having a baby but become regular after delivery. Conversely, others are perfectly predictable before childbirth but become erratic afterward, sometimes developing extremely severe premenstrual tension. Doctors are unable to predict these changes.

Causes of Ovulatory Abnormalities

CONTROL-CENTER MALFUNCTION

> *The only way to avoid stress would be to do nothing at all. Virtually all human activity involves stress—from a game of backgammon to passionate embrace. But this can be defined as the stress of pleasure, challenge, fulfillment. What we all want is the right kind of stress for the right length of time—at a level that is best for us. Excessive or unvaried stress, particularly frustration, becomes distress. And this, in turn, can lead to ulcers, hypertension, and mental or physical breakdown.*
>
> HANS SELYE, *Stress Without Distress*

Some patients fail to ovulate because their hypothalamus does not function properly. Not much bigger than the end of your thumb, the lower brain is constantly on the alert, regulating a cascade of bodily functions. Weighing only a quarter of an ounce, the lower brain's duties include regulating hunger, thirst, temperature, sleep, growth, and reproduction. The hypothalamus indirectly controls thyroid and adrenal function. The thyroid gland regulates metabolic rate, and the adrenal glands secrete the hormones that help us respond to stress, all of which influence the ovulatory process.

When the hypothalamus is affected by chronic stress, ovulation can stop even though the woman's reproductive system is otherwise normal. A certain amount of stress is invigorating—without any we would be dead—but excessive stress, especially if it exceeds our ability to cope, can be harmful.

It has been proved in animals that stress stops ovulation. A rat exposed to a bright light or to loud noises will cease ovulating. Although we know that infertility can be associated with chronic stress, it can be difficult to eliminate because it often stems from the patient's family or job. Airline stewardesses and high-altitude skiers, for example, frequently have irregular periods. A stewardess has a stressful job, dealing with the public; in addition, her hypothalamus is continually bombarded by noise pollution and changes in the light cycle. Long flights across time zones where the sun rises at different hours affect the hypothalamus and, consequently, have an impact on ovulation.

There are other, extremely rare causes of dysfunction of the hypothalamus leading to anovulation (lack of ovulation) that a doctor has to keep in mind. For example, a few patients are born with a lower brain that does not function properly; they cannot get pregnant. These people are often extremely short and underdeveloped; they are not difficult to diagnose. Other rare causes of anovulation are benign or malignant lesions near or within the hypothalamus, which can be picked up by a CT scan or MRI.

DIETARY CAUSES

Overexercise, inadequate diet, and tremendous weight fluctuations also can stop ovulation dead in its tracks. I see women who feel so good from jogging that they overdo it. Others diet and lose thirty to forty pounds and stop their periods. Some young women actually carry dieting to the point where it not only stops ovulation but also becomes deadly.

Occasionally a patient with an ovulatory disturbance will start infertility testing but refuse to bring her weight up to normal. Although she professes to want a baby, she either secretly or subconsciously does not want to get pregnant. *Not* getting pregnant may be important to her because if she loses her body image she may have severe psychological problems. This woman can be difficult to care for if she does get pregnant. As we will discuss later in the context of preanorexia, I have had longtime infertility patients become pregnant and ask to be aborted when they start losing their figures. These patients need the help of a psychiatrist.

I think that blood sugar also plays a role in ovulation. I see quite a few women with hypoglycemia (low blood sugar) who have irregular menstrual cycles. They often seem stressed. Although it is difficult to tell which came first, the stress or the low blood sugar, I have found that it helps these patients to organize their food intake. If they distribute their caloric intake over six or eight small meals and avoid refined sugar, they do much better. Refined sugar gets into the bloodstream too fast, causing the pancreas (specifically the beta cells of the islands of Langerhans) to overact and pump too much insulin into the bloodstream. This causes the blood-sugar level to plummet, affecting every cell in the body. Not only does the person become ravenously hungry, but the feedback along the hormonal axis can be interrupted.

Illegal drugs also have an adverse impact on ovulation. In animals, marijuana has been shown to inhibit ovulation and is associated with depressed LH. In humans, one of the few studies on the effect of marijuana on female reproductive function shows that users have two-day-shorter menstrual cycles and a shorter luteal phase than nonusers. Marijuana users also have more cycles without ovulation.

Patients on illicit drugs do not eat properly. I see infertile drug users who are so underweight that their hypothalamus is affected, causing them to quit ovulating. This may be one of the main ways in which illegal drugs adversely affect fertility.

Patients who smoke marijuana often drink considerably more alcohol than nonusers. Since alcohol is associated with menstrual irregularities, it is difficult to isolate which substance causes the menstrual problems.

Whatever the exact cause, I frequently see heavy marijuana users who stop ovulating and menstruating. Once they stop using pot, their periods generally return within three to six months.

Even excessive use of aspirin or aspirinlike products can cause a woman to miscarry. Normally, after the egg pops out of the ovary, the follicle left behind fills with blood. If the woman takes too much aspirin, the newly forming corpus luteum can hemorrhage and die, because aspirin adversely affects the blood's clotting ability. Without the pregnancy-supporting effect of progesterone produced by the corpus luteum, the woman will lose the embryo, unless she is given the hormone by her physician.

PROLACTIN HORMONE ELEVATION

Women with elevated levels of prolactin circulating in their bloodstream frequently do not ovulate and may have either irregular or no periods. Prolactin is the pituitary hormone that stimulates and sustains lactation in nursing mothers. Although an unreliable birth-control method, elevated levels of this hormone indirectly provide nursing mothers with limited protection against pregnancy.

Stress, alcohol, tranquilizers, high-blood-pressure medication, low thyroid level, low blood sugar, or a pituitary tumor can elevate the level of prolactin. Secretion of this hormone is so sensitive to stress that a doctor can tell a woman that he is going to draw her blood for a test, and, unless she is lying down, her fear of the needle will cause her prolactin level to rise.

How does prolactin stop ovulation? Simply put, doctors think that the hormone suppresses secretion of gonadotropin-releasing hormone (GnRH), the key hormone from the hypothalamus that sets the ovulatory process in motion. Unless stimulated by GnRH, pituitary sex-hormone levels of FSH and LH will fall. As you know, without sufficient stimulation from these sex hormones, the ovaries cannot mature a follicle and release its egg.

EXCESS MALE HORMONE

I think that even the stress of everyday life—if it exceeds our ability to cope with it—can overstimulate the adrenal glands and indirectly cause some women not to ovulate. Simply put, stress causes the adrenal glands to secrete more cortisol and more male hormones called androgens (testosterone and DHEA-sulfate) into the bloodstream. Testosterone is the male hormone that weightlifters foolishly take to gain weight and build muscles. If a woman has too much androgen circulating in her blood, she may ovulate poorly or not at all.

Most people think of adrenaline rather than cortisol as the hormone that helps the body handle stress. Although it is true that adrenaline helps you handle the urgency of the moment, it is cortisol that sustains you throughout the battle. If a one-thousand-pound bear is charging you, adrenaline speeds up your heart, enabling it to pump more blood to your muscles, simultaneously raising your blood sugar so that you can run away. But if you are foolish enough to stay and fight, you had better have plenty of cortisol to build up your muscles and keep you going. This is the well-known fight-or-flight response.

In women, as the body calls for more cortisol to handle stress, the accompanying rise in adrenal androgen negatively affects ovulation. In addition, the ovaries also contain androgen-producing cells, and when ovulation ceases these cells increase in number. This causes the woman to have too much male hormone, coming not only from the adrenal glands but also from the ovaries. If this process remains untreated, the woman may develop a complicated endocrine disorder that we discuss later called "polycystic ovarian disease" (PCO). Although PCO usually develops after years of interrupted ovulation, it can occur sooner.

Lack of ovulation, however, does not always cause excess male hormone to be produced. Women who fail to ovulate because the hypothalamus is not communicating with the ovaries do not produce extra androgen. Birth-control pills, for example, do not cause this problem, because they suppress the pituitary sex hormones FSH and LH that stimulate the ovaries. Although menopausal women usually do not ovulate, they also do not produce excess male hormone. They do show some of the effects of androgen, however, because they lack the balancing influence of ovarian estrogen. This is why some older women have increased hair growth on the upper lip unless they take replacement hormones.

Determining the Cause of Irregular Menstruation

One obvious reason a woman misses her period is that she is expecting. It is extremely important to pick up pregnancy early, because some patients need help to prevent a miscarriage. Furthermore, the doctor would not want to miss a dangerous ectopic pregnancy in a fallopian tube or give a fertility drug to a patient who is already pregnant! Palpating the thyroid gland is one of the best ways to diagnose early pregnancy, because the thyroid becomes enlarged when a woman is expecting. In pregnancy, the breasts are full, the cervix is soft, and the doctor can feel the pulsating uterine arteries. By observing these clues and by running a beta-hCG test, I can tell within a week of conception if the woman is pregnant.

Once pregnancy is ruled out, I have to make certain that my patient's erratic periods are actually caused by an ovulatory disorder. Charting ovulation with the basal thermometer, as I did with Annie, is the easiest way to do this.

There are excellent baseline tests available to help doctors rule out pathological causes of amenorrhea (lack of menstrual periods). You will recall that normal thyroid function is generally necessary for normal ovulation. An underactive thyroid gland can cause menstruation to cease by secreting insufficient thyroid hormone or by elevating the prolactin level. When the thyroid is underactive, the hypothalamus, sensing the need for more thyroid, tells the pituitary to secrete more thyroid-stimulating hormone (TSH) in order to increase thyroid production. But, as a side effect, the hypothalamus also stimulates the pituitary to release more prolactin. This, of course, can stop ovulation. Fortunately, once the thyroid condition is treated with supplemental thyroid, the prolactin level will drop and menstruation will return, if other factors are normal.

Another cause of amenorrhea is premature ovarian failure (early menopause). At birth, a woman's ovaries contain approximately two million oocytes (cells that develop into eggs). As she ages, the number of egg-containing follicles in her ovaries decreases. Eventually either the woman runs out of follicles or the few that are left become resistant to the hormone that causes oocyte maturation and ovulation. The last menstrual period is known as "menopause" and normally occurs between the ages of forty-five and fifty-five; fifty-one is the average. Sometimes the ovaries still produce enough hormones so that the woman doesn't require estrogen replacement. Often, however, the level of this hormone drops so low that the patient has hot flashes, insomnia, and other symptoms. Such a patient may benefit from hormone-replacement therapy— taking estrogen and progesterone. Although it is rare, the ovaries may be depleted of follicles earlier than normal—for example, in the mid-thirties. When this happens, the woman experiences early menopause (called early ovarian failure) and usually can no longer have biologically related children.

No matter when it occurs, menopause is diagnosed with a blood test that measures plasma levels of FSH and LH. If these pituitary hormones are elevated, it means the brain is trying to force the ovaries to ripen a follicle but they are unable to do so.

Menopause is not always an all-or-nothing situation. Although menopausal patients think that they cannot ovulate anymore, they may still have some follicles. Stress or some other factor occasionally causes their ovaries to release an egg. This is why postmenopausal women occasionally get pregnant if they discontinue contraception.

If the patient is under thirty-six years old, wants a baby, and has mildly elevated FSH and LH, it may be worthwhile to do an ovarian biopsy to see if she has sufficient follicles to conceive. I do this only in the rare instance where I am trying to decide if the patient has enough follicles to be pushed into ovulation with medication. As a rule, I try to avoid operating on ovaries unless they are diseased because scar tissue can form after surgery. Sometimes, however, the patient has only a short time before she will run out of eggs. A decision has to be made whether to push her ovaries. If she has no eggs, it would be wrong to give her an expensive fertility drug.

If the ovarian biopsy shows that a woman has follicles, I sometimes prescribe Pergonal. A powerful fertility drug, this medication provides additional FSH and LH directly to her ovaries, which may overcome their resistance to ovulate. Premature menopause is not always a hopeless situation, but it does require more study to see if the woman has follicles. If she has none, she will not be able to have a biological child—doctors cannot create eggs where there are none.

All the above baseline studies give a complete picture of the patient's hormones. Tests show not only the serum levels of the female hormones estrogen and progesterone but also the amounts of male hormones in the blood. By checking serum levels of testosterone and DHEA-S (adrenal androgen), I can tell if the male hormone is coming from the ovaries, from the adrenal gland, or from both. As we will discuss later, if adrenal androgen is normal, the patient may be a candidate for the fertility drug clomiphene citrate (Clomid or Serophene). If DHEA-S is high, the patient may need to be treated with a cortisonelike hormone to lower adrenal androgen before taking clomiphene.

Treatments

Time and Reassurance

If my patient is under twenty-five, has been trying to have a baby for only six months, and has no underlying disease, I explain to her that it often takes six months to a year to conceive. Other than a few baseline tests and an analysis of the husband's semen, she may need only a little time and reassurance.

This is the time, however, to start talking with her to determine if her eating habits are good and if she is under too much stress. Such stress may cause the adrenal glands to overact. Without relief, a woman's menstrual cycles may become irregular. Sometimes, by resetting her priorities or giving herself more time to reach her objectives, a patient can lighten her daily responsibilities. Once her stress is manageable, her ovulatory mechanism may become more regular.

Empiric Treatment

If my patient has been trying to conceive for over six months, is over twenty-five years old, and has no evidence of endometriosis on pelvic examination and normal baseline tests, I sometimes prescribe clomiphene citrate (Clomid or the less expensive Serophene) for several months, as I did with Annie. If, after a few months, she still fails to conceive, I often suggest a complete medical infertility workup. This includes an X-ray to see if at least one fallopian tube is open and if the uterus is normal, a laparoscopy to rule out endometriosis and pelvic adhesive disease, and an endometrial biopsy to study the effect of progesterone on the uterine lining.

Sometimes doctors are unable to pinpoint the exact reason for a patient's failure to ovulate regularly. What we can do, however, is to rule out underlying diseases and other problems. Once we do this, we sometimes have to treat empirically with clomiphene to induce ovulation. You will recall that empiric treatment is based on past experience instead of exact scientific evidence proving the cause of the problem. But clomiphene can hurt rather than help the woman with endometriosis, especially if the disease is in the ovary. Hence, if I suspect endometriosis, I look inside the pelvic cavity with the laparoscope before treating with clomiphene for any length of time.

Although the goal in medicine is specific diagnosis—the less empiric the diagnosis the better for the patient—sometimes empiric treatment is necessary to prevent the progression of disease. Since over time lack of ovulation can lead to the complicated and potentially devastating endocrine disorder called "polycystic ovarian disease" (PCO), it is better to treat empirically rather than allow the patient to develop this condition.

Empiric treatment with clomiphene can often regulate erratic menstrual cycles, making more invasive testing and treatment unnecessary. By simply making a woman regular, Clomid probably reduces the risk of a misplaced pregnancy or early pregnancy loss. The effect of late ovulation is seen in Catholic women who use the rhythm method. They abstain from sexual relations around ovulation, sometimes becoming pregnant in the late phase of a long menstrual cycle that, for example, is forty-five days instead of twenty-eight days. Doctors have noticed a higher incidence of ectopic pregnancy and miscarriage among such patients. Although the usual tests show nothing abnormal, these women probably had some kind of ovulatory disturbance.

Fertility Drugs

CLOMIPHENE CITRATE (CLOMID OR SEROPHENE)

The fertility drug clomiphene citrate has enabled many women such as Annie, with ovulatory disorders, to conceive. Often referred to as "Clomid," this much-discussed drug can help stimulate regular ovulation in women who otherwise fail to mature and release an egg on schedule. If the woman's menstrual periods are irregular, clomiphene often synchronizes her reproductive clock so that, when she does ovulate, the endometrial nest is at the right stage of development to support a pregnancy. By making erratic periods regular, clomiphene also helps pinpoint the exact time of ovulation, thereby increasing a couple's chances of correctly timing intercourse. Furthermore, by helping an irregular woman ovulate every month, clomiphene increases the opportunities for conception.

First successfully used to induce ovulation in the early 1960s, clomiphene yields ovulation rates of approximately 75 percent and conception rates of about 35 percent. The drug helps women whose ovaries make some estrogen but fail to produce a sufficient estrogen surge so that the pituitary hormones FSH and LH are released. As you now know, these hormones are necessary to stimulate ovulation.

Unfortunately, clomiphene yields poor results if the patient's ovaries produce insufficient estrogen. Doctors can test for adequate estrogen with a vaginal smear, an assay of blood or urinary estrogen, or an endometrial biopsy, or by giving a shot of progesterone or an oral progestin (a synthetic progesterone) such as Provera. If the patient fails to bleed following the shot—indicating a lack of estrogen—clomiphene usually will not work.

The exact way clomiphene works is unknown. One theory is that the medication, which has a chemical structure similar to that of estrogen, works by competing with estrogen for receptors in the hypothalamus. It is difficult to prove, but it appears that Clomid causes FSH and LH to be released from the pituitary. One recent study suggests that the drug may increase the number of pituitary or ovarian receptors.

When the patient stops taking clomiphene, the receptors are released, causing an outpouring of FSH and LH. This hormonal surge often causes several follicles to ripen. As the follicles mature, they pump increasing levels of estrogen into the bloodstream. The brain subsequently senses the rising estrogen level and sends a burst of LH to the ovary. This triggers ovulation.

In patients with monthly periods, Clomid sometimes lengthens the menstrual cycle, because it often is started on day 5 rather than on day 1 (day 1 is the first day of bleeding). The drug also can be given from the first day of the cycle and continued for ten days to build up the follicle. If the woman does not have periods, clomiphene is started on the fifth day after withdrawal bleeding or menstruation is induced with progestin. Ovulation usually occurs about one week after taking the drug, and menses follow two weeks later. If the patient becomes pregnant on Clomid, her BBT will remain elevated for more than fourteen days, and menstrual flow usually will not start.

There is controversy over whether clomiphene can cause luteal-phase defects, resulting in inappropriate levels of progesterone. (See chapter 2 for a review of luteal-phase defects.) Women with luteal-phase problems abort more often than normal. In the past, we felt there might be a relationship between luteal-phase defects, spontaneous abortion, and the use of Clomid. But since we use Clomid to regulate irregular cycles and to push abnormal ovaries into ovulation, the increased incidence of luteal-phase problems and abortion is probably the fault of the abnormal ovaries rather than clomiphene. If the patient has a progesterone deficiency, I give her progesterone vaginal suppositories or oral micronized progesterone to try to prevent miscarriage.

Not all patients ovulate on the minimum dosage of clomiphene. For this reason, doctors generally follow a detailed plan of increases in the dosage until the drug works. We begin with one tablet (50 milligrams) daily for five days, starting between days three and five of the patient's menstrual cycle. We carefully follow the patient's reaction to the medication by taking her basal body temperature and by measuring serum-progesterone concentration after ovulation. If she fails to ovulate on the minimum dosage, I sometimes increase the dosage to 100 milligrams daily for five days in the next cycle. The maximum dose of Clomid that should be given is 250 milligrams a day for five days. About 10 to 20 percent of women treated with clomiphene will not ovulate, even on the maximum dosage.

For women who are resistant to clomiphene and fail to ovulate on two, four, or even five clomiphene a day, I sometimes prescribe a drug called "bromocriptine." This medication, combined with just one clomiphene per day, makes some of these patients suddenly ovulate (see page 146 for further information on bromocriptine).

Depending on the couples' wishes and their ages, I usually give Clomid for about four to six months, occasionally as long as a year. If the ovulatory pattern is unsatisfactory on clomiphene, I sometimes suggest the powerful fertility drug Pergonal for three months (see below).

Clomiphene can cause side effects, but they are seldom severe enough to interfere with treatment, especially at the lower doses. Doctors prescribing Clomid, however, must watch for the occasional patient whose ovaries become overstimulated by the drug. PCO patients, or women who experience pelvic pain, must be followed with particular care. If clomiphene is given in too high a dose or for too long, enough follicles can be stimulated to cause the ovaries to swell and hurt. This usually can be avoided, however, by examining the patient every month that the drug is given.

There is controversy over the effect of Clomid on cervical mucus.

Since the quality of cervical mucus is estrogen-dependent, clomiphene—
which has primarily an antiestrogenic effect—may decrease the quantity
and the quality of the mucus. This adversely affects the sperm's chances
of reaching the egg. The higher the dosage of Clomid, the more serious
the problem becomes. We sometimes get around this by giving a supplemental estrogen marketed as Premarin (0.625 to 2.5 milligrams a day
for seven to ten days before ovulation is expected). Sometimes, however, we have to use intrauterine insemination, where the sperm are
washed free of semen and are placed directly in the uterus, or low doses
of the powerful fertility drug Pergonal, to overcome cervical mucus
problems.

One of the first questions patients ask about clomiphene is: Will it
cause me to have multiple births? Although the incidence of multiple
gestations on clomiphene is approximately 7 percent, most of these are
twins, with deliveries of three or more babies accounting for fewer than
1 percent. With the early use of ultrasound, the doctor can tell the
patient how many babies she is carrying.

About 11 percent of patients on Clomid have vasomotor symptoms
that resemble the well-known hot flashes of menopause. Another 7.4
percent have abdominal discomfort, and a few patients complain of mood
swings, nausea, blurred vision, afterimages, and light flashes. Although
the symptoms disappear when the drug is discontinued, if the patient
has vision problems I seek a consultation with an ophthalmologist. Furthermore, preliminary unconfirmed studies have reported a slight increase in the incidence of ovarian cancer following the use of ovulation
induction drugs.

The question of greatest concern to most women is: Will my baby
have an increased risk of having birth defects if I take Clomid? Over
thirty-five years' experience with this drug has shown that the rate of
birth defects is not increased over that of the general population.

TRIGGERING OVULATION WITH
SUPPLEMENTAL hCG

In some patients on Clomid, the egg ripens but fails to pop out of
the ovary. These women may need a shot of human chorionic gonadotropin (hCG) in order to ovulate. You will recall that hCG, which is
secreted by the developing placenta, is the hormone that is measured
to determine if a woman is pregnant. Extracted from the urine of pregnant women, hCG, which has a chemical similarity to LH, sometimes is

used during Clomid cycles to trigger the release of the egg from its follicle, much the way the monthly midcycle LH surge probably triggers ovulation normally. With the aid of the urine test for LH, we can tell if this hormone has surged.

PERGONAL

Unfortunately, not every woman is helped by Clomid. For the patient with a deficiency of the pituitary sex hormones FSH and LH whose ovarian follicles are adequate but understimulated, doctors sometimes prescribe the fertility drug Pergonal. With ovulation rates over 90 percent and pregnancy rates of 60 percent, this expensive medication has helped hundreds of my patients have babies. Without this powerful drug most of these women probably would have never conceived. If no factors other than irregular ovulation are causing infertility, the pregnancy rates are higher.

By providing replacement therapy for women lacking sufficient FSH and LII with low estrogen levels, Pergonal usually stimulates the ovaries to mature and release several eggs. Originally extracted from the urine of postmenopausal nuns, Pergonal known to doctors as "human menopausal gonadotropin" (hMG)—supplies an equal combination of FSH and LII directly to the ovaries, bypassing the brain.

Capable of stimulating the maturation of more than one estrogen-producing follicle, Pergonal has a multiple-birth rate of about 20 percent. Although 15 percent of these are twins, the drug is responsible for the well-publicized cases of deliveries of three, four, and five babies at a time.

Pergonal not only often causes the ovaries to release multiple eggs each cycle, but also has the potential to overstimulate the ovaries—sometimes to the point where they might rupture! Women with low FSH, LH, and estrogen are not as likely to have this reaction as the patient who has been a candidate for Clomid with an intact hormonal system. It is imperative, however, that the doctor conscientiously follow any patient on this medication and that he be experienced in its use. Requiring *daily* monitoring of follicular development to avoid hyperstimulation of the ovaries, treatment with Pergonal is time-consuming and expensive. Doctors have found that, by suppressing the ovaries with the amazing new LH-RH agonist Lupron before giving Pergonal, they can reduce the chances of hyperstimulation significantly.

Since the more follicles are stimulated, the higher the estrogen levels, physicians can assess whether the ovaries are becoming hyperstimulated by measuring the level of estrogen in the blood. Interestingly, the closer the ovaries are pushed toward hyperstimulation, the more pregnancies occur. We also carefully monitor development of the ovarian follicles with ultrasound, a noninvasive technique by which the developing follicles can be seen on a computerized TV-like screen. These tests are absolutely necessary and have led to a reduction in multiple births and potentially serious side effects.

With Pergonal, ovulation is always triggered with a shot of hCG. If the serum estrogen level is too high, we avoid hyperstimulation by withholding the hCG injection. If hyperstimulation does occur, it usually is noticed three to seven days after the hCG shot and progresses for another seven to ten days. If the problem is severe, the patient must be hospitalized so that fluid intake can be carefully monitored.

Before taking Pergonal, the patient must have a complete infertility workup, including an X-ray of the fallopian tubes and a laparoscopy. A semen analysis of the husband also is required. These tests are done to look for other problems that might interfere with fertility.

Unlike Clomid, Pergonal has a beneficial effect on the cervical mucus. Since multiple follicles ripen on Pergonal, the estrogen level increases. This stimulates the production of mucus, making it more watery so that the sperm can swim through the cervix more easily. Sometimes Pergonal is given with clomiphene to improve the cervical mucus.

The side effects of Pergonal are extremely variable. The drug throws the ovaries into high gear, making them more sensitive. Patients sometimes have bloating, abdominal pain, nausea, insomnia, hot flashes, and depression. These symptoms increase at the time of ovulation but slowly diminish until menstruation, when they disappear. If the woman conceives, the symptoms may last for three or four weeks, because the ovary continues to be extremely active.

No increases in birth defects are associated with Pergonal above those found in multiple pregnancies. There is, however, a 25-to-30-percent increased chance of miscarriage, especially in cases of multiple gestations. All Pergonal pregnancies must be closely monitored because they have a high ectopic-pregnancy rate of about 3 percent. I have had patients with both an intrauterine pregnancy and a dangerous tubal pregnancy at the same time!

If a woman is going to get pregnant on Pergonal, she usually does so within the first four treatment cycles. This is also true for clomiphene. If she fails to conceive during the first few menstrual cycles, it usually means that something else is wrong besides ovulatory dysfunction. If she has at least one fallopian tube open, this may be the time to follow superovulation by Pergonal with intrauterine insemination (IUI), whereby large numbers of "washed" sperm are injected directly into the uterus. If I think that she might be helped by one of the assisted reproductive technologies (ART), I may recommend *in-vitro* fertilization (IVF), also called "test-tube" fertilization, a procedure in which conception occurs outside the body. A few patients may benefit from GIFT, a procedure in which the eggs are retrieved from the ovary and injected with the sperm directly into the fallopian tubes (see chapter 9 for details).

AMAZING NEW FERTILITY DRUGS

Doctors now have an amazing new drug with which to treat infertility called "synthetic gonadotropin-releasing hormone" (GnRH). Depending on how GnRH is administered, it can either induce ovulation or as discussed earlier temporarily stop it. The effect of GnRH is contingent upon whether the drug is given in a pulsatile manner (in regular intermittent bursts) or in a sustained manner. If GnRH is given in a pulsatile fashion, it acts as a fertility drug by stimulating ovulation. Administered this way, GnRH is equal to or better than Pergonal in treating women with irregular ovulation—as long as they have an intact pituitary. GnRH is especially effective in inducing ovulation in patients with polycystic ovaries. In contrast, if GnRH is given in a sustained manner, the drug has the reverse effect: after an initial surge of the sex hormones FSH and LH, daily or monthly injections of GnRH will bring ovulation to a screeching halt. As a potent ovulation inhibitor, GnRH can be used in the treatment of estrogen-dependent endometriosis and fibroid tumors.

In nature, GnRH—also called "LH-RH" or "LH-releasing hormone"—is secreted by the hypothalamus in bursts occurring approximately every ninety minutes. This pulsatile release of GnRH is crucial to reproduction. If all women suddenly started secreting this hormone in a sustained manner, the human race would eventually end. As you now know, without GnRH the pituitary gland will not secrete the sex hormones FSH and LH to set the ovulatory process in motion.

It makes sense that, in order to induce ovulation with synthetic GnRH, the drug must be administered in a fashion that generally mimics nature's rhythmic ninety-minute GnRH pulses. Unfortunately, at present the only way to do this is by using a portable mini-infusion pump. This computerized pump, which must be worn by the woman for about six to eight days, automatically releases the drug every ninety minutes into a vein. After the follicles have matured, an injection of hCG can be given to trigger ovulation in women who fail to release an egg.

Recovery from the Pill

The year after Paula quit taking oral contraceptives so that she could have a baby, she had only two extremely light menstrual periods. By the time she came to see me, she had been off the pill for almost eighteen months, had seldom menstruated, and was eager to find out what was wrong.

Paula told me that she had gone through puberty late and that her periods had never been regular. She had been given a birth-control pill with a high dosage of estrogen and had switched back and forth between the pill and an IUD (intrauterine device) three times in seven years. Many doctors think that the pill, when taken at an early age, may suspend the maturation of the hormonal axis. I wondered if this might have happened to Paula.

How the Pill Works

Most oral contraceptives (OCs) prevent pregnancy by suppressing ovulation. Today's pill usually contains a combination of a progestin (a progesteronelike hormone) and an estrogen, both in lower doses than in the past. Ovulation is stopped because these hormones act together to suppress the pituitary sex hormones FSH and LH, which stimulate the ovary to mature a follicle and release its egg. The pill also works by making the cervical mucus dry and scant and by inhibiting the growth of the uterine lining. After the pill is discontinued, normal ovulatory cycles generally resume within three to six months.

Causes of Failure to Menstruate Postpill

If a teenager has too much stress when her hormonal axis is starting to cycle at menarche—and many do—she may have irregular ovulation and erratic periods. If her menses become so irregular that she continually spots, or if she is sexually active, her doctor may put her on the pill. Sometimes, instead of alleviating her stress, unnecessary worry within the family about the safety of the pill adds to the problem.

Although today's low-dose pill is widely accepted as a safe form of contraception, 0.2 to 3.1 percent of women discontinuing oral contraceptives fail to resume menstruation after six months. Doctors call this problem "postpill" amenorrhea. In these women, the pituitary does not start cycling again. The problem sometimes occurs if the patient takes

OCs before her reproductive system has matured, or if she shocks her hormonal axis by continually starting and stopping the pill.

Since Paula had been trying to conceive for one year, I suggested that she have a complete infertility workup. After checking to see that all of her baseline tests were normal, I gave her the fertility drug clomiphene, and within a few cycles she was cycling normally again. I continued giving her Clomid for two cycles, and then let her rest one month before restarting the drug. During her next Clomid cycle, Paula became pregnant.

Since the pill might interfere with the maturation of the hormonal axis, I feel that it is better not to give OCs—especially those with a high dose of estrogen—to a young woman until her hormonal system has finished maturing. Sometimes merely giving the hormone progesterone will help an immature axis begin cycling. Nevertheless, there are times when a doctor needs to prescribe the pill to a teenager: for example, if she is bleeding constantly and becoming a "pelvic cripple" or if she is sexually active and refuses to use other forms of contraception. Furthermore, if a teenager is headed toward polycystic ovarian disease, oral contraceptives can help prevent the buildup of male-hormone-producing cells that sometimes occurs with time in an ovary that fails to ovulate. A potentially devastating disease, PCO is discussed in detail in the following section.

Polycystic Ovarian Disease (PCO)

Martha was a likable woman with an incredibly active mind. An extremely intense person, she always had at least six irons in the fire at all times. When she came to see me at age twenty-six, she was working full-time as a highly successful stockbroker and was going to night school to finish her master's degree in finance. Martha had been married to a mechanic named Larry since high school and had been trying to conceive for slightly over six months. She had had only four or five periods the previous year.

Martha had been overweight for years. She had gained forty additional pounds during the preceding two years. By the time I saw her, she was obese, carrying most of the excess weight around her waist.

Although she had many friends and was happy about her career and her progress in school, Martha was extremely depressed about her appearance and seemed to have a poor self-image. She asked me if I could cure her severe acne and help her get rid of the excessive hair on her face and other parts of her body.

My clinical impression of this patient was that she probably had polycystic ovarian disease (PCO), also called "Stein-Leventhal syndrome." An extremely complicated endocrine disorder, PCO is associated with long-term lack of ovulation and excess androgen circulating in the blood. Each month that an ovary fails to release an egg, cysts form inside the gland, so that over time both ovaries become filled with cysts— hence the name, "polycystic" ovaries (see fig. 2.15).

The classic patient suffering from full-blown PCO is overweight— often obese—and has the male-pattern hair growth associated with excess androgen. She may have a period approximately every forty-five to sixty days and often is infertile. In about two-thirds of cases, the ovaries are enlarged; in advanced stages, each ovary is frequently larger than the uterus.

Not all patients with PCO, however, fit this classic pattern. In fact, only about 10 to 20 percent of my patients with polycystic ovaries have all the classic symptoms of the disease, as Martha had.

Since full-blown PCO is the result of failure to ovulate, usually over a long time, doctors see patients in various stages of the disease. Although this condition progresses in an S-curve, not everyone gets worse at the same rate. Typically, the woman headed toward PCO at first can maintain her weight by dieting. But, over time, the sustained elevated level of androgen makes it increasingly difficult to lose weight. Eventually the woman loses the battle.

Stress and the Adrenal Glands

Like many PCO patients, Martha looked as if she had been under stress her entire hormonal life. I felt that she had constantly pushed her adrenal glands.

When a young woman has too much stress—especially when her pituitary and ovaries are beginning to cycle at puberty—her chances of ovulatory disturbances are increased, because excessive stress causes the adrenal glands to increase androgen production. Some studies indicate that the problem may start as early as in the womb. If a pregnant woman has too much stress, it may affect her unborn baby's hypothalamus, so that it may not cycle properly at puberty. Unfortunately, time often makes this problem worse.

Martha's condition can be understood better if we look at a related but more serious disease called "congenital adrenal hyperplasia." People with this condition have an enzyme defect affecting the production of cortisol. This problem can be life-threatening. Simply put, the brain senses a lack of this vital chemical and causes the pituitary to overproduce a hormone called "ACTH" (adrenocorticotropic hormone). ACTH stimulates the adrenal glands to raise the cortisol level back to normal. Unfortunately, the extra ACTH also causes the adrenal glands to secrete too much androgen.

Like Martha, some women have only mildly overactive adrenal glands. Doctors call this condition "adult-onset adrenal hyperplasia." When we try to measure an enzyme defect in these women, we often are unable to detect it. One theory suggests that such patients actually may not have an enzyme defect but that instead their adrenal glands have been repeatedly overstimulated, causing them to become overactive. Regardless of the cause, this condition can lead to excess male hormone. Over time, many of these patients suffer from some or all of the symptoms of full-blown PCO, such as irregular periods, weight gain, acne, excessive hair growth, and infertility.

The big question is whether PCO can be caused or at least exacerbated by stress—and I think that it sometimes can. In the laboratory setting, researchers can stimulate the adrenal glands of rats into overactivity by frightening them with repeated loud noises. A similar situation can happen to the adrenal glands of patients who, like Martha, have lived under too much stress for many years.

There probably are other predisposing factors leading to PCO besides stress. Heredity and years of poor eating habits can also play a role. The daughters of PCO patients are at a higher risk of becoming overweight and of getting the disease.

Although doctors do not know for certain whether PCO starts with the adrenal glands, the brain, or the ovaries, we do know that the disease sets up a vicious cycle in its victim. A likely hypothesis of what happens is that under stress the patient's adrenal glands become overactive, androgen production increases, and the woman quits ovulating. This lack of ovulation causes her ovaries also to secrete too much androgen, mainly testosterone. She now has excess male hormone coming from her adrenal glands and her ovaries. The more androgen the woman produces, the more weight she gains. The more weight she gains, the more androgen she produces. The problem snowballs.

One likely effect of elevated androgen in the female is that the hormone hinders the release of the egg. Although nobody knows for certain what causes the egg to be extruded from its follicle, ovulation almost always follows a spurt of estrogen into the bloodstream, followed one or two days later by a spurt of LH. Doctors think that the androgen has a dampening effect on the estrogen spurt so that LH from the control center in the brain does not surge and the egg is not released.

PCO is an exceedingly complicated disorder, but basically what

happens is that the excess androgen from the adrenal glands and the
ovaries is converted into estrogen in fatty tissue. The brain, sensing
the elevated levels of estrogen in the blood, depresses FSH and sometimes increases LH, throwing the LH:FSH ratio out of balance. This
sends a mixed-up signal to the ovaries. Since the signal from the brain
is out of kilter, the follicles start to mature but fail to ripen properly.
Without the LH surge, the eggs are never released, and the ovary
produces excess androgen. Over time, more and more trapped follicles
build up in the ovaries so that they become filled with cysts and hard
fibrotic areas. The woman is set up for obesity, male-pattern hair growth,
and endometrial carcinoma (cancer of the lining of the uterus).

Why Precise Diagnosis Is a Must!

Although this disease should be discovered by physicians in its
early stages, Martha's condition had never been diagnosed. This was
extremely unfortunate, because the vicious cycle leading to her obesity and enlarged ovaries might have been broken if the disease had been
properly treated sooner. Moreover, PCO patients are in danger of hyperplasia (overgrowth) of the lining of the uterus and, as just stated,
endometrial cancer because of the high levels of estrogen unopposed
by progesterone. Furthermore, their ovaries also seem to be at higher
risk of abnormal cell development, sometimes leading to ovarian cancer.

Although Martha's symptoms of obesity, acne, and excess hair
growth immediately made me think of PCO, not all patients with these
problems have PCO; and not all PCO patients have all of these symptoms. Before I could make the diagnosis, I had to rule out early menopause and a prolactin-secreting pituitary tumor (see the section on
"Pituitary Tumor" later in this chapter).

Although it is extremely difficult to do a pelvic examination on an
obese patient, my impression was that both of Martha's ovaries were
enlarged. Her laboratory tests also pointed to PCO. Her adrenal glands
and ovaries were producing excess androgen. An elevated DHEA-S level
(a kind of androgen that comes from the adrenal glands) suggested that
some of the excess male hormone was coming from these glands. Her
testosterone level was also elevated, indicating that part of the androgen
was produced in the ovaries.

Further laboratory tests ruled out premature ovarian failure, because
her serum FSH was about normal. Her blood tests did indicate, however,
that, although her circulating prolactin and LH levels were rather high,
the ovulation-triggering LH surge was missing. This was suggestive of
PCO. Luckily, further investigation suggested that we did not have to

worry about a prolactin-secreting pituitary tumor. Furthermore, an X-ray (HSG) of the fallopian tubes indicated that Martha did not have tubal disease.

Since the LH level was elevated and poised to surge, I felt that Martha, like many PCO patients, probably would be extremely sensitive to Clomid. Before suggesting a laparoscopy, I prescribed three cycles of this drug, along with a weight-reducing diet.

Martha, however, did not conceive, and I recommended a laparoscopy. At the time of the 'scope, I performed a D&C to check for carcinoma of the endometrium. Although the uterine lining was overgrown, Martha did not have cancer. Along with an endometrial biopsy, the X-ray, and the laboratory tests, the 'scope gave a complete picture of Martha's reproductive system. (I wanted to make certain that her ovaries weren't malfunctioning because she had a "chocolate cyst"—see fig. 2.17 and fig. 2.18.)

When I looked at Martha's ovaries through the laparoscope, I noticed that each ovary was covered with a thick capsule, which may help to explain why polycystic ovaries have unruptured progesterone-producing follicles. Under pressure from inside, each ovary was smooth, with small, visible blood vessels running across it. There was no doubt that Martha had PCO.

Treatment: Breaking the Vicious Cycle

EXERCISE, MEDITATION, AND DIET

My job as Martha's doctor was to convince her that, if she wanted to conceive, she must lose weight. Large amounts of estrogen were being metabolized from androgen in her body fat. I wanted her to work with me before giving her more clomiphene, because I felt that without her help her chances of conceiving on Clomid were not very good.

Martha not only wanted a baby but also wanted desperately to be thinner and was extremely frustrated because, although she was not eating excessively, she was getting heavier. As we will explain, the extra fat cells she had accumulated over the years were making it increasingly difficult for her to shed pounds. In order for her to accomplish her goals, her stress had to be reduced and her androgen production lowered.

Since Martha lived in Houston, I suggested that she attend the weight-control clinic at Woman's Hospital of Texas or Methodist Hospital. She needed guidance and support, in the same way an alcoholic needs Alcoholics Anonymous. By following a sensible diet of six small meals each day that were low in refined sugars, she could normalize her low blood sugar. Over time, her appetite would gradually decrease, so that she would slowly lose weight.

A patient with polycystic ovaries also needs increased activity—it can help her start to reduce. If she diets without exercise, she usually will be unable to reduce her caloric intake over the long haul, because it is just too hard on her. She is fighting hormonal causes of weight gain; when a woman's testosterone level is high, she tends to retain fluid and hold body fat.

I encouraged Martha to do smooth aerobic exercises such as bicycling, swimming, or walking. Walking can provide almost the same amount of aerobics as jogging, without jarring the uterus, breasts, and joints.

Many people think that exercise must be strenuous to do any good—that they must jog rather than walk. But I think that jogging probably has been oversold to the whole population. I do not believe that women in particular are built to jog, and even in men it can cause problems. Many of my running friends have aching backs, hips, knees, joints, and ankles.

Exercise, however, affects each person differently. If a woman has been jogging all her life, I am not going to tell her to quit unless she has problems. Jogging definitely lifts a person's spirits. The well-known "runner's high" occurs because the brain releases the body's natural opiates—the endorphins—during exercise. I would hesitate, however, to recommend that an overweight PCO patient run, even though I have had a few of these young patients start jogging, lose weight, and become pregnant.

Connie, one of my PCO patients, changed her brain chemistry and her life through exercise. When she first moved to Houston from Dallas, she knew no one and was lonely, unhappy, and depressed. At five feet eight inches and 162 pounds, she had not had a menstrual period for almost six months. She felt that she looked "big" and said that her social life was "the pits." The more depressed Connie became, the more she ate, often eating a pint of ice cream in the middle of the night.

Then one day Connie met a marathon runner and started getting up an hour earlier in the morning and walking with him as he warmed up. Before long, she started jogging—at first only a half-block. Slowly she worked up to a quarter-mile, then a half, and by six months she was running one to two miles a day. A year passed.

Although Connie had jogged six days a week for an entire year, she had lost only ten pounds. Nonetheless, she had dropped a dress size, and her menstrual periods had returned. And, most important, she was no longer depressed. In fact, for the first time in several years—Connie was happy.

Instead of giving up because she still had not reached her desired weight, Connie faithfully kept up her exercise program for another year, slowly decreasing her caloric intake. During this time, she watched her weight fall seventeen more pounds. Finally, two years after she started jogging, she reached her goal. Connie weighed 135 pounds and looked terrific—like a different person!

Connie's romance with the marathon runner eventually ended. A year later, she fell in love, and soon married. When Connie and her husband wanted a baby, she had no problem conceiving.

Connie believes that exercise can contribute to a person's health and well-being if it can be incorporated into one's lifestyle easily. She says: "Exercise can refresh your mind. I exercise to the point where it benefits me, but I don't overdo it so that it causes another problem."

If a woman gets her heart rate up and keeps it there for a half-hour to an hour, something unknown but good happens to her brain's chemistry that helps her work on her weight. It is the feeling of well-being that makes the difference, more than the calories burned during exercise. Women with PCO appear to have a peculiar type of body chemistry. If they have no way of burning up the excess adrenaline and cortisol through exercise, they feel stressed and they overeat. This is just what we do not want.

Walking is particularly good for PCO patients because it calms them down. Over the years, I have observed that women with PCO are in high gear most of the time—their minds are constantly racing ninety miles an hour. If I can convince my PCO patient to take the time to do it, walking may well be more valuable to her than jogging because the former slows down her mental activity. I think that it is better for this woman to spend an hour walking than ten minutes running. She needs to give the time to herself—and to recognize that she deserves every minute of it!

Although exercise is the best, cheapest, and most practical way to calm down a PCO patient and at the same time to help her lose weight, not everyone can exercise. If increased activity is impossible, meditation or psychotherapy—when the woman really gets into the sessions and tries to understand herself—may be helpful. The goal is to change the brain's chemistry.

Of utmost importance to this patient is her realization that she must follow a diet-and-exercise program that she can live with for the *rest of her life*. She must *not* fast or go on fad diets!

Most PCO patients have tried a dozen or more crash diets. At first they lose weight rapidly. But then the body throws in all of its defenses and they hit a plateau. Soon they get discouraged—and gain back every pound, and more.

One diet program promoted by some diet centers that can be particularly harmful uses the hormone hCG to reduce the appetite. Although we are uncertain why hCG works, some doctors think that it causes a feedback to the satiety center of the brain, which makes a person feel full. Other doctors think that the drug has only a placebo effect. HCG is a protein, and if it is used weekly, over time a woman can become allergic to it. Even worse, repeated hCG shots can permanently damage a patient's hormonal system! I have known women who were given hCG weekly who developed antibodies against it and never were able to become pregnant. When infertility specialists use hCG to trigger ovulation, we give only one shot a month for a short time.

Once a patient sees that there is no quick fix, we can help her change her whole body image, partly with medications but mainly through understanding. And understanding means that we know she is having an extremely difficult time losing weight but that she must not use PCO as an excuse.

I sometimes compare these patients' situation to that of the married man who is going through a mid-life crisis. He hears that everybody experiences this, and so he goes out and buys a fast car and chases the girls like the middle-aged actors in the movies. He is using the mid-life crisis as an excuse. His minister, priest, or rabbi can advise him, but in the final analysis only he controls his actions. Similarly, an overweight patient's doctor can encourage and help her, but she can do more for herself than anyone else. I cannot say to her: "You have got to be thinner."

What I try to do for her, although it seldom works the first time, is to show her how her excess weight affects her hormones and her ability to get pregnant. I have had patients who have weighed 180 to 200 pounds lose 50 pounds, conceive, gain the weight back during pregnancy, and deliver a healthy baby. But when they wanted to have a second child, they had to start the weight-loss program all over again in order to ovulate. The point is that an obese patient with polycystic ovaries has to modify her behavior. Over time, she must change her body image and the way she perceives food.

MEDICATION

Besides diet and exercise, Martha needed drug therapy to suppress the excess adrenal androgen. Low doses of prednisone, a cortisonelike drug, make the adrenal glands stop producing too much androgen. This is important, because Clomid and Pergonal stimulate production of more male hormone from the ovaries, which makes acne worse, causes growth of more unwanted hair, and increases emotional instability.

Some women will resume ovulation naturally once they have lost weight. Martha, however, needed a fertility drug such as clomiphene to begin cycling again. Clomid helps 95 percent of PCO patients ovulate, although only 40 to 50 percent conceive. If a patient fails to become pregnant on clomiphene, I sometimes suggest Pergonal. But, as I mentioned earlier, Pergonal is extremely expensive, and the patient must make many visits to the doctor.

The outcome of Martha's case was tremendously rewarding for both of us. With determination and hard work, she was able to overcome many of the problems associated with PCO. Eighteen months after she started her diet-and-exercise program, Martha had lost sixty-five pounds and was pregnant! Since she had totally changed her eating habits, she gained only twenty-five pounds during her pregnancy. By exchanging the destructive habit of overeating for the healthy habits of proper diet and exercise, Martha has maintained her normal weight for over five years. She now has two healthy children.

SURGERY

Sometimes women who have had PCO for a long time do not ovulate with medication. Nowadays, fertility specialists have a new laparoscopic treatment that helps some patients. To reduce the number of male-hormone-producing cells, the doctor makes multiple punctures in the polycystic ovary with the Yag or Argon laser. In other words, the surgeon puts the laser in the ovary and destroys four millimeters of tissue with each five-second laser blast, "drilling" at least fifteen deep holes in each ovary.

Since tissue handling and bleeding are reduced, this new procedure causes fewer adhesions than "ovarian wedge resection," the surgery doctors used to perform to try to help PCO patients. In the past, a pie-shaped wedge was cut out of each ovary. Although this older surgical technique sometimes helped PCO patients ovulate, probably because ovarian androgen was reduced, I haven't performed this operation for over ten years.

Prevention Through Early Diagnosis

Since PCO usually is the end of the road of long-term anovulation, early diagnosis is crucial to prevent this devastating disease. If the androgen production is stopped early, the ovaries will function properly so that the woman can conceive when she desires pregnancy.

Doctors need to monitor the daughters of PCO patients carefully because they sometimes also develop this condition. Physicians must accept the difficult challenge of trying to help teenage patients reduce stress and improve their eating habits.

For the PCO-prone patient not desiring pregnancy, I often prescribe an estrogen-dominant birth-control pill. The pill rests the ovaries by suppressing the irregular stimulation of the pituitary sex hormones FSH and LH. This decreases both ovarian and adrenal androgen production. The estrogen counteracts the androgen, and acne gets better. Treated patients are less likely to become obese or develop enlarged, cystic ovaries. The progestin in the pill helps prevent the overgrowth of the endometrium because it causes regular menstrual bleeding.

Anorexia and Preanorexic Behavior

> *Lacking inner guide posts, they have relied excessively*
> *on the praise and good opinion of those around them.*
> *They feel safe from blame and criticism only when they*
> *can maintain the image of perfection in the eyes of*
> *others.*
>
> HILDE BRUCH, M.D., *The Golden Cage*

Explanation and Diagnosis

Ruth, an only child of older, well-to-do parents, had spent the first sixteen years of her life trying to please everyone but herself. Although she made excellent grades, she had little self-confidence and few friends. Starved for a sense of self-worth, Ruth felt ineffectual and believed that she was incompetent to pursue life on her own. When her psychiatrist asked her to draw a picture of herself, she drew a formless body—she seemed to lack a well-defined sense of who she was.

A fastidiously groomed girl with huge sunken blue eyes and dull blond hair, Ruth was extremely concerned about her appearance, especially about staying "fashionably thin." At five feet six inches and ninety-two pounds, she considered herself "overweight" and felt that she had extremely large hips.

Much of Ruth's family's conversation centered around cooking and dieting. At age fifty-two, Ruth's well-meaning but constantly hovering mother, Nancy, had been obese for many years. This had caused tremendous friction between Ruth's parents. Determined to remain thin and "acceptable," Ruth ate as little as possible, often chewing laxative gum when she felt "bloated."

When trying to be "perfect" to please her parents, her teachers, and the world in general became too much, Ruth's quest for thinness took over her life. She started jogging to the point of exhaustion and lost weight precipitately. She felt that her eating habits were the one area where she had control. Her unspoken attitude toward bringing her weight up to normal was that she would rather suffer the gnawing pain of hunger than continue to be controlled by others. The defiant look in her eyes said: "You can't make me eat!"

Nancy had brought her daughter to see me because at age sixteen Ruth had never had a menstrual period. Nancy expressed great concern because Ruth refused to eat regular meals. Although Ruth denied ever being hungry and insisted that her fanatical desire to lose weight was "normal," the truth was that she was obsessed with food. Placing a premium on self-denial and self-discipline, she was in horror of "yielding" to her voracious hunger. When Ruth did "give in" to her intense craving for sweets, she would induce vomiting.

Ruth's case paints a picture of the classic anorexic, who needs intensive psychiatric help from an expert in treating this devastating condition. A dangerous disease—an estimated 10 to 15 percent of patients starve themselves to death—anorexia plays havoc with the body, causing hypothyroidism (low levels of thyroid), decreased heart rate, partial diabetes insipidus (a disorder of the pituitary resulting in tremendous thirst and excretion of huge amounts of urine), and lack of menstruation.

When a young woman refuses to eat to the point where her weight drops 25 percent below normal, she will fail to start menstruating at puberty; or, if her periods have started, they will cease. Her ovaries stop ovulating and making estrogen, and her breasts either fail to develop or shrink; her genitals become withered, rather like those of an elderly woman. She usually appears much older than her age and suffers from extreme sensitivity to cold.

Although classic anorexia is rare, I see many preanorexic young women who just overdo the weight loss. Even though these patients are preoccupied with staying thin, they do not have the profound psychological problems of the anorexic. Preanorexics diet to excess because they want to measure up to society's constant pressure to be slender. They think that, if they are extremely thin, they will be loved.

Although preanorexics are often otherwise normal, they have a distorted attitude toward eating. Even as they lose weight, their fear of fat stays with them. Failing to realize that moderation is the true quintessence of control, they often have an "all-or-nothing" attitude toward food. Lacking the developed internal governors of adults that can help keep weight within a normal range, teenagers can easily go in one direction or the other—they can become either too skinny or too fat.

Long-distance runners can create the same kind of problems with their bodies that anorexics do. The psyches of the two groups appear rather similar, in that they seem to think that, if a little bit is good for them, a lot is better. The overzealous dieters eat less and less; the joggers become four-, six-, and eventually twenty-five-milers. Carried to excess, jogging can cause a loss of calcium from the bones and stress fractures similar to those found in older women with osteoporosis.

Treatment

A teenager who feels comfortable when she is far enough below her normal weight to quit ovulating and producing estrogen is going to get into trouble. I have noticed over the years that girls with anorexic tendencies are often inflexible and need someone rigid to organize their diet. If, as their doctor, I can gain their confidence—provided that nothing else is wrong with them—and put them on a well-balanced diet to bring their weight up to normal, they will start menstruating and avoid the menopauselike symptoms of anorexia.

Sometimes these patients need to take supplemental estrogen to help them gain weight and to regain their secondary sexual characteristics. Once they attain their ideal body weight, ovulation and menstruation usually return. Furthermore, estrogen can help protect underweight women from stress fractures. Sometimes, however, the patients refuse to take this hormone, because it gives them the body image that they are trying to avoid: estrogen makes them rounder. They have been brainwashed with the idea that being as thin as a New York model is the ultimate. This is wrong.

When a woman with anorexia says that she desires pregnancy, the infertility specialist has to make certain that her psychiatrist feels she can handle the pregnancy emotionally. Often an anorexic should not get pregnant! Sometimes she really doesn't want to carry a child but is under pressure from her husband to conceive. What the doctor has to do is to guard against helping a woman get pregnant who really doesn't want to. I have had anorexic patients carry a baby for three or four months and then request an abortion. For anyone who works with women who are desperately trying to have babies, this is a nightmare! But when the psychiatrist says that the woman will commit suicide, there is no choice— the pregnancy must be terminated.

If the patient is preanorexic and the psychiatrist feels pregnancy is safe, Pergonal may make such a woman ovulate. Clomid will not help a woman achieve pregnancy as long as her estrogen level is low. If she is a true anorexic and her reproductive system is totally shut down, there is little the doctor can do to make her ovulate until she gains weight. The question I keep asking such a patient is: "Can you accept the physical changes of pregnancy?" If she can, then I go ahead and treat her. Occasionally having the baby will change the focus of her life.

Pituitary Tumor

Suddenly, at age twenty-seven, Jane found that her normally regular menstrual periods ceased. She occasionally complained to her husband of headaches. When her menses failed to return after three months, she came to see me. She was considering attempting pregnancy and wondered why her periods had stopped.

On physical examination, I noticed that Jane's breasts seemed firm, as in early pregnancy, and that they produced a milky discharge. Although she had no other physical signs of pregnancy, she had missed three periods, making it necessary to rule out pregnancy with an hCG urine test. The results quickly confirmed that she was not expecting.

Causes of Elevated Prolactin

When a patient's breasts produce fluid, it is essential to do a baseline test to measure the level of prolactin in her blood. As you know, prolactin is the pituitary hormone that stimulates and sustains lactation in nursing mothers. In the presence of other hormones, excess prolactin can cause the breasts to leak. Not unexpectedly, Jane's test for prolactin disclosed that the level of this hormone was significantly elevated. Since too much prolactin inhibits ovulation, the increase probably had caused her to quit ovulating and menstruating.

There are several causes of milky discharge from the breasts (galactorrhea) in patients who are not pregnant. In the majority of cases, galactorrhea does not point to a serious medical problem, especially if the patient has regular menses. Breast discharge can occur in women who have had children or who have taken oral contraceptive. Although breast stimulation, fibrocystic disease, or polyps in the mammary ducts also can cause breast discharge, in approximately half of women with galactorrhea no definite cause can be found. If the discharge is bloody, it can suggest a malignancy—occasionally the polyps become cancerous.

Unfortunately, galactorrhea can be a symptom of a prolactin-secreting pituitary tumor called a "prolactinoma." A gray-colored mass, this type of tumor develops out of a cell in the pituitary gland that synthesizes prolactin. Doctors do not know the exact cause of prolactinomas, but we do know they are benign and almost never adversely affect a patient's thinking ability, though they sometimes pose other problems.

The rate of growth of prolactinomas varies considerably. Many remain small for life and are never noticed. Some slowly grow, taking many years to become symptomatic, whereas others expand rapidly. Once these tumors become large, they can be dangerous! If left untreated, an expanding prolactinoma eventually can compress the optic nerve, causing blindness. The tumor can also cause diabetes insipidus. The prolactinoma can even replace the whole master gland, significantly decreasing production of other important pituitary hormones. This is debilitating and may become life-threatening.

Making the Diagnosis

The more I investigated Jane's case, the more I became worried that she could be harboring a prolactin-secreting pituitary tumor. There were several clues that, together, pointed toward this preliminary diagnosis. When a patient has a prolactinoma the serum-prolactin level can shoot up so high that the breasts leak. Not only did Jane have a significantly elevated serum-prolactin level and a milky discharge from her breasts, she also had noticed that her sex drive had decreased. She complained of pain during intercourse and vaginal dryness. This was caused by a low estrogen level, which usually occurs as a result of the effect of high prolactin on ovarian hormone secretion.

Jane's history helped me rule out some of the other factors that can elevate prolactin at least mildly. She was under no unusual or chronic stress. She seldom drank and used no antihypertensive drugs to lower high blood pressure or psychiatric drugs such as phenothiazine—any of which could have raised her prolactin level.

Another cause of an elevated prolactin level is an underactive thyroid gland. Some women have a low level of thyroid circulating in their blood and are unaware of it. They just don't feel good. Sometimes galactorrhea is their only symptom. Consequently it was important to evaluate Jane's thyroid function. The same hormone (dubbed "TRH" or "thyrotropin-releasing hormone" by doctors) that orders the pituitary to signal the thyroid gland to increase thyroid production also causes the pituitary to release prolactin. In other words, there is a crossover effect.

Here is what happens. If a patient's thyroid gland is not releasing enough thyroid hormone, her hypothalamus, detecting insufficient thyroid in the blood, sends a special hormone signal (TRH) to the pituitary, telling it to release thyroid-stimulating hormone (TSH). Reaching the thyroid through the blood, pituitary TSH tries to stimulate the thyroid gland to increase thyroid production. The problem is that TRH not only stimulates the release of TSH but also stimulates the pituitary to release more prolactin. This makes the patient's serum-prolactin level shoot upward, often causing her to quit ovulating. Jane's thyroid tests, however, were normal, indicating that her excess prolactin was not caused by an underactive thyroid gland.

Another problem that could have stopped Jane's periods was a failure of her ovaries, causing her to experience early menopause. Jane, however, was only twenty-seven years old. Furthermore, menopausal women do not have a milky discharge from the breasts. Laboratory tests showed that Jane's problem was not caused by premature ovarian failure, because her pituitary sex hormones FSH and LH were within a normal range. (Remember, when a woman's ovaries fail, these hormones elevate, in a fruitless attempt to stimulate maturation of an egg-containing follicle.)

An MRI was necessary to check for a prolactinoma of the pituitary and to rule out other problems. Unfortunately, the results showed that my suspicions were correct—the MRI revealed a five-millimeter prolactinoma. Since it is less than one centimeter in diameter, doctors call a small tumor like this a "microadenoma." Those larger than one centimeter are referred to as "macroadenomas."

Treatment

The treatment of prolactinomas is somewhat controversial. As a general rule, the choice of therapy depends on the size of the tumor, the amount of prolactin secreted, the woman's age and symptoms, and the rate of tumor growth. Depending on the patient, therapies include medication, surgery, or no treatment at all.

Interestingly enough, asymptomatic prolactinomas can go unnoticed for a lifetime—at autopsy, tumors are found in approximately 22 percent of the general population in patients who have died from other causes.

If the tumor is minute—and the majority remain small—the patient may need to be watched by a specialist and have her prolactin level measured every six months. A very few tumors disappear spontaneously.

Although the size of the prolactinoma correlates to some extent with the level of prolactin in the blood, the amount of this hormone secreted by tumors of similar stages of development can vary. Says a study headed by Milam E. Leavens, M.D., published in *International Advances in Surgical Oncology*: "Unless the basal prolactin level is extremely high, one could not predict the stage of development of the adenoma [tumor] on the basis of prolactin level alone." A drastically elevated prolactin level, however, does indicate that the tumor is invasive.

MEDICATION

Although some infertility specialists follow the smaller prolactinomas themselves, I work with a team of doctors, seeking the consultation of an endocrinologist, a neurosurgeon, and a radiologist. Nowadays, endocrinologists overwhelmingly recommend a drug called bromocriptine (marketed as Parlodel or Pergolide) to manage these tumors. This medication, which was mentioned earlier, usually causes a decrease in tumor size and density. Since bromocriptine in proper dosage always lowers prolactin level, ovulation and menses may return—frequently allowing pregnancy, if all other reproductive factors are normal.

Once bromocriptine is withdrawn, the prolactin level rises again, indicating that the patient is not permanently cured. Thus, except for a few tumors that spontaneously resolve themselves, medically treated patients have to take bromocriptine for life.

Unfortunately, bromocriptine is not without its side effects, although only approximately 10 percent of patients discontinue treatment for this reason. Some women complain of nausea, dizziness, and vague headaches. Other, less common complaints are fatigue and abdominal cramps. In the majority of cases, the side effects diminish after the first few weeks. (It should be noted that the FDA no longer permits obstetricians to give bromocriptine to suppress lactation after childbirth. Articles in the lay literature have reported maternal deaths following use of the drug for this purpose.)

NEUROSURGERY

In the past, highly skilled neurosurgeons have removed expanding prolactinomas that were visible on an X-ray. Formidably named "transnasal transphenoidal resection," this microsurgical operation had a mortality rate between 0 percent and 2 percent in expert hands. Today, however, few neurosurgeons have the expertise to remove these tumors successfully and completely.

Depending on the size of the tumor before surgery and the level of the experience of the surgeon, the tumor can recur. Unfortunately, tumor remnants sometimes grow back, or a new tumor forms. If this happens and the patient is symptomatic, additional treatment may be necessary.

Pregnancy Following Therapy

Once a woman is expecting, treatment with bromocriptine is discontinued. Fortunately, the mother generally does well and her baby usually is healthy. It is absolutely imperative, however, to monitor this patient carefully during and after delivery. Although pregnancy causes some enlargement of the pituitary in women without prolactinomas, a great increase in the size of the gland may indicate that the tumor is growing. Doctors should watch for symptoms of pressure, headaches, and visual problems. If the prolactinoma starts expanding during pregnancy, the doctor may have to put his patient back on bromocriptine. In Europe, patients take the medication throughout pregnancy, even if they don't have symptoms of tumor expansion.

Jane's case had a happy ending. Treatment with bromocriptine caused the tumor to decrease in size, and her prolactin level dropped to normal within a few weeks. Two months later, her periods returned; within six months, she was expecting. Followed closely by her doctors during her entire pregnancy, Jane delivered a healthy seven-pound girl. After the birth of her baby, her endocrinologist continued to measure her prolactin level every six months to make certain that the level remained normal.

Turner's Syndrome: A Genetic Abnormality

Making the Diagnosis

Once in every twenty-five hundred to twenty-seven hundred births, a female baby is born with Turner's syndrome, a genetic abnormality characterized by shortness of stature and "streak" ovaries of white tissue containing no eggs. Lacking follicles and thus normal ovarian hormones, these patients fail to go through puberty and do not develop secondary sexual characteristics. They have no menstrual periods and are unable to have children by normal means.

In the past, the only way a Turner's patient could start a family was by adopting a child. Nowadays, however, with the recent advances in reproductive technology and the aid of donor eggs, some of these patients can give birth. Using the techniques learned from *in-vitro* fertilization, doctors mix an egg donated by another woman with the sperm of the husband of the Turner's patient. The resulting embryo is then frozen, later to be thawed, examined, and transferred to the hormonally prepared uterus of the childless patient. If the fertilized egg attaches to the uterine lining, the patient becomes pregnant with her husband's child and will require supplemental hormones to support the pregnancy (see chapter 9 for further details on embryo transfer). She will require a cesarean section because of her small size.

I usually can tell if a patient has Turner's syndrome when I first meet her, although the diagnosis must be confirmed with blood tests. Some of the physical characteristics typical of this syndrome are extreme shortness (the patient is usually under five feet tall), a shieldlike chest, a thick neck with a low hairline at the nape, and prominent, low-set ears. Although the statistics say that 10 percent of these women are mentally retarded, I have yet to encounter a retarded Turner's patient in my practice.

Since Turner's patients usually have normal though infantile-appearing external genitals, 40 percent are not diagnosed until they fail to go through puberty. Sometimes, however, the condition is noticed at birth. Puffiness of the hands and feet and low birth weight should alert the physician that further investigation may be necessary.

About 20 percent of Turner's patients suffer from congenital cardiovascular abnormalities, especially coarctation (narrowing) of the aorta. These patients are also at increased risk of diabetes mellitus, thyroid and kidney problems, red-green color blindness, loss of calcium from the bones, and hearing difficulties. Regrettably, even with the latest advances in medical technology, pregnancy is inadvisable for some of these patients. For example, patients with cardiac abnormalities or those who might suffer obstetrical complications because of their small size should not give birth.

To begin to understand Turner's syndrome, which is caused by an abnormality in the patient's genetic blueprint, one has to look at the basic chromosome patterns of normal individuals. Found in the nucleus of every human cell are twenty-three pairs of chromosomes that carry the genes of inheritance contributed by both parents. These genes determine not only such traits as our eye and hair color and our height but also our sex. Babies destined to be female have two "X" sex chromosomes with a genetic blueprint of "46 XX." Males have one "X" sex chromosome and one "Y." The "Y" chromosome carries a gene that is responsible for the development of the testes, which secrete the male sex hormone testosterone. Thus a normal male-chromosome pattern of "46 XY" simply means that each cell has forty-six chromosomes and that the person is male.

Babies born with Turner's syndrome have a genetic abnormality in their sex chromosomes. Instead of the normal "46 XX" female pattern, these patients often have only a single sex chromosome, written with one "X." This is reflected in a genetic pattern of "45 X," also written "45 XO," where the "O" indicates the absence of the second sex chromosome (see fig. 4.2).

To make the final diagnosis of Turner's syndrome, a study of a person's chromosomal pattern or karyotype is needed. This test is done

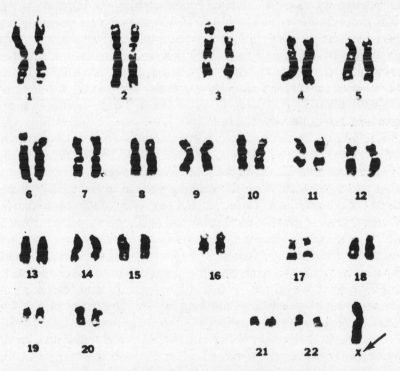

FIGURE 4.2. Chromosome pattern for Turner's syndrome. (Reproduced with permission from R. W. Kistner, Gynecology: Principles and Practice, 4th ed., copyright © 1986 by Year Book Medical Publishers, Inc., Chicago.)

by examining the white blood cells as they divide under a microscope. In patients with Turner's syndrome, the second "X" sex chromosome is either missing or defective.

Without a normal second "X" sex chromosome, the patient's ovaries consist of streaks of white tissue with no egg-containing follicles to produce ovarian hormones. Since the ovaries lack ripening follicles, which secrete estrogen, Turner's patients generally never go through puberty. Even though the pituitary attempts to initiate puberty by signaling the ovaries to increase hormone production, without follicles the ovaries cannot respond. In the absence of normal amounts of ovarian estrogen and progesterone, breast development and menstruation fail to occur.

Treatment: Hormone Therapy

Many of the fifty or sixty Turner's patients in my practice are able to have normal sex lives and are happily married. Some have adopted children and are devoted mothers. Patients with a "45 XO" and "45 XO/46 X" genetic makeup can receive tremendous psychological benefit from hormone therapy, because it allows them to go through puberty. Estrogen will bring about sexual development. In combination with progestin (a progesteronelike hormone), estrogen causes the buildup of the uterine lining and menstruation. Progestin also is necessary to counteract long-term estrogen exposure, especially since Turner's patients are at increased risk of endometrial cancer.

The goal of these patients, however, is not only to achieve puberty but also to reach their maximum potential height. Yet hormone therapy can terminate growth, although in small amounts estrogen actually may cause a growth spurt. When the growing portions at the end of the long bones (called epiphyses) close, growth stops. If X-rays show that the epiphyses haven't closed, the best treatment is to give growth hormones until the girl's maximum potential height is achieved, followed by estrogen. In large amounts, however, estrogen may cause a spurt of growth and then terminate it permanently by causing the epiphyses to seal.

So, to promote secondary sexual development while avoiding premature fusion of the ends of the long bones, the dosage of estrogen should be kept low until the patient has finished growing. Once full height is reached, the dosage of estrogen can be increased to maintain female sex characteristics if necessary.

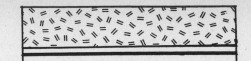

Part II

Male Infertility: Evaluation and Treatment

Repair of an Obstruction of the Duct System and a Varicose Vein of the Testicle

LARRY I. LIPSHULTZ, M.D., AND
DOROTHY KAY BROCKMAN

Ed and Elizabeth had tried repeatedly during the first eighteen months of their marriage to conceive a baby but without success. Ed, thirty-seven, had been married before, but he and his first wife had never tried to have children. Elizabeth had also been married earlier and had a three-year-old daughter by her first husband. Wondering why she hadn't gotten pregnant, Elizabeth, twenty-five, went to Dr. Franklin.

Dr. Franklin's physical examination of Elizabeth turned up no explanations. He then suggested a routine screening semen analysis for Ed because in up to 50 percent of infertility cases the problem lies with the husband. It is extremely important to do this simple, inexpensive test early in the medical workup to determine if the husband's semen is of adequate quality to initiate a pregnancy. Doctors study the sperm count (concentration or density of sperm per cubic centimeter of fluid), sperm motility (their swimming ability), and sperm morphology (their shape and structure). Ed's semen analysis told the story: at least one reason Elizabeth wasn't pregnant was that Ed's sperm count was zero.

When Dr. Franklin reported this, Ed looked at him in total disbelief. Stunned, Ed refused to accept that there was anything wrong with his semen. What was wrong, he angrily told the infertility specialist, was that the laboratory wasn't worth the powder to blow it to hell.

After giving Ed a chance to get over his initial shock, Dr. Franklin suggested that the semen analysis be repeated in a couple of weeks. Since a man's sperm count typically varies over time (although a drop to zero isn't normal), the study usually is repeated two or three times (see fig. 5.1). Ed agreed to another test but only to prove his point about the lab. He was certain the outcome would be different next time. The semen analysis two weeks later, however, produced the same results. But by this time, although Ed was still angry, he had stopped denying the facts and had started asking questions.

A distinguished-looking man with prematurely graying temples, heavy black eyebrows, and a stocky build, Ed was president of a large construction company and was used to confronting difficult problems. He also was accustomed to getting tangible results when he gave orders. Before Dr. Franklin had a chance to offer any suggestions, Ed demanded to know what was causing his problem and what could be done about it.

Dr. Franklin replied with several possible causes for the azoospermia (no sperm in the semen). He explained that the lack of sperm in Ed's semen didn't necessarily mean that his testes weren't making sperm. An obstruction in the ductal system of his reproductive tract might be blocking delivery of the sperm to the egg (see fig. 1.6). This sometimes can be repaired with surgery. If indeed there was an intrinsic problem in sperm production in the testes, it could be diagnosed with hor-

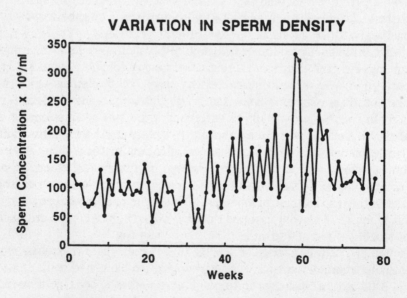

VARIATION IN SPERM DENSITY

FIGURE 5.1. Variations in one patient's sperm concentration over time. (Courtesy of Dr. L. I. Lipshultz.)

mone tests or by looking at a tiny sliver of testicular tissue under the microscope. (For review of the male reproductive system, see chapter 1.)

Dr. Franklin suggested that Ed might learn more about his azoospermia from an andrologist, a urologist who specializes in male infertility. Since I have spent years working with men's fertility problems, Dr. Franklin referred Ed to me.

Risk Factors: Looking for Clues in the Medical History

During our first visit, I began Ed's evaluation by exploring his medical history for the known risk factors that can cause male infertility. I hoped my questions would yield clues to the absence of sperm in his semen: Had his sperm production been impaired by some illness or infection? Was he born with an undescended, "hidden" testicle—a testis that had failed to drop down into the scrotum? (See fig. 5.2.) If so, had the problem been surgically corrected? Had Ed had any other operations? Had his scrotum ever been injured? Did he use any medications or illegal drugs—some of which can affect sperm production? Was he under great stress? Had he ever been exposed to any environmental toxins?

One chronic systemic illness that sometimes leads to infertility is diabetes mellitus, a disease of metabolism characterized by the presence of excessive sugar in the urine and in the blood. Over time, diabetes can cause peripheral neuropathy, a deterioration of the "sympathetic" nerves that cause the bladder neck to close and the sperm ducts to empty during orgasm. This can cause retrograde (backward) ejaculation of the semen into the bladder, instead of out of the body through the penis. Unlike Ed, who didn't have diabetes, patients with retrograde ejaculation may have significant numbers of normal sperm but a reduced semen volume. Eventually some patients have total lack of emission. Fortunately, doctors can sometimes correct this problem by prescribing antihistamines and other medications such as the antidepressant imipramine. In fact, following treatment, forward ejaculation returns in up to 20 to 30 percent of patients.

Ed also had no history of mumps after puberty, venereal diseases, or epididymal infections, any of which might have damaged his testicles. Theoretically, any illness or blood-borne virus infection that causes a fever can temporarily lower semen quality. The damage can be permanent but only if an obvious orchitis (an inflammation of the testis

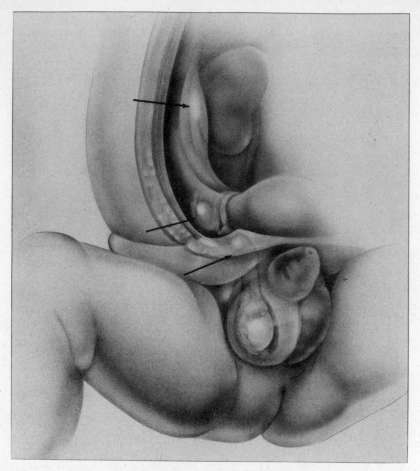

FIGURE 5.2. Male infant with "hidden" testicle. Shows descent of testicle and locations where descent sometimes stops. (Courtesy of Carol Donner, from Dr. L. I. Lipshultz and Dr. Irvin H. Hirsch, from Masters in Urology, vol. 1, no. 2, 1985, published by CPC Communications, Greenwich, Connecticut.)

marked by pain and swelling) eventually leads to testicular atrophy. An infection's impact on semen may appear rapidly or take weeks or months to occur. Sperm take about three months to form and mature. Thus, if the virus attacks sperm forms in their early stages of development, the negative effect on the semen will appear later than if the virus invades the more mature sperm in the epididymis.

You will recall from chapter 1 that the epididymis is a long coiled canal located behind and attached to each testis (see figs. 1.6 and 5.3). Although sperm are produced in the testes, it is in the epididymis, which has both absorptive and secretory properties, where the sperm gain the

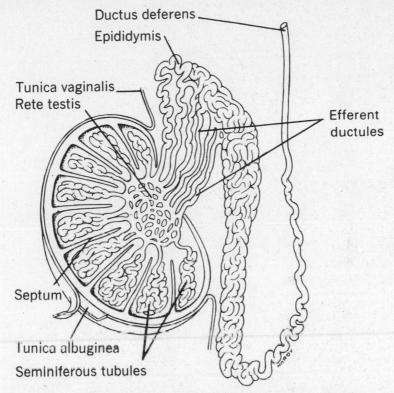

FIGURE 5.3. A cross-section of the testis. Note the position of the epididymis and the ductus deferens or sperm duct. (From E. E. Chaffee and I. M. Lytle, Basic Physiology & Anatomy, 4th ed., Philadelphia: J. B. Lippincott, 1980.)

ability to move actively and where most are stored. The number available at any one time depends on how many are produced and the frequency of ejaculation. After a viral illness, it may take several months for the quality of the sperm in the epididymis to return to normal.

The mumps virus can have a devastating effect on fertility if it attacks the testicles of an adult. Although the infection doesn't seem to affect the testes before puberty, afterward the virus viciously invades the rapidly dividing reproductive cells. Thirty percent of males over age eleven or twelve infected with mumps will have one testicle affected; 10 percent will have both affected. As long as one testicle remains healthy, the man can usually still father a child. But if the virus destroys all of the spermatogonia (the sperm-generating mother cells) in both testes (see fig. 5.4), the disease will leave its victim sterile. Keep in mind that recovery from mumps of the testicles usually takes more than a year, often much longer.

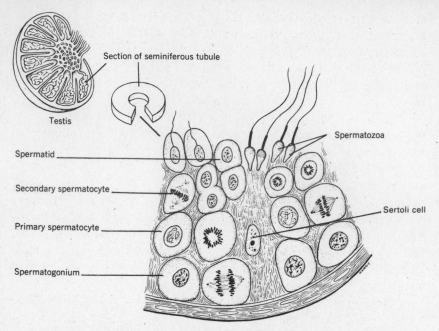

Section of seminiferous tubule

Testis

Spermatozoa

Spermatid

Secondary spermatocyte

Sertoli cell

Primary spermatocyte

Spermatogonium

FIGURE 5.4. *A section of a seminiferous tubule of the testis that shows the stages of the birth of a sperm. (From E. E. Chaffee and I. M. Lytle,* Basic Physiology & Anatomy, *4th ed., Philadelphia: J. B. Lippincott, 1980.)*

The venereal disease gonorrhea can cause infertility in men as well as women. In the advanced stages, this sexually transmitted disease can scar and partially or totally obstruct the epididymis. The blockage often affects both testicles. Sometimes the man's fertility is damaged even though the infection is treated with antibiotics.

The venereal disease chlamydia—which, as you know, can destroy a woman's fertility—also is common in sexually active men, especially those with multiple partners. In males, chlamydia can cause an inflammation of the urethra called "nongonococcal urethritis." If a man has no symptoms and his doctor finds that he has chlamydia, will this infection make him infertile? Our data does not adequately prove that it does. If, however, the patient is symptomatic and has a serious bacterial infection, or if he has many white cells in his semen, the infection could be contributing to his infertility. If an infection reaches the epididymis and causes an inflammation, it must be treated with antibiotics. If left untreated, or not treated long enough, epididymitis can cause sterility.

Ninety percent of men suffering from chlamydia have sufficient symptoms to prompt them to get medical care. Unfortunately, some patients stop taking the medication after the symptoms disappear but before they are cured. Although chlamydia may not cause infertility in such a patient, he becomes a carrier, giving the infection to his partner. Since chlamydia can destroy a woman's fallopian tubes—often before she even knows she is infected—it is extremely important to treat the male with antibiotics until he is cured. This may take a long time.

Many men have another kind of infection, caused by bacteria but with viruslike qualities, called "mycoplasmas." Often these patients are unaware that they have this sexually transmitted disease. Although the exact role of mycoplasmas in causing infertility is unknown, one study suggested that they may impair sperm motility. But if a man has no symptoms, doctors have been unable to prove that these microorganisms cause infertility in the male. Nevertheless, if a patient with mycoplasma has impaired sperm motility, and no other causes are known, antibiotic therapy may help. When Dr. Franklin finds this infection in a woman, he treats it in her and also in her husband, so that they don't reinfect each other.

It is important to ask an infertile patient like Ed if he has ever had a cryptorchid (undescended) testicle. Research has shown that 3 or 4 percent of full-term babies have some impairment of testicular descent, although only 0.7 to 0.8 percent still have a "hidden" testis at age one. When undescended testicles fail to drop down spontaneously, surgery to bring them into the scrotum often is recommended. Called "orchiopexy," this operation usually is performed around age one to reduce the risk that the child's future sperm production will be adversely affected. Unfortunately, regardless of when the testicle is relocated, overall semen quality at puberty will often be considerably less than normal.

When I asked Ed about stress, he said his business was a pressure cooker filled with countless deadlines. He added, however, that he loved his work, had learned to cope with its stresses, and, in fact, thrived on the challenge. To Ed, doing nothing was much more stressful than topping out a towering office building.

The effect of stress on infertility in the male is controversial. In women, we known that stress can affect fertility by stopping ovulation. But does stress cause infertility in the male? We know that the pressure to perform sexually at ovulation time can cause some husbands who had no prior sexual dysfunction to become impotent during their wives' fertile time. We know that the stress of combat and surgery can depress the level of the male hormone testosterone circulating in the blood. We also know that some animal studies have shown that sperm production drops during periods of stress.

But although some doctors think that stress might have a delayed effect on sperm quality, we haven't proved that stress diminishes sperm production. I think that the sheer numbers of a normal man's sperm production probably make stress relatively unimportant to male fertility. A man produces millions of sperm every day, making literally billions during his life. In general, at any time he has about 425 million sperm waiting to be released. If stress does lower sperm count, and I think that it might, sperm production may be affected in such a subtle way that the man never has an infertility problem. In contrast, a woman releases only one egg each cycle. If she fails to ovulate one time, she loses a whole month.

Even if stress does play a role in men, how do you measure it? It is extremely difficult to relate a stressful event to the semen analysis. One problem is separating the effect on sperm production of the stress itself from the negative effects of poor health habits that may be stress-related. When people are under a great deal of stress, they often react by doing things that aren't good for their general health: they may be unable to sleep, they may not eat properly, or they may use cigarettes, alcohol, or drugs. All these habits can harm the body and thus impair sperm production.

Severe obesity may also be associated with male infertility. Extremely overweight men may have significantly reduced levels of the male hormone testosterone and elevated levels of the female hormone estrogen circulating in their blood. Excess estrogen, which is converted from testosterone in fatty tissue, is thought to be responsible for subfertility in these men. Such patients may have low sperm counts or impaired sperm motility. If the patient can lose weight, his estrogen level should drop to a normal level and his semen analysis may improve.

Your doctor will ask if you have been exposed to environmental toxins because the rapidly dividing sperm cells are especially vulnerable to toxic insults. Some pesticides, such as DBCP and industrial compounds, may harm sperm production. Certain medications, such as those used to treat colitis (inflammation of the colon), peptic ulcers in the stomach, high blood pressure, and other common illnesses can also be detrimental. Chemotherapy and radiation can damage the sperm-producing mother cells. Following treatment for a malignancy, some patients may be temporarily infertile or permanently sterile. The more radiation a man has received, the more likely it is that his sperm production will be arrested. Over time, if sufficient spermatogonia survive, a man's sperm count may recover. Some doctors worry that the DNA code of the spermatogonia may be rearranged, putting the man's offspring at increased risk of birth defects, but "DNA damage" has not been proved. Before I do any therapy or other procedure that might cause sterility or possible DNA damage, I advise patients that their sperm can be frozen and stored in a sperm bank.

Some physicians think that prolonged exposure to excessive heat, such as working around a hot furnace, may depress sperm production, but we really don't know for certain. Articles in the lay press have reported that wearing tight clothing also might decrease sperm production, but this hasn't been shown to be of clinical significance. Some investigators have suggested that wearing a testicular cooling device could increase sperm production. Water circulating through such a device, which is worn like a jockstrap, is used to cool the testes. Unfortunately, testicular coolers don't seem to be effective. There are no concrete data to support the theory that applying cold to the testes is an efficacious way of treating male infertility.

Alcohol and illegal drugs probably impair fertility too. How much alcohol is too much? How little is safe? We just don't know. We do know, however, that daily consumption of large quantities of alcohol for relatively short periods of time can reduce serum levels of the male hormone testosterone. We also know that alcohol can cause impotence. Furthermore, by damaging the liver and also by causing an elevation in the pituitary hormone prolactin, continued use of alcohol can decrease sperm production.

Marijuana is retained in the testicles for weeks and can temporarily lower semen quality. When my infertility patients smoke marijuana, I ask them to stop. If they cannot, I suggest that use be cut to a minimum.

Anabolic steroids, widely abused by competitive athletes, harm semen quality. When used by youngsters, steroids can actually stunt growth. These drugs depress the secretion of the pituitary sex hormones FSH and LH and thus interfere with sperm production. But if an adult male who takes anabolic steroids had a normal sperm count before using these drugs, he often can initiate a pregnancy afterward, even though his sperm count is lower.

Another cause of male infertility is scrotal injury. The sperm-producing cells can be damaged by any trauma, such as a kick in the scrotum or a motorcycle accident. Testicular damage and even sterility can also be caused by surgery. If the blood supply to a testis is damaged during a hernia operation or during repair of a scrotal varicose vein, the sperm-manufacturing plant can malfunction. Even an operation to remove stones from the lower ureter can cause infertility if the vas deferens (sperm duct) is injured.

A sexual history is an important part of your infertility workup. Sometimes a couple haven't conceived simply because they are using a coital lubricant containing a spermicide. In other cases, the husband and wife don't understand that the egg is normally available for fertilization only around the middle of the menstrual cycle. Such couples may fail to have intercourse at this time; consequently the sperm never come in contact with the egg. In still other cases, the man has erectile or ejaculatory problems that preclude fertility until they are treated. Erectile dysfunction (impotence) can be broadly classified as organic or functional. The latter requires psychotherapy. Physical causes of impotence may be related to testosterone hormone deficiency, diabetes mellitus or atherosclerosis (a narrowing of the arteries caused by plaque formation on the inner arterial walls). A penile prosthesis can be used if impotence fails to respond to hormonal treatment or if psychotherapy does not help. Failure to ejaculate is a more difficult problem to treat. One new technique stimulates ejaculation with a rectal probe. Although this sounds dreadful, it may be of great importance to this group of patients.

Ed, fortunately, had none of these problems. In fact, his history gave no clues to the lack of sperm in his semen.

Physical Examination: Another Step in the Long Diagnostic Trail

Like many men his age, Ed didn't have a regular physician and hadn't had a complete physical since college, so that was the next step. He appeared in good physical health and had no operative scars from previous surgery. Careful examination indicated that his liver and thyroid gland were normal. An enlarged liver is sometimes associated with faulty sex-hormone metabolism. The thyroid gland regulates cell metabolism by secreting thyroid hormone. Either an over- or an underactive thyroid can affect sperm production. In a patient with delayed puberty, it is important for the doctor to ask if his sense of smell is normal. Infertile patients with anosmia (no sense of smell) can have a rare condition called "Kallmann's syndrome," which we will discuss later. Occasionally I see an infertility patient with impaired visual fields, milky discharge from the breasts, or loss of libido. In such a case, the doctor should do a special hormone test to determine prolactin levels, to help rule out a pituitary tumor. In still other patients, an androgen deficiency appears to exist. I measure the arm span of such men, because lack of androgen during development causes prolonged growth of the extremities. The arm span will exceed the norm for the height of these patients.

Up to this point in Ed's physical, I found nothing that gave me any clues to his sterility. But while examining his reproductive organs, I noticed that Ed's testes were slightly smaller than usual. Normally each testis is moderately firm and about the size of a hen's egg, measuring more than four by two centimeters in length and width. When the testes are smaller than this, the patient often has a problem with sperm production. Seventy to 80 percent of each testis is involved in the manufacture of sperm. Small or extremely soft testicles are indicative of damage to the mother cells within the seminiferous tubules (the "seed-bearing" tubules in which sperm develop). (See figs. 5.3 and 5.4.) Extremely firm testes suggest a genetic abnormality called "Klinefelter's syndrome" as well as some other diseases. Hard or irregular testicles are indicative of an abnormal growth or a malignancy.

Ed also had a scrotal varicocele (a varicose vein or enlarged, dilated vein) around his left testis. It was of moderate size. Like a varicose vein of the leg, a varicose vein of the testicle occurs when the valves in the vein are damaged. When you stand up, these leaflike retaining valves normally allow blood only to return to the heart. In other words, the blood flows in just one direction, away from the testes. If the valves are damaged, the blood falls backward into the scrotal veins, causing them to swell until they look rather like a blue "bag of worms."

Even though about 20 percent of all men have a varicose vein of the testicle, most affected men are fertile. In an infertile man, however, a varicocele sometimes can be an important clinical finding, because some damaged veins affect semen quality. In fact, a varicose vein is the most common surgically correctable abnormality found in subfertile men. Between 20 and 40 percent of infertile men have scrotal varicose veins, a frequency almost twice that of the general population.

When a man has a varicose vein of the testicle, the warmer blood from his abdomen collects in a stagnant pool in his scrotum. This elevates the temperature around the testis, which is extremely sensitive to heat. Doctors think that heat has a negative effect on the sperm-manufacturing plant. Some physicians also think that poor circulation resulting from the abnormal vein might reduce the oxygen supply to the testicle.

Although the first case to draw attention to the relationship between infertility and a varicocele involved a man with no sperm in his semen, a varicose vein, when causing testicular damage, is often the cause of impaired semen quality but not necessarily quantity. In other words, sperm shape and swimming ability are more often affected than sperm count or concentration.

Varicoceles occur more frequently on the left side than on the right. Reports now describe a solitary left-sided varicose vein in 50 to 60 percent of patients examined and found to have varicoceles. Both testicles should be checked for these swollen veins, because they are found on both sides more commonly than previously thought. About 40 to 50 percent of men with these vasculature abnormalities have a varicose vein on both sides. About 2 percent of patients have swollen varicoceles on the right side only.

Although large varicoceles can easily be seen and those of moderate size can usually be felt, diagnosis of a small varicose vein requires more careful examination. Often the size doesn't correlate with the extent of semen abnormalities. To detect varicoceles, the doctor asks the patient to stand up and bear down or cough to put increased pressure on the vein. Small varicose veins sometimes can be palpated at this time. The physician can also detect small veins with the Doppler Ultrasonic Stethoscope by listening for the characteristic sound of the blood regurgitating in the abnormal vein. In some cases, thermography is used to detect a small hidden testicular vein. This technique measures the warmer-than-normal temperature of a varicose vein, which photographs bright blue on the thermogram. Nowadays, with the aid of high-resolution or color-flow Doppler ultrasonography, doctors can sometimes detect small, non-palpable varicoceles.

The significance to fertility of a small varicose vein that cannot be felt remains in question. Enlarged veins usually can be palpated by a urologist if they are at least three millimeters in diameter. "Subclinical" varicoceles can only be diagnosed with venography, an X-ray of the testicular veins, or ultrasonography. Although venography can be performed on an outpatient basis, it is an invasive study. Since the advent of noninvasive ultrasonography, I have reserved venography for patients who might benefit from further therapy to close the vessel. Often such a patient has already undergone repair of a varicocele, but it may have persisted or recurred.

Further examination of Ed showed that both of his spermatic cords, which contain the sperm ducts, were thickened, but that his epididymis seemed normal. A rectal examination was necessary to evaluate the chestnut-sized prostate gland and the two seminal vesicles, which produce most of the seminal fluid (see fig. 5.5). Normally the seminal vesicles aren't palpable and the prostate is firm. Although Ed's prostate seemed normal, an enlarged or boggy prostate may indicate prostatitis (inflammation of the prostate), which usually is the result of an infection. This patient may have symptoms of pain, frequent urination, fever, and chills, and subsequently is treated with antibiotics. Although a prostate infection, which takes a long time to cure, can affect semen quality, prostatitis is an uncommon cause of infertility in an asymptomatic patient.

Some infertile men will have round cells in their semen that look like white cells or pus cells, but these don't always signal an infection. Some-

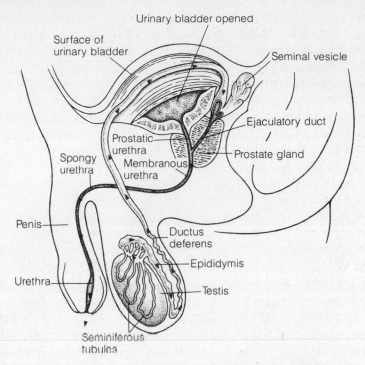

Urinary bladder opened

Surface of
urinary bladder

Seminal vesicle

Ejaculatory duct

Prostatic
urethra

Prostate gland

Spongy
urethra

Membranous
urethra

Penis

Ductus
deferens

Epididymis

Urethra

Testis

Seminiferous
tubules

FIGURE 5.5. *A cross-section of the male reproductive system. Note the ejaculatory duct and the ductus deferens or sperm duct. (From E. E. Chaffee and
E. M. Greisheimer,* Basic Physiology & Anatomy, *3rd ed., Philadelphia: J. B. Lippincott, 1974.)*

times the round cells aren't white cells at all but, rather, round, immature
sperm. With an ordinary light microscope, it is difficult to differentiate
between white cells and immature sperm unless special diagnostic techniques are used. For this reason, some infertile patients are misdi-
agnosed as having prostatitis. These men actually have a higher incidence
of immature sperm cells in their semen, released prematurely by a
damaged testicle.

By the end of Ed's physical examination, we had valuable clues
pointing to the cause of his azoospermia (sterility). One important finding
was that each of the two vasa deferentia (plural of "vas deferens") was
thickened. The vas deferens or sperm duct ("ductus deferens" in fig.
5.5) is a long tube located within each of the two spermatic cords. As
a means of male birth control, the sperm ducts can be severed during
a vasectomy operation, thus making the man sterile. (Later doctors can
perform an operation called "vasovasostomy" in which the sperm ducts
are sewn back together with microsurgery in an attempt to restore

fertility.) A thickened vas can point to either an inflammation or an obstruction. If the vasa deferentia had not been palpable, it would have indicated that they were absent from birth. Because testes lose their size as they lose their sperm-making ability, the rather small size of Ed's testicles suggested that he might have a problem with sperm production. Perhaps the varicocele was causing reduced testicular size.

At the end of Ed's physical examination, but without the benefit of further semen analyses, I was thinking: Is Ed's varicocele causing his lack of sperm? Does he have some intrinsic problem with sperm production? Or does he have an obstruction?

Laboratory Tests

Semen Analysis: A Question of Quantity and Quality

Obviously, because Ed's screening semen analyses indicated a sperm count of zero, he had no chance of initiating a pregnancy without treatment. Generally, however, a semen analysis isn't a test for fertility, although it often is highly predictive of the importance of the male factor in an infertile couple. The normal range of sperm concentration is twenty million to three hundred million per milliliter. The average is sixty million per milliliter or a hundred million per ejaculate, but these numbers don't set limits of fertility. In other words, a sperm count of forty million, which is below average, often is adequate to establish a pregnancy. If the sperm count is below twenty million, however, or above three hundred million, the chances for pregnancy decrease tremendously.

A key point in a semen analysis is the quality of the sperm, of which sperm movement is the easiest criterion to measure. Hence semen analysis studies sperm motility (forward progression). By watching sperm move under a microscope, an examiner estimates the percentage of motile sperm. The quality of their forward progression is evaluated using a scale of 0 to 4, with 4 indicating the best progression. Since results are based on the subjective observations of a technician, it isn't difficult to understand why this test is prone to error.

Some research centers use a video camera to record pictures of moving sperm, and a personal computer to count the number of sperm and to track their speed. Called "videomicrography," computer-assisted semen analysis (CASA) is as yet only a research tool. We don't currently know how much these expensive systems are going to aid in the clinical management of patients. Computers should make semen analysis less subjective, though at present they often cannot differentiate between sperm-sized debris and the actual sperm. Thus the computer overestimates the sperm count and underestimates the motility. In other words, the machine perceives the debris as sperm and then notes that the debris aren't moving.

Your doctor will also study the morphology (structure or shape) of your sperm under a microscope. At least 60 percent should be properly formed and mature, each having an oval head and one tail (see fig. 1.7). This means that as many as 40 percent of the sperm can be abnormally formed before the semen analysis is considered below par. The oval-shaped head of normal sperm is aerodynamically designed to move through the woman's cervical mucus. If its head is malformed, the sperm doesn't move well through the female reproductive tract. Not only are misshapen, immotile sperm incapable of swimming through cervical mucus, they also seem to be unable to penetrate an egg.

Another property of semen studied by the doctor is its viscosity or thickness. Special enzymes added by the seminal vesicles cause the semen to coagulate immediately after ejaculation. Twenty to thirty minutes later, other enzymes, added earlier by the prostate gland, cause the semen to reliquefy. Some doctors think that, if the semen remains too thick, the sperm may become entrapped. This theory is controversial, however, because in some animals the semen never liquefies. The only time I worry about hyperviscosity is if the sperm cannot swim through receptive cervical mucus at ovulation. As we will discuss in detail later, this is studied by a special test called the "Sims-Huhner postcoital test." If results of this study show that the sperm can penetrate your wife's cervical mucus, semen viscosity isn't a concern.

TABLE 5.1. LIMITS OF "ADEQUACY"

On at least two occasions:

Ejaculate volume	1.5–5.0 mL
Sperm density	Greater than 20 million/mL
Viability	Greater than 60 percent
Motility	Forward progression greater than 2 (on 1–4 scale)
Morphology	Greater than 60 percent are of normal oval shape

and   No significant sperm agglutination (no clumping)
        No significant pyospermia (no white cells in the semen, indicating infection or inflammation)
        No hyperviscosity (not too thick)

When discussing semen analysis, your doctor may speak of minimal limits of "adequacy." Below these somewhat arbitrary limits, the patient's chances of fathering a child decrease significantly, but not absolutely (see table 5.1). Keep in mind that men with high-quality motile sperm may be fertile despite a very low sperm count or density.

Proper semen collection is crucial if your test results are to be correct. It is important to abstain from ejaculating for two to three days before the semen is collected. The specimen should be collected in a clean, wide-mouthed container to avoid loss. The total volume usually equals about one teaspoon. Remember that generally most of the sperm are concentrated in the first half of the ejaculate. Some patients collect semen in a special condom that is a Silastic sheath devoid of any spermicidal agent. The container should be kept at room temperature (not in the refrigerator or in the sun) and must be brought to your doctor's office within two hours. Semen analyses are usually conducted on specimens obtained once a week for three weeks, because sperm counts and quality can vary with time.

Urinalysis

A complete urinalysis sometimes leads to further clues in the evaluation of a patient such as Ed. White blood cells in the urine may suggest a urinary-tract or prostate infection. If the semen volume is low but the urine sample contains many sperm, retrograde ejaculation into the bladder may be the problem. A urinalysis immediately after ejaculation can confirm this diagnosis. Occasionally the urinalysis detects an undiagnosed disease, such as diabetes or kidney failure.

In Ed's case, the three semen specimens and the urinalysis were telling: Not only was the sperm count repeatedly zero, but the volume was low. He had no sperm or white cells in his urine. Although the results of these tests told me much about my patient's fertility status, I still couldn't give Ed a definitive diagnosis.

A Problem of Production or Transport?

Since Ed had no sperm in his ejaculate, it was important to determine whether he had a problem with sperm production, a blockage in the ductal system of his reproductive tract, or a combination of both. I already knew that Ed was producing only a small amount of semen, which indicated that he had either poorly functioning or nonemptying seminal vesicles. The other possibility, retrograde ejaculation, had been ruled out when, after ejaculation, his urine contained no sperm.

Since Ed's semen contained no sperm, it was necessary to test his semen for fructose. Sometimes called "fruit sugar," fructose is added to the semen by the seminal vesicles and serves as a source of energy for sperm movement. Ed's fructose test showed that there was no fructose in his semen. Since his ejaculate volume was low and his fructose test was negative, I thought that he might have either no seminal vesicles or an obstruction of the ejaculatory ducts. The ejaculatory ducts are one-inch-long canals leading from the seminal vesicles to the upper end of the urethra in the prostate (see figs. 5.5 and 5.6).

A Basic Hormonal Profile: Laboratory Clues

It was now necessary to do a basic hormonal profile for Ed. We needed to study his blood levels of the male hormone testosterone and the sex hormones from the pituitary gland—luteinizing hormone (LH) and follicle-stimulating hormone (FSH). About 5 percent of infertile men have too few or no sperm because of hormonal abnormalities. Testos-

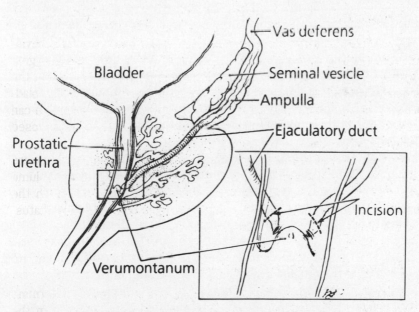

FIGURE 5.6. This diagram illustrates the procedure of transurethral resection of the ejaculatory ducts. After loop resection of the verumontanum (see inset), a special knife is used to incise a portion of the prostatic urethra along the esti-mated location of the ejaculatory ducts (dotted lines). (Courtesy of Dr. L. I. Lipshultz and Dr. Irvin H. Hirsch, from Masters in Urology, vol. 1, no. 2, 1985, published by CPC Communications, Greenwich, Connecticut.)

terone, which is synthesized from cholesterol in the Leydig cells in the testes, is responsible in part for a man's sex drive and the development of his secondary sexual characteristics—all the changes associated with puberty, such as his deep voice and his masculine appearance. Measurement of serum testosterone is especially useful in patients with a history of delayed puberty, decreased libido, or impotence. This hormone fluctuates widely during the day, reaching its highest levels in the early morning. As I expected, Ed's blood tests showed that his testosterone level was normal.

The body has an amazing control mechanism to keep this powerful male hormone in balance. The messenger hormone LH, which travels through the blood from the pituitary gland to the testes, stimulates the Leydig cells to make testosterone. When blood-borne testosterone reaches a certain level and feeds back to the brain, the control center in the man's head automatically decreases production of LH. This in turn causes a reduction in testosterone output by the Leydig cells.

Excess androgen in the male, rather like too much estrogen in the female, can suppress pituitary sex-hormone secretion. In fact, if serum testosterone levels get too high, the testes will shut down sperm production, causing a problem that doctors call "secondary testicular failure."

For Ed, however, a study of FSH—the messenger hormone necessary for sperm production—was the most critical hormonal test. Doctors can tell a great deal about how the testes are working by measuring blood levels of this key pituitary hormone. Although scientists don't really know how FSH works, we do know that the site of FSH activity is on the Sertoli cells, the nurse cells that nourish the sperm (see fig. 5.4). Perhaps FSH acts through the initiation of growth-promoting substances from the Sertoli cells that are necessary for normal sperm production. In a sterile patient, a very high FSH level suggests a sperm-production problem in the testes, rather than a blockage in the ductal delivery system. As sperm production drops, FSH levels usually rise. Hence, by the time there is a marked reduction in the more mature sperm forms, FSH is almost always elevated. In fact, if serum FSH is elevated more than three times normal and the testes are small, there is only a slight chance that any type of therapy will help. Fortunately for Ed, his FSH level was normal, indicating that his testicles were producing sperm. All his other hormone tests also were within their normal ranges.

A man can have relatively low levels of the messenger hormones FSH and LH circulating in his blood and still initiate a pregnancy. As long as sperm production and testosterone levels are normal, depressed

FSH and LH secretion is unimportant. Such patients don't need treatment.

Occasionally, however, low levels of FSH and LH indicate that the man has Kallmann's syndrome, a rare condition in which sexual development is incomplete as an adult. This problem occurs when the hypothalamus fails to stimulate the pituitary to release enough of its sex hormones to cause sexual maturation. Such men usually produce no sperm. As mentioned earlier, they often have no sense of smell even as boys. Some of these men also are deaf and color-blind. Treatment with the powerful fertility drug Pergonal, which contains FSH and LH, and with hCG, which, like LH, causes the testicles to make testosterone, allows sexual maturation to progress and frequently establishes fertility.

In a sexually mature man, low levels of serum FSH and LH may be caused by too much of the pituitary hormone prolactin in the blood. In men as in women, severe or chronic stress, alcohol abuse, and certain medications can elevate serum prolactin. High levels of this hormone, particularly if the patient has a milky discharge from the breasts, may suggest the prolactin-secreting tumor of the pituitary gland called a "prolactinoma." This tumor develops out of a cell in the master gland that synthesizes prolactin, and the tumor's presence is marked by an increase of the hormone in the blood. Although these tumors aren't cancerous, they not only can cause infertility but can be dangerous, especially if they become large. On clinical examination, such a patient may have visual-field changes and decreased sex drive. Although treatment with bromocriptine can reduce serum prolactin and thus increase the sperm count, some patients may require neurosurgery to remove the tumor (see "Pituitary Tumor" in chapter 4).

Special Diagnostic Studies

Examining the Prostate with Ultrasound

At this point, I thought that Ed's sterility probably wasn't caused by markedly impaired sperm production because his FSH levels were within normal limits. The next step was to evaluate his seminal vesicles and ejaculatory ducts. We scheduled him for transrectal ultrasonography of the prostate, which is used to detect prostatic disease. Although the report showed that Ed's seminal vesicles and prostate appeared normal, we couldn't see his ejaculatory ducts or further evaluate his ductal system.

Scrotal Exploration: More Than Just a Biopsy

Since Ed had no sperm in his semen, and his physical examination showed that his testes were slightly smaller than normal, I suggested that he have scrotal exploration. In Ed's case, this would include a biopsy of one testicle, vasography (an X-ray of the sperm ductal system), and an inspection of the variococele. The biopsy would enable us to study Ed's sperm-production plant to see if his testes were adequately manufacturing sperm. This surgery is performed only if the man is sterile or has marked oligospermia (a low sperm count), particularly if the semen volume is low. The biopsy helps the doctor decide whether medical therapy might be worthwhile. If, for example, the biopsy specimen shows severe scarring around the sperm-producing seminiferous tubules, it is unlikely that medical therapy would be effective.

At first, Ed was hesitant to have a testicular biopsy, because he thought that it would be painful. I assured him that he could be asleep during the entire procedure, although it can be done with a sedative and local anesthesia. After this surgery, which takes about fifteen to thirty minutes, most patients have only minimal pain, which they say feels like a headache in the testicle. If the surgery is performed by a well-trained urologist, there usually are no significant side effects, although swelling, pain, and infection can occur.

During Ed's scrotal exploration, a small incision was made in the scrotum and a tiny snip of the delicate testicular tissue was removed. Before sending this biopsy to the laboratory, the tissue was "touched" to a sterile glass slide so that the excess cells could adhere. The slide was sprayed with fixative and immediately stained. With this test, I knew within five minutes that mature sperm were present. The biopsy specimen also was permanently fixed and stained. The resulting slides included a cross-section of many sperm-producing seminiferous tubules, which normally contain the germ cells (sperm precursors and sperm) and the interstitial tissue between those tubules. The latter contain the testosterone-producing Leydig cells.

When the pathologist looked at the biopsy specimen through a microscope, he immediately saw that Ed's sperm factory was normal. All the elements of sperm production were present: the sperm-generating mother cells and the immature and mature sperm were laid out in perfect assembly line fashion (see fig. 5.4). We would have good news for Ed when he woke up—there was a chance that his problem was correctable. Since Ed's testes were making mature sperm, I knew that he had a blockage rather than an intrinsic deficiency in sperm production.

In some patients, the biopsy shows that sperm are present but their development is arrested. This means that somewhere along the sperm assembly line, maturation is completely halted. The Leydig cells, however, are usually normal. Still other patients have a condition called "hypospermatogenesis" in which all the elements of sperm production are present, and the Leydig cells appear normal, but few sperm are produced. Sometimes this condition coexists with abnormal maturation. Medical treatment is only rarely effective. Varicoceles, if present, can produce either of these microscopic pictures.

In a few patients, the biopsy report shows a total lack of germ cells. This is the worst possible finding for ultimate fertility. If no mother cells are present, the doctor obviously cannot create new ones. Occasionally the biopsy also indicates that the testosterone-producing Leydig cells are abnormal. More often, however, even though a patient has no sperm, he still has functioning Leydig cells. In rare instances, an unsuspected testicular malignancy is found.

In Ed's case, since his testicular biopsy showed normal sperm production, vasography was indicated to determine whether the ejaculatory ducts were open. I began this procedure, which I perform with an operating microscope, by making an incision in the left sperm duct, one inch from the epididymis. The duct was very dilated at this level, although the epididymis was not. Fluid coming from the testicular side of the incision contained abundant amounts of sperm. A radio-opaque contrast medium was injected into the abdominal side (away from the epididymis) of the incision in the sperm duct. The dyelike substance could be seen moving up the duct and down through the seminal vesicles. When the contrast medium reached the ejaculatory ducts, there was resistance. This indicated an obstruction. When the dye didn't flow freely into the bladder, I knew instantly what Ed's problem was: he had an obstruction of the ejaculatory ducts.

Apparently, sperm were leaving Ed's testes, moving through the epididymis, and distending the sperm duct, the ampulla (enlarged ending) of the sperm duct, and the seminal vesicles. The backup of sperm, however, was not causing the epididymis to become dilated. I used to think that an obstruction would always cause the epididymis to become dilated. But this is not true. Some men can absorb this back pressure. Although a dilated epididymis means an obstruction, a normal-appearing epididymis doesn't rule out an obstruction.

Following the biopsy and X-ray, Ed, like most patients, required only a mild pain-relieving medication and was able to go home the same day. He had no significant side effects. Within two to three days after surgery, Ed was back at work, although we advised him to wear a scrotal support for one week.

Treatments

Surgical Therapy

It was time to meet with Ed and Elizabeth to explain our findings and offer a treatment. When I told them that Ed had an ejaculatory duct obstruction, he wanted to know what had caused it. I explained that it is unclear whether this type of obstruction is present at birth or acquired. Although I think that it usually is congenital, there is some evidence that such a blockage might result from an inflammatory process. Venereal disease usually causes a blockage in the tail of the epididymis and the adjacent portion of the sperm duct rather than in the ejaculatory ducts.

I said the only way to open the obstructed system was to perform an operation called a "transurethral resection of the ejaculatory ducts." I also carefully explained that the overall success rate with this procedure is low. Even if it was unsuccessful, however, it would not make matters worse. Since Ed and Elizabeth were eager to do whatever possible to increase their chances of pregnancy, Ed decided to have this surgery.

UNBLOCKING THE EJACULATORY DUCTS

On the morning of Ed's surgery, after he was asleep, I examined the urinary bladder with an instrument called a "cystoscope" that had been inserted through the urethral opening in the tip of the penis. The entire anatomy seemed normal. Using a special telescopic endoscope used for cutting, called a "resectoscope," I resected the verumontanum, a landmark in the prostatic urethra indicating the exit site of the prostatic and ejaculatory ducts (see fig. 5.6). Since the two ducts enter the prostate close together, one bite opened both. I had hoped that I would see a burst of milky fluid gushing out of the incision site, telling me that I had opened the obstruction. I didn't. Although disappointing, the lack of fluid didn't mean, as I later told Ed, that I hadn't "unroofed" the obstruction. Perhaps there was only a small amount of fluid in the system. Only time would give us the answer.

Although not a difficult operation to perform, transurethral resection of the ejaculatory ducts has a low success rate because the surgeon can only estimate where the ejaculatory ducts should be—in other words, where they enter the prostate.

LOOKING GOOD—AT FIRST

About five weeks after surgery, after an uneventful recovery, Ed came to my office for his first postoperative semen analysis. At this time, his sperm density was eighteen million per milliliter; many were of normal shape. Sperm motility was 65 percent, but forward progression was poor. Based on a scale of 0 to 4, with 4 indicating active forward movement, forward progression was only 1.5. Two months passed. At this time, I was glad to see that Ed's semen density was markedly increased, to fifty-eight million per milliliter. Unfortunately, however, his sperm motility had dropped to 30 percent, and forward progression was only 1. Although later semen analyses did show an improvement in sperm motility, forward progression remained poor.

Why did my patient have sperm of decent quantity but poor quality? There were two possibilities: his previously diagnosed varicocele could be adversely affecting semen quality. Or, perhaps, he could be allergic to his own sperm. In other words, he might have developed an autoimmunity against his sperm in which sperm-killing autoantibodies were attacking and immobilizing sperm as if they were foreign invaders. This could explain his sperm's poor forward progression. It isn't uncommon to see this problem in patients who have had a ductal obstruction, especially if the blockage has been present for many years. For example, men who have had a vasectomy of long-standing often produce autoantibodies against their sperm.

Doctors use a special test called the "immunobead assay" to check for antisperm antibodies. Ed's test confirmed that his immune system was causing his sperm to agglutinate (clump together) and become immotile. I told Ed that, as with allergy, there are therapies that might help but that doctors are unable to treat every case effectively.

REPAIR OF THE VARICOSE VEIN

Six more months passed, and Ed's wife still wasn't pregnant. My feeling was that we might be able to improve the quality of Ed's semen by surgically repairing his varicose vein of the testicle. This is the most common problem contributing to poor semen quality. After surgery, 67 percent of patients produce sperm that are better formed and more lively. About 40 percent may father a child within six to nine months following surgery. In patients showing no sperm, however, the success rate is much lower. Furthermore, not every patient with a varicocele should have it corrected. Rather, surgery generally is reserved for the man with poor sperm motility or density for which no other explanation can be found.

Ed was depressed at the prospect of having another operation. Although he was an unusually strong person, he had been through a lot, and the stress of infertility was taking its toll. I told him that a varicocele operation usually is performed on an outpatient basis under general or regional anesthesia. Most men go back to work in three to four days and, if the procedure is in expert hands, the side effects are few. Ed decided to go ahead with the surgery.

Repair of a varicocele, which doctors call "varicocelectomy" or "spermatic vein ligation," involves tying off the affected veins with a nonabsorbable suture so that the blood in the abdomen cannot back-flow into the scrotum. Afterward the blood returns to the heart from the testicle through collateral (secondary) drainage routes; hence the varicose vein characteristically decreases in size but often will not disappear entirely.

I told Ed that, if all went well, we might see a slight improvement in semen quality in about three months; it takes that long for new sperm to mature and work their way through the epididymis. Full recovery, however, would take at least six months. My hope was that by this time Ed's sperm would be much better swimmers.

Unfortunately, surgical repair of one varicose vein doesn't ensure that another cannot develop. In the 5 to 10 percent of cases in which this happens, an alternative to a second operation is to block the vein using a sclerosing agent, a coil or a balloon. Such relatively new radiological techniques may have a few more side effects than surgery, may take longer to perform, and may have a slightly higher recurrence rate.

Medical Therapy for Antisperm Antibodies

After repairing Ed's varicose vein, I prescribed high-dose prednisone therapy (a tapered regimen lasting for one month) to try to reduce the high concentration of circulating antisperm antibodies. Although the importance of the immune factor is difficult to pinpoint, suppression of sperm-killing and immobilizing antibodies sometimes seems to improve semen quality. Some of my patients have initiated a pregnancy after this treatment.

Unfortunately, prednisone therapy has admitted side effects that must be carefully explained to the patient. These include indigestion caused by increased stomach acid, insomnia, and acne of the back—all of which go away when the drug is discontinued. As I told Ed, there is an extremely rare but serious side effect that doctors call "aseptic necrosis of the femoral head." Basically, this means that the head of the femur, or thighbone, that fits into the hipbone can be severely damaged. This complication is not entirely dose-dependent, and doctors cannot predict who will be affected. Ed, fortunately, had no serious side effects, although he did have some difficulty sleeping.

The Sims-Huhner Postcoital Test

Several more months passed. It was now time to do another semen analysis to see if the varicocele operation and the prednisone therapy had improved Ed's semen quality. If the results were good, we would do the Sims-Huhner postcoital test to see if Ed's sperm could swim through his wife's cervical mucus at ovulation. The timing of this study is crucial, because the mucus changes during the menstrual cycle. If the test is performed at any other time except around ovulation, the cervical mucus will be of poor quality.

You will recall that the cervical mucus serves as an amazing filter that guards the entrance to the womb against bacteria and sperm. Around ovulation, however, the mucus is miraculously transformed. Under the influence of the female hormone estrogen released from the ripening follicle (remember, the follicle usually contains the egg), the cervix opens. At the same time, the mucus changes from a thick, sticky, pluglike barrier to a clear, watery liquid with remarkable stretchability (*Spinnbarkeit*). Thus, for a brief time around ovulation, the mucus becomes copious and serves as a vehicle that allows the best-swimming sperm to enter the uterus.

For two days before the postcoital test (but not longer), the couple should refrain from sex, so that the man's sperm will not be depleted. On the day of the test, the couple should have intercourse two to four hours before the wife's appointment with her gynecologist, although for some studies relations should occur the night before the test. Her doctor will examine the cervical mucus under a microscope to determine how many motile sperm per high-power field succeed in swimming deep into the cervix. This *in-vivo* test (occurring in a living organism) not only indicates the quality of the mucus at ovulation but also shows the sperm's ability to penetrate the mucus in order to enter the uterus.

The results of Ed's semen analysis and the couple's postcoital test were extremely encouraging. Ed's semen count was now fifty-five million, with 55-percent motility and a forward progression of 3. The Sims-Huhner test showed that the sperm were penetrating the cervical mucus. When I told Ed this, the expression on his face said it all.

When Ed left my office, he was more optimistic about his chances of becoming a father than I had ever seen him. He had overcome a number of fertility problems, including a blockage of his reproductive system, a varicose vein of the testicle, and autoantibodies against his own sperm. As this case so clearly shows, just because a patient has one fertility problem doesn't mean that he might not have others as well. Although I haven't visited with Ed since his last semen analysis, I received a short note from him about fourteen months later. Enclosed was a picture of his two-month-old son.

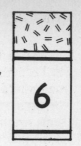

"Low" Sperm Count—Cause Unknown

LARRY I. LIPSHULTZ, M.D., AND
DOROTHY KAY BROCKMAN

After a thorough medical examination by an expert in male infertility, 30 to 40 percent of infertile men still will not know why they have a low sperm count because their doctor has found no clues. Idiopathic oligospermia ("idiopathic" means "of unknown cause" and "oligospermia" means "few or insufficient sperm") is a problem that is difficult to treat and frustrating for all concerned. These patients, who represent the largest group of men treated with medical therapy, generally have a sperm concentration of fewer than twenty million per milliliter, or fewer than fifty million per ejaculate. They usually have a normal sex drive and are virile. They have a normal hormone profile and normal genitalia. They have never had a "hidden" testicle or an inflammation of the testis, epididymis, or prostate. There is no evidence of a varicocele (varicose vein in the scrotum) or a ductal obstruction.

Other patients have a poor semen analysis because they have a problem called "idiopathic asthenospermia," an unexplained decrease in sperm motility or movement. Some patients have sperm with low motility but high sperm concentration, or vice versa.

In general, sperm motility is the best indirect predictor of sperm function. Sometimes excellent motility can compensate for low sperm count or concentration; and, to a limited extent, sperm density can make up for sluggish sperm movement. If a man has many sperm with poor motility, the count becomes a less effective predictor of fertility. If the semen volume is large but low in sperm density, even though there will be many sperm in the ejaculate, the potency will be reduced. Concentrating semen and placing it directly in the woman's uterus may help men with overly diluted semen produce a pregnancy.

Not all patients with poor motility improve after surgical treatment: some are unable to initiate a pregnancy after repair of a varicose vein of the scrotum; others don't achieve adequate semen quality following reversal of a vasectomy, despite the presence of sperm in the ejaculate. When surgical treatments fail, are there any other options? What can be done if a patient's semen analyses still show a low sperm count or poor motility and the reason is unknown? Will empiric treatment (therapies based on past experience rather than direct scientific evidence) with fertility drugs improve the fertility potential of these men?

Treating Male Infertility with Fertility Drugs

Men with a low sperm count of unknown cause often are treated empirically with clomiphene citrate (Clomid or Serophene), the fertility drug used to induce ovulation in women. The goal is to improve sperm density and motility. Doctors debate, however, whether it works. I think that it does, in selected cases. The problem is that we cannot predict in advance who will respond. About 20 percent of my patients show improvement in sperm density, but clomiphene seldom increases motility. Patients may have to take the drug for at least six months before we can tell if it is working. During this time, each man must be followed closely, because, instead of increasing his sperm count, the drug can have the opposite effect—it can act as a male contraceptive!

When clomiphene works, how does it improve a man's sperm count? It increases the pituitary hormones FSH and LH—key blood-borne hormones that work together to stimulate sperm production in the testes. Normally the female hormone estrogen, which is converted from testicular testosterone, feeds back to the brain and down-regulates the secretion of FSH and LH. But when a patient takes clomiphene, it blocks the uptake of natural estrogen by the brain. By blocking estrogen's "shut-off" effect on the pituitary hormones, clomiphene causes serum levels of FSH and LH to increase. Together with LH, elevated levels of FSH theoretically can stimulate the testicles to increase sperm production.

One reason clomiphene doesn't always work in men is that the drug can cause the level of male hormone in the blood to get too high. By indirectly causing an increase in LH, clomiphene stimulates testosterone production by the testes. Excess levels of this male hormone and its conversion to estrogen can cause sperm production to fall.

Sometimes doctors use the fertility drug tamoxifen citrate to treat subfertile men. This medication seems to have fewer side effects than the better-known clomiphene, although results with tamoxifen are generally no better than with the more widely used drug. Like clomiphene, tamoxifen increases serum levels of the hormones LH and FSH and may be used to treat idiopathic oligospermia. Results, however, are varied. Depending on which medical study one reads, tamoxifen increases sperm density in 11 to 100 percent of patients, with no significant increase in motility. Pregnancy rates have ranged from 11 to 30 percent.

Another drug, human chorionic gonadotropin (hCG), also has been used to treat men with low sperm counts. This is the hormone that is produced in increasing amounts during pregnancy. HCG, which, like LH, can stimulate the testes to increase testosterone production, has been prescribed for many years to initiate puberty in teenage boys and to treat men with "hidden" testicles. But in treating male infertility, the effectiveness of nonspecific hCG therapy is debatable. Studies report that the drug increases sperm density by 11 percent to close to 70 percent. Pregnancy rates are 9 to 36 percent.

HCG offers some hope for patients with sperm densities of fewer than ten million per milliliter who haven't responded to varicocele repair. The problem is that, once again, the results aren't uniformly reproducible. Like clomiphene, hCG can not only increase serum testosterone to the point where sperm production drops but also increases the conversion of testosterone to estrogen.

HCG also is used to treat Kallmann's syndrome, a rare condition in which sexual development is incomplete as an adult. Such patients fail to go through puberty, because the hypothalamus doesn't stimulate the pituitary to release enough FSH and LH. By using hCG as a substitute for LH, doctors can stimulate testosterone production, thus allowing the sexual maturation characteristic of puberty and, in some cases, limited sperm production. To get a complete stimulation of sperm production, we add FSH in the form of the drug Pergonal (human menopausal gonadotropin or hMG). It's the drug mentioned in chapter 4 that is often used to induce ovulation in women.

Gonadotropin-releasing hormone (GnRH), which is secreted in pulsatile (pulselike) bursts by the hypothalamus, stimulates the pituitary to secrete the gonadotropins FSH and LH. The use of this hormone in treating male infertility as yet has produced no uniform data.

Let's assume that we put a patient with unexplained oligospermia on clomiphene for six months and that his sperm count increases from ten million to thirty-five million per milliliter with fairly good volume. Unfortunately, however, sperm motility remains poor. Although his wife is diagnosed as normal, she doesn't become pregnant. What other options does medical science have to offer this couple? How can they decide whether they are good candidates for one of the new assisted reproductive technologies (ART)?

Artificial Insemination by Husband (AIH)

Artificial insemination by husband (AIH) is a basically simple procedure in which the husband's semen is placed near or in the wife's cervix or within her uterus, using a syringe or a narrow tube. By concentrating the sperm in these areas, we may increase the chances for pregnancy. In general, AIH may be recommended for cases involving impotency and premature ejaculation unresponsive to treatment; retrograde ejaculation, which sometimes is a complication of diabetes; and low semen volume of unknown cause. Although AIH has helped some men with sperm-delivery problems, results in patients with poor-quality sperm have been disappointing.

In the past, the split-ejaculate method of artificial insemination was used to help oligospermic men with or without poor motility. This technique uses only about the first one-third of semen. Since the more concentrated, higher-quality sperm are found in the first portion of the ejaculate, this insemination method sometimes increases the chance for pregnancy. Split-ejaculate insemination, however, is now out of date. Currently the sperm can be processed (mechanically concentrated) before being placed within the uterus.

Treating Male Infertility with Assisted Reproductive Technologies (ART)

Couples with male infertility unresponsive to surgical or medical therapies may wish to consider one of the new assisted reproductive technologies (ART) such as intrauterine insemination (IUI) by husband, superovulation and IUI, *in-vitro* or "test-tube" fertilization (IVF), "gamete intrafallopian transfer" (GIFT), or "zygote intrafallopian transfer" (ZIFT). Of particular interest to men with reproductive failure is a new micromanipulation technique called "intracytoplasmic sperm injection" (ICSI).

During IUI, a few droplets of washed and concentrated semen containing large numbers of motile sperm are placed deep within the cavity of the uterus around ovulation. This procedure may be performed to bypass cervical mucus that is hostile to sperm activity. To make more eggs available to the sperm, the woman can be "superovulated" with fertility drugs to stimulate increased egg production. During IVF, the eggs are removed from the ovaries via a vaginal probe and fertilized with the husband's sperm in a "test-tube." Later, any resulting pre-embryos are placed in the woman's uterus or frozen for subsequent uterine transfer. During GIFT, the eggs are harvested from medically stimulated ovaries via laparoscopy, placed in a catheter, and, together with the husband's sperm, immediately injected through the 'scope into the outer end of each fallopian tube. During ZIFT, which is a combination of GIFT and IVF, a *fertilized* egg is transferred into the oviduct under laparoscopic direction. During ICSI, a single sperm is injected directly into the center of the tiny egg, often setting the stage for fertilization by men formerly labeled "sterile."

Success rates with IUI following fertility drugs have ranged from 8 to 10 percent per cycle, with the outcome highly dependent upon the reason for treatment. Generally, this procedure is recommended for women with a cervix damaged from a previous inflammation, with cervical stenosis (a narrowed cervix), or with inadequate or hostile cervical mucus, and for some couples with unexplained infertility. Those with a cervical problem but no other infertility factor have the best results. In fact, if a cervical factor is the only known problem, the success rate may approach 40 percent. For patients with unexplained infertility, success rates range from 5 percent to 25 percent within three to six cycles. Unfortunately, results with superovulated IUI for male infertility have been disappointing, with the outcome highly dependent upon how much the semen specimen improves after processing in the laboratory. Although IUI may help some women with antisperm antibodies that kill or immobilize sperm, it won't help men with autoantibodies against their own sperm.

Before IUI, motile sperm are separated from the semen and mechanically concentrated, using special washing techniques. The sperm are then capacitated, a biochemical process by which enzyme inhibitor is stripped from the sperm head. Unless capacitated either in the woman's body or in a special culture in the laboratory, the sperm cannot fertilize the egg. Once processed, the sperm can be used not only for intrauterine insemination but also for IVF, ZIFT, or GIFT.

With IVF, ZIFT, or GIFT the sperm don't have to swim through the female reproductive tract. Hence, with these ART procedures the sperm need not be as vigorous as when deposited by intercourse. Furthermore, *in-vitro* sperm processing may expose the egg to an optimal concentration of high-quality, motile sperm. Since the sperm can be washed, concentrated, and placed right next to the egg, these procedures sometimes allow a man with an unusually low percentage of active sperm to initiate a pregnancy. Despite washing and concentration, however, sperm with poor activity often cannot fertilize an egg.

Unfortunately, in our experience GIFT hasn't been an effective procedure for male infertility. If patients are unable to get pregnant with superovulation combined with IUI—which is easier on the woman and cheaper—they generally don't conceive with GIFT. Hence, we rarely use GIFT anymore, unless the patient needs a laparoscopy for other reasons. Sometimes we may combine GIFT with IVF. Unlike GIFT, IVF enables us to document fertilization. Once the eggs are fertilized, they can be transferred to the uterus or the tubes.

Although ART therapies offer some hope for subfertile men, IVF success rates at clinics around the country are cut approximately in half if the problem is associated with the man rather than the woman. Doctors generally agree that infertility in couples with a significant male factor is usually caused by a decrease in the ability of the sperm to enter an egg—not by the ability of the resulting embryo to implant in the uterus. The exciting news is that ICSI is enabling more subfertile men to father children, thereby rapidly changing these statistics. (See chapter 9 for further details concerning ART.)

Can Your Sperm Fertilize an Egg?

The Sperm Penetration Assay (Hamster Egg Test)

How do doctors predict if a patient's sperm can fertilize an egg? One way is to study sperm function with a test called the "sperm penetration assay" (SPA) or "hamster egg–sperm penetration assay." A hamster egg with its outer coat removed serves as a surrogate for a human one. This laboratory study of sperm performance may be used to determine the fertility potential of severely oligospermic men before *in-vitro* fertilization and to evaluate sperm function in seemingly normal males with unexplained infertility. Some centers routinely use SPA to screen all patients prior to entrance into *in-vitro* fertilization programs. Although the sperm penetration assay may shed light on egg-sperm interaction, the test doesn't evaluate the sperm's ability to migrate through the female reproductive tract.

To determine sperm viability, about one million are incubated with twenty or more hamster eggs that have been stripped of their species-specific zona pellucida. The gelatinlike zona is the membrane surrounding the egg that keeps more than one sperm from entering. When the zona is removed, functioning sperm often can penetrate the hamster egg, although it isn't fertilized.

The results of this *in-vitro* test often correlate with the sperm's ability to fertilize a human egg. Some laboratories say that if fewer than 10 to 14 percent of the eggs are penetrated, the SPA suggests—but does not prove—that the sperm are incapable of initiating a pregnancy. In other laboratories, with more sensitized testing, all the eggs are routinely penetrated, and the number of penetrations per egg defines a normal versus a subfertile sperm population. In the latter test, five penetrations per egg is the lower limit considered normal; this result is known as the "Sperm Capacitative Index."

We have learned from "test-tube" fertilization (IVF) that some sperm incapable of fertilizing a zona-free hamster egg can penetrate a human egg when placed right next to it in a laboratory dish. Nevertheless, the SPA is a good test for a couple who can't decide whether to try *in-vitro* fertilization. If the assay shows that the man's sperm can penetrate a hamster egg, his sperm usually will fertilize his wife's eggs *in-vitro*. Hence IVF might be worth the couple's investment in time and money. For some people, IVF is just too expensive to attempt if the SPA indicates a low fertilization rate. In other words, we use the assay as a guide; we don't use it to exclude people from IVF. Embryos fertilized with sperm from males with semen of reduced quality seem to have at least as good a chance of implanting in the uterus as embryos from men with normal semen.

The Hemizona Assay

A new test called the "hemizona assay" (HZA) or "sperm binding test," which is too complicated to have widespread clinical application, is now being used at some of the medical centers to study sperm function.

The ability of sperm to bind to a split nonliving human egg helps doctors predict the sperm's fertilizing potential.

Egg-Sperm Micromanipulation: Getting the Sperm into the Egg

Yet another barrier to fertility has been broken. Amazing new IVF breakthroughs are helping infertile men initiate pregnancies, even though their sperm are unable to penetrate an egg. "Intracytoplasmic sperm injection" (ICSI) is allowing some men with nonswimming sperm, poorly shaped sperm, few sperm, or sperm with other abnormalities to have children. In order to induce normal fertilization with ICSI, a single sperm is injected directly into the center of an egg, thereby bypassing all the egg's natural physical barriers.

Nowadays, even men with *no obvious* sperm in their semen are becoming biological parents. Using an ICSI technique referred to as MESA or "microscopic epididymal sperm aspiration," urologic microsurgeons can obtain mature sperm from the epididymis or even from a testis biopsy specimen. By injecting sperm obtained during MESA into the cytoplasm of the egg, doctors have helped men with surgically irreparable obstructions of the reproductive tracts. In fact, some patients with no sperm ducts from birth (congenital absence of the vasa) now are able to father babies.

Couples need to know all the details before attempting any of these new assisted reproductive technologies. ICSI results in fertilization of approximately 60 percent of the eggs injected, with conception rates varying widely depending on the quality of the eggs and sperm. With some couples, all of the eggs fertilize; with other patients none do. Unfortunately, at this time approximately 10 percent of eggs are irreversibly injured during the ICSI procedure. At present, over one thousand babies have been born following fertilization with ICSI, with no identified increase of birth defects. Subtle problems, however, may not become apparent until a much larger population of ICSI-conceived babies has been born.

As you might imagine, all of these complicated high-tech IVF procedures are time-consuming, expensive, and stressful. MESA immediately followed by "test-tube" fertilization using intracytoplasmic sperm injection can cause the most significant strain because doctors not only must recover and fertilize the eggs but also must retrieve the sperm with microsurgery. The results nevertheless have been gratifying to both patients and their physicians.

With the thin covering of the dot-sized egg at last a broken barrier, men who formerly had little hope of ever having a child are finally becoming fathers. At last, after years of disappointment, they too have the opportunity to be somebody's dad—a privilege most "infertile" parents say is worth all the effort.

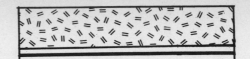

Part III

Important
Issues
in
Infertility

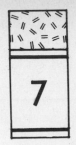

7

Unexplained Infertility

Between 10 and 15 percent of patients completing an infertility workup are told that nothing abnormal can be found. These couples are said to have "unexplained infertility" or "infertility cause unknown," a diagnosis arrived at by ruling out all the known causes of infertility. Doctors sometimes call such patients the "normal" infertile. This, however, is a misnomer that gives the false impression that, if allowed enough time, many of these couples eventually will have a baby.

Unexplained infertility is an extremely frustrating diagnosis for both the couple and their physician. The couple go home not knowing what to do next. Should they consult another doctor? Should they adopt? Or should they just keep trying year after year?

What such a couple should not be told is, "Go home and relax," as if infertility is their fault because they are too uptight. As their doctor, I tend to place the responsibility for failing to pinpoint the cause of infertility on myself. I know that there obviously is a reason the couple haven't had a baby but that medical diagnostic testing is as yet unable to solve the mystery.

I want as few of my patients as possible to end up in this category. Although doctors can treat these patients empirically, when treatment is not based on a specific diagnosis the results often are disappointing. In fact, if, after exhaustive testing by an infertility expert, the cause of infertility remains unknown, the prognosis for pregnancy by conventional means is poor. Happily, some couples have surprised me, but if the diagnosis is indeed "cause unknown," the chances of getting pregnant are extremely low.

When a couple with unexplained infertility are referred to me, I begin by doing a detailed review of every step of their previous medical workup. I think that they deserve a thorough investigation, leaving no stone unturned. When reviewing the results of earlier tests, the doctor has to keep in mind that the factors influencing fertility change over time: sperm counts fluctuate; tiny spots of endometriosis often grow; women with normally regular menstrual cycles can quit ovulating regularly because of the stress of infertility.

With state-of-the-art tests and tireless effort, we have been able to reduce the number of our patients with unexplained infertility to between 3 and 5 percent. The laparoscope, though an invasive procedure, is the most informative diagnostic test. If a laparoscopy hasn't been performed (and sometimes even if it has), I often find a plausible cause of infertility when I look directly at the pelvic organs through the 'scope. Endometriosis, for instance, can be underdiagnosed by doctors inexperienced in treating infertility. The appearance of the disease varies tremendously during the menstrual cycle. In fact, I'd estimate that endometriosis has twenty to thirty different faces. Thinking that the amount of misplaced endometrial tissue looks insignificant, physicians sometimes ignore the disease. The same is true of adhesions. This is unfortunate because either could be the unknown cause of infertility, and both often can be treated with laser laparoscopy.

Once a patient who has had an infertility workup is told that she and her husband are normal, it is difficult for a new doctor to establish rapport with them. Repeating a diagnostic procedure performed by a previous physician can be extremely upsetting to a patient. Hence it is important for her to know exactly why redoing a particular test is necessary. If she and her husband are to make educated choices about their treatment, they need to understand precisely how further investigation might help them.

Drs. Edward E. Wallach and Kamran S. Moghissi provide an excellent analysis of the diagnosis of unexplained infertility in their book for doctors entitled *Progress in Infertility*. These experts say, "The adequacy of an evaluation varies considerably among different centers and depends to a large extent on the competence and expertise of the physicians, availability of clinical and laboratory facilities, and perseverance of the patients in completing an extensive evaluation. The more exhaustive the evaluation of the infertile couple, the greater the probability of uncovering etiologic factor(s) [the causes] responsible for the couple's inability to achieve pregnancy."

Further Diagnosis

The Egg in Its Follicle

In some women with unexplained infertility, the maturing egg isn't released from its follicle at ovulation. Called "luteinized unruptured follicle" (LUF), this problem can be diagnosed with serial ultrasound scanning of the ovaries. In these women, a cystic follicle still appears on the ultrasound screen after the upward shift in the BBT. Patients with this condition often have abnormal eggs. Although LUF should be discovered during the regular infertility workup, it is possible that the diagnosis could be missed. IVF may help some of these women. As described in detail in chapter 9, the eggs can be aspirated via a hollow needle that is passed through the vaginal wall. By examining the eggs in the "test-tube," doctors can determine if they are fertilizing.

A few patients with unexplained infertility may have an undetected luteal-phase defect, although this usually is diagnosed during the original workup. This problem should be suspected when the ovulation or temperature chart is abnormal. It is possible, however, to miss an inadequate luteal phase and the resulting insufficient progesterone. Malfunction of the corpus luteum following ovulation is not an all-or-nothing situation. During some cycles, the corpus luteum may produce enough progesterone to prepare the uterine lining for pregnancy, whereas during other months hormone production may be erratic. Repeating the tests for progesterone twice during the original workup usually picks up this problem. But what if, for instance, the patient happens to have a luteal-phase defect seven months a year—but during the test cycles the luteal phase is adequate? In such a case, her blood test for progesterone and her endometrial biopsy would appear normal even though pregnancy was unlikely in over half of her cycles. Generally this shows up on the BBT ovulation chart—but not always.

It is possible for the corpus luteum to secrete enough progesterone to make the temperature chart appear normal, yet not enough to allow pregnancy. In other words, insufficient progesterone can be produced even though the length of the luteal phase on the temperature chart appears normal. If a dated blood test for progesterone and an endometrial biopsy are not performed, this type of luteal-phase problem might remain undetected.

Incorrect dating of the endometrial biopsy may cause inaccurate test results. You will recall that this study is used to determine if the uterine lining is at the proper stage of development around the time the pre-embryo normally would implant. Although the endometrial biopsy is a simple test, it can be poorly done and inaccurately interpreted. Either the doctor or a specially trained pathologist should examine the slide. Since the endometrium changes throughout the menstrual cycle, the doctor must date the sample correctly. To do this, we calculate the day of the cycle by counting forward from the first day of the current period and then backward from the start of the next period.

Sometimes follicles fail to ripen properly because the pituitary hormones that stimulate the ovaries into production are off balance. The follicular phase of the menstrual cycle, before ovulation, may be slightly too long, and the following luteal phase a little too short. Some patients conceive on fertility drugs such as clomiphene citrate (Clomid or Serophene) or human menopausal gonadotropin (Pergonal). But if there is indeed an abnormality in the follicle, clomiphene won't help. When a patient has a luteal-phase defect, we treat it with progesterone suppositories. Some medical centers prefer to use synthetic GnRH (gonadotropin-releasing hormone).

The Fallopian Tubes

Sometimes the cause of unexplained infertility lies with the fallopian tubes (oviducts). You will recall that each fallopian tube resembles a flexible pencil-sized arm with a little fernlike fimbriated end that looks like a horn of plenty. The other end of each tube is attached to the uterus. A muscular organ that can move around the pelvis, an oviduct in search of an egg can completely cover the ovary or sweep the cul-de-sac. Even though both tubes appear normal on the HSG X-ray, they still might have subtle abnormalities in shape or secretory function that prevent the egg and sperm from meeting. Sometimes the egg is fertilized but fails to travel through the tube to the uterus. The hairlike cilia that line the inside of the oviducts may be inadequate to propel the fertilized egg toward its goal. Unless the pre-embryo dies because of poor tubal blood supply and is absorbed by the body, a fertilized egg stuck in an oviduct can become a dangerous ectopic pregnancy.

A low-grade pelvic infection can destroy the cilia, but this diagnosis sometimes is missed, especially if the patient has a chlamydial infection. And there are a few patients, with Kartagener's syndrome, who are born with no cilia in their bodies. Suffering from upper-respiratory problems, they also are unable to get pregnant, because they lack cilia to move the fertilized egg through the fallopian tubes. IVF might help some of these patients.

Undiagnosed tubal adhesions, especially those affecting the end of the tube near the ovary, may keep the fingerlike fimbriae from picking up the egg. These interlacing cobweblike adhesions can be difficult to see. Sometimes the only way we can detect such filmy adhesions is to try to pick up the tube. Unlike adhesions inside the oviducts, weblike scar tissue on the outside of the oviducts is easily repaired through the 'scope with microsurgery.

The Endometrium

A patient with unexplained infertility might have chronic undiagnosed endometritis, an inflammation of the endometrium or uterine lining. Since the uterus cleans itself by sloughing the endometrium at menstruation, chronic endometritis is rare. Nevertheless, this problem, which usually is detected with an endometrial biopsy, should be considered in women who have used an IUD (intrauterine device), especially if they have had multiple sexual partners. Such patients are more prone to pelvic inflammatory disease (PID), an inflammation of the upper reproductive tract involving the uterus, the fallopian tubes, and the ovaries. An infection such as chlamydia, which can be chronic as well as acute, can travel up the wick of an IUD to the reproductive organs with few warning symptoms. Besides destroying the oviducts, infections also can lead to chronic low-grade endometritis. If undiagnosed, an inflammation of the endometrium can prevent the fertilized egg from implanting. Even if the egg does manage to implant, the woman often miscarries. (For further information on PID, see chapter 3.)

Mycoplasma infections also might be the cause of some cases of unexplained infertility, although the relationship is tenuous. Certainly the doctor must look for these infections in patients with infertility of unknown etiology and, if such organisms are found, treat with doxycycline.

The big unknown in infertility is the role of viral infections. There may be some PIDs that still remain undescribed. It is possible that an undiagnosed viral infection of the uterine lining could lead to unexplained infertility by causing a woman to abort before she even knows that she is pregnant.

At laparoscopy, doctors sometimes find small blebs, or blisters, that look inflamed, but biopsy proves that they aren't endometriosis. Even though the usual diagnostic cultures for infections are negative, it is our feeling that these patients might have one of the prevalent sexually transmitted viral infections. Those that can be specifically diagnosed, such as the papilloma virus, can be eradicated with the laser. Others may be undiagnosed genital herpes infections that can be treated with oral acyclovir.

The Cervix

The cervix, or mouth of the womb, can be the cause of unexplained infertility if the cervical mucus keeps the sperm from entering the uterus. Part of the job of the amazing cervical mucus filter is to weed out faulty sperm. Sperm with abnormally shaped heads, for example, are detoured into the cervical crypts and are absorbed by the body.

By bypassing the cervix, intrauterine insemination, especially when combined with fertility drugs, sometimes helps patients with cervical mucus problems if their oviducts are open. "Test-tube" fertilization, which bypasses not only the cervix but also the fallopian tubes, may help women with undetected abnormalities of the oviducts, abnormal cervical mucus, or both.

Faulty Sperm

The sperm often are the "unexplained cause" of infertility. In the normal male, sperm concentration (count or density), motility (swimming ability), and morphology (shape) vary considerably over time. For this reason, the semen analysis must be repeated several times. In addition, some of the newer methods of evaluating semen, such as computer-assisted videomicrography, may detect subtle differences in sperm movements not picked up by ordinary tests (see chapter 5).

If the husband's semen analysis shows over 30 to 40 percent abnormally formed sperm, he is less likely to initiate a pregnancy; remember that poorly shaped sperm are weak swimmers. But analysis of sperm shape is subjective. Thus it is possible for results to vary among laboratories.

It is important for the laboratory to study the shieldlike acrosome that covers the sperm head. The acrosome contains an enzyme that is thought to be necessary for penetration of the gelatinlike membrane that surrounds the egg. Known as the zona pellucida, this membrane prevents cross-species fertilization and keeps more than one sperm from entering an egg. Men with normally shaped sperm appear to have a higher level of the sperm-penetrating enzyme acrosin than those with poor sperm morphology. The poorly shaped sperm may lack the acrosome cap and thus the acrosin needed to pass through the egg's membrane.

The hamster egg–sperm penetration assay (SPA) is used to discover if the sperm can fertilize an egg. A hamster egg stripped of its species-specific zona pellucida is used for this test. The results often correlate with the sperm's ability to penetrate a human egg, but we have learned from *in-vitro* fertilization that some sperm incapable of fertilizing a hamster egg can penetrate a human egg when placed right next to it in a petri dish. A study by Marilyn L. Poland and colleagues published in 1985 in *Fertility and Sterility* showed that about 20 percent of men with sperm incapable of penetrating a hamster egg *can* fertilize a human egg. Considering this, *in-vitro* fertilization should *not* be ruled out for men with a poor hamster test.

Even though the husband's semen analysis indicates an adequate concentration of a high percentage of perfectly shaped, straight-swimming sperm, they still may be unable to penetrate the cervical mucus filter. Doctors suspect that, even though sperm may appear normal on some tests, the sperm actually may lack sufficient forward-propelling force to penetrate the cervical mucus or the egg.

Will ART Help?

After unsuccessfully attempting pregnancy for years, some couples with unexplained infertility may wish to try the new assisted reproductive technologies such as superovulation with fertility drugs combined with intrauterine insemination (IUI) or *in-vitro* fertilization (IVF), which are explored fully in chapter 9. Since these procedures can be stressful, patients should be carefully monitored by their doctor. Many couples with unexplained infertility have fertilization problems. During the *in vitro* process, physicians sometimes can pinpoint an undiagnosed cause of infertility, such as faulty eggs or sperm which are incapable of initiating a pregnancy. By mixing the sperm with the human egg in a laboratory dish during IVF, doctors can tell if the sperm are capable of penetrating the zona pellucida surrounding the egg. If they aren't, the couple may wish to consider intracytoplasmic sperm injection (ICSI). You will recall from chapter 6 that during this new procedure a sperm is injected directly into the egg.

Furthermore, a combination of GIFT and IVF called ZIFT (an acronym for "zygote intrafallopian transfer") also may help selected couples with unexplained infertility, especially those with immunologic infertility. Such couples appear to have trouble conceiving because the sperm are attacked either by the male's immune system while in his reproductive tract or by the woman's immune system while in the cervix, uterus, and oviducts. During the ZIFT process, the results of conception, the pre-embryos (instead of eggs and sperm) are placed in the fallopian tubes via the laparoscope. Once again, in cases in which the sperm cannot penetrate the eggs, intracytoplasmic sperm injection can be added to the ZIFT procedure. (See chapter 9 for further details about ZIFT.)

Depending on the couple's stress level, I sometimes suggest that my patients with unexplained infertility take a break from trying to have a baby. Although this approach may not be based on scientific evidence, I have noticed over the years that, when couples refocus their lives away from the constant push to conceive, the woman sometimes becomes pregnant. This doesn't mean that infertility is their fault because they are too tense but, rather, that the medical workup itself is stressful.

Repeated Spontaneous Abortion

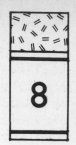

8

Two years after the surgical repair of my fallopian tubes, my pregnancy test finally was positive. At last Mark and I were going to have our first baby—or so we thought.

In retrospect, the eight weeks that followed seem like a long-awaited dream turned into a nightmare. On hearing the exciting news, my husband instantly phoned both sets of soon-to-be grandparents, his brother, and my sister. The whole family had been praying for us, and even our little nieces and nephews were overjoyed; everyone knew that infertility had run our lives for seven frustrating years.

Two months passed. Not dreaming that anything could go wrong, Mark and I decided to share our good fortune with four of our dearest friends over dinner. Right before dessert, my husband proudly announced that we were going to have a baby in April. Mark's best friend immediately ordered champagne, and everyone except me—I, of course, dared not drink— toasted the happy news. Soon thereafter I told Mark that I was exhausted and wanted to go home.

At 3:00 A.M. I was awakened by a cramping pain in my abdomen. Half asleep, I felt as if I might be starting my period. The thought made me open my eyes with a start. Stunned, I lay frozen in my bed, afraid to move.

Then I remembered that my mother had spotted throughout four successful pregnancies. Perhaps, I reassured myself, I had just stayed out too late. I would get out of bed, go to the bathroom, and see what was happening.

As I inched my way off the mattress, the cramping became a churning dagger in my side. I could not believe what I saw! Blood was gushing from my body. Helplessly I struggled to stop the red current, but I had no control. Fear now shook me to the bone. With my life crumbling under me, I called out to my husband.

He instantly jumped up, threw on the light, and frantically dialed my doctor. As I stared at the tissue coming from my womb, my mind refused to accept the loss that my body already had detected and was automatically expelling. Our cherished baby—that tiny spark of life that briefly flickered within me—was no more. Drained of all hope, I ached with a desperate emptiness beyond endurance. "Dear God!" I cried. "Can I do nothing right? What terrible deed have I done to deserve this? Have the past seven years not paid for my mistakes? Why have You sent us this gift of love— the answer to our unending prayers—only to reclaim it? Why have You taken my baby away?"

—Alice

Many people fail to realize how traumatic pregnancy loss can be for a family. They think that since the woman will soon be pregnant again, miscarriage (pregnancy loss before viability) is only a minor event. Friends and relatives often offer condolences, saying that spontaneous abortion (the medical term for miscarriage) is just nature's way of rejecting a deformed baby. Although nearly half of all miscarriages are caused by genetic abnormalities in the baby, those statistics usually fail to ease the woman's grief over her loss. An ordeal for any woman, for patients like Alice—who doubt their ability to get pregnant ever again— losing a confirmed pregnancy can be devastating.

Alice felt that her miscarriage was not merely a fatal mistake of nature but, rather, the loss of a tiny life that had burrowed its way into her heart. She feared that if she ever did get pregnant again she would lose that baby also. When I saw Alice several weeks after her miscarriage, she said: "After my daddy died, I felt as though I had a hole in my heart, but I could at least talk about my grief. But now I hurt so much that I don't want to talk with anyone—not even my husband."

It wasn't good for Alice to keep her emotions bottled up inside her. She needed to talk about her feelings. This is when the doctor can spend a little time and listen to the patient. Sometimes a caring friend also can help, if she knows how to listen and what to say. Occasionally professional counseling is necessary.

When a patient starts talking about the negatives of her miscarriage, the doctor can help her see the positives. I reminded Alice that, to get pregnant, her reproductive system had to have worked reasonably well.

Many unknowns had been eliminated. She obviously had ovulated, the egg had been fertilized, and the embryo had attached to the lining of the uterus. It is well known in animals that pregnancy makes pregnancy. Although this remains unproved in humans, it is thought that once a woman conceives it is easier for her to become pregnant a second time— that is, unless the loss becomes such an emotional ordeal that her hormones are affected.

Traditionally, habitual abortion is defined as three consecutive pregnancy losses. The implication of this definition is that the first two miscarriages are nonrecurring events and probably don't need further investigation. But, as with everything else in medicine, the way miscarriage is handled depends to a great extent on the individual patient. Not only is the woman's attitude toward the loss important, but also her age, her fertility history, and her physical examination. If a patient conceives easily or already has one child, her first miscarriage, although an unhappy event, usually doesn't affect her as much as it did Alice. This is particularly true if the loss occurred during the first six weeks of pregnancy. If a woman's general health, her hormones, and her pelvic examination appear normal, there is nothing wrong with letting her try again. But once she loses a second pregnancy, she will worry that something is seriously wrong and that she might miscarry a third time. Such a patient deserves a thorough investigation to try to discover the reason for the spontaneous abortions.

If the patient has a long history of infertility, the doctor should do everything possible to discover why she miscarried. Alice desperately wanted me to find out why she had been unable to carry her long-awaited pregnancy to term. Unfortunately, some doctors in the country won't do studies on a patient who has miscarried just once unless there is something obviously wrong, such as endometriosis.

Doctors subscribing to this school of thought do little or nothing to discover the reason for the first and often the second spontaneous abortion. These doctors take the fatalistic attitude that the reason their patients are losing babies is probably a genetic problem with the fetus. The assumption is that miscarriage is just nature's way of getting rid of a genetic mistake—and that nothing can be done about it. Sometimes this is true, and sometimes it is not!

No one would argue that over half of early spontaneous abortions do occur because the fetus isn't forming properly, often because of a genetic defect. But what about the other half of the babies, who are normal? Some of these babies might be saved. Should the doctor allow his patient to keep losing babies without looking for an explanation until she reaches the "approved" definition of repeated spontaneous abortion?

I think not! One hundred percent of patients deserve studies because 30 to 50 percent might be helped. I think doctors should worry about the miscarriages they might have prevented but didn't.

Obviously the management of patients who miscarry is controversial. Physicians with a "conservative" mind-set tell patients who have aborted to "just keep on trying," in hopes that statistics will work in their favor. These doctors don't consider one or two miscarriages to be an indication of a hormonal or physical problem. For this reason, they fail to look for other causes until their patients have lost three babies. If a woman is miscarrying because the fetus is abnormal, it is true that she sooner or later may succeed in carrying a healthy baby to term. Unfortunately, not all patients are so "lucky." Some infertility patients never conceive again. Others get pregnant but keep losing babies.

For Alice, it would have been wrong to hesitate to offer diagnosis and treatment when subsequent miscarriages might be prevented. Although unnecessary tests must be avoided, the patient can suffer if the physician is too conservative. The doctor has to decide whether the information gained from a diagnostic test is worth the cost. Tests are expensive and sometimes stressful for the patient—but so are miscarriages.

When pregnancy loss isn't associated with a defective embryo, subsequent miscarriages sometimes can be prevented if a probable cause can be diagnosed and properly treated. Although chromosomal abnormalities are the only *proven* cause of miscarriage, doctors see many other problems associated with recurrent fetal loss. We think that as many as a third to a half of all spontaneous abortions may be related to problems such as endometriosis, adenomyosis, hormonal imbalances (primarily luteal-phase defects), malformations of the uterus, infections, immune-system abnormalities, or an incompetent (weak) cervix. Although after one or two miscarriages a high percentage of patients eventually deliver, a higher percentage carry to term if a specific cause can be found and treated.

Genetic Abnormalities

Of clinically confirmed pregnancies, at least 10 to 15 percent end in miscarriage. Many more go unnoticed by the woman, the only clue being a heavy period that is one or two days late. The rate of spontaneous abortion increases with maternal age to 23 percent at age thirty to thirty-four, and 48 percent at age thirty-five to thirty-nine. With each ensuing natural abortion, the chances of a future pregnancy loss increase significantly. After three miscarriages, the risk of losing another fetus approaches 75 percent.

Studies show that about half of early spontaneous abortions are associated with chromosomal abnormalities of the embryo. Found in the nucleus of every human cell, the chromosomes carry the genes of inheritance contributed by both parents. Such traits as eye color, hair color, and height are known to be determined by messages encoded in our genes. According to the Genome Database, of the 100,000-odd genes in the human body, scientists have identified only 5,236.

In the complicated process of creating a human baby, genetic errors can occur. As the genetic code is transferred to the embryo, a chromosomal defect can arise that is so severe the fetus eventually dies and is expelled by the body. Sometimes the embryonic cells simply fail to divide correctly. Not all errors in the genetic blueprint are lethal. Babies can be born with chromosomal abnormalities that cause sterility, physical handicaps, mental retardation, or premature death. Down's syndrome or mongolism, characterized by mental retardation, is a tragic example of a genetic error in which an extra chromosome number 21 appears in the cells of the body.

The best diagnostic tool is the fetus itself. Since Alice's husband had the presence of mind to bring the aborted tissue with them to the hospital the night of her miscarriage, the laboratory was able to look for genetic abnormalities. No major chromosomal defects were found, so other causes had to be considered. If the laboratory report *had* indicated an abnormal genetic picture, that would have been assumed to be the cause of the miscarriage.

Occasionally the genetic problem lies with the parents, although the incidence is low compared with the number of aborted fetuses that have genetic defects. To check for this problem for Alice and Mark, we examined the chromosomes in their white blood cells under a microscope. Known as "karyotyping," this test studies the chromosomal makeup of a cell as it divides. Alice's and Mark's test results were negative. Had the genetic blueprints of either parent been abnormal, I would have recommended genetic counseling.

When a couple has a genetic problem, they want to know if their next baby will be healthy. The dilemma is: What do you tell them? The geneticists cannot totally predict. With some couples, the experts can foretell that the odds are against their having a normal baby. In such cases, patients may wish to consider *in-vitro* fertilization and pre-implantation genetic testing of the fertilized egg (see chapter 9). In other cases, the statistics are in the couple's favor. Often the genetic defect is a nonrecurring event.

One theory is that some genetic abnormalities may be caused by the environment inside of the uterus. If the baby fails to get the proper food supply from the lining of the uterus, embryonic cell division may go awry. If, for example, the woman has an abnormal luteal phase, inadequate progesterone may be produced. When this happens, the endometrium—which provides the sustenance for the early embryo—will be inadequate. It makes sense, although we can't prove it, that if the environment can be improved, some of the genetic problems may be avoided.

Amniocentesis

Many genetic defects can now be diagnosed before birth with amniocentesis, a minor procedure in which a small amount of the fluid surrounding the fetus is removed and the cells are analyzed (see fig. 8.1). Doctors suggest this test for patients with a family medical history that puts the baby at increased risk of severe abnormalities. Pregnant women thirty-three years of age or older also may wish to consider prenatal diagnosis because the incidence of Down's syndrome increases significantly over this age (see table 8.1).

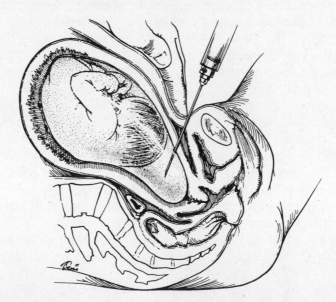

FIGURE 8.1. *Amniocentesis late in pregnancy. (Reproduced, with permission, from J. A. Pritchard, P. C. MacDonald, and N. F. Gant, Williams Obstetrics, 17th ed., copyright © Appleton-Century-Crofts, 1985.)*

In addition to chromosomal abnormalities such as Down's syndrome, amniocentesis can also detect rubella, hemophilia, sickle-cell anemia, Tay-Sachs disease, neural-tube defects such as spina bifida, and some metabolic disorders such as an inherited tendency toward excess serum cholesterol. Although this procedure diagnoses many additional problems, hundreds of birth defects still cannot be pinpointed before birth.

In highly skilled hands, amniocentesis is a relatively safe, minor procedure that doesn't appear to increase the risk of fetal loss significantly. The test has helped several hundred thousand women learn more about their pregnancies. Experts in prenatal diagnosis at Baylor's Kleberg Prenatal Genetics Center say: "For standard amniocentesis, the most common complications are vaginal spotting or bleeding, severe cramping, or miscarriage. Infection occurs in less than 1 in 1,000 cases.

TABLE 8.1. FREQUENCY OF DOWN'S SYNDROME AS RELATED TO MATERNAL AGE*

Maternal Age	Frequency of Down's Syndrome Infants among Births
30	1/885
31	1/826
32	1/725
33	1/592
34	1/465
35	1/365
36	1/287
37	1/225
38	1/176
39	1/139
40	1/109
41	1/85
42	1/67
43	1/53
44	1/41
45	1/32
46	1/25
47	1/20
48	1/16
49	1/12

*From Lindsjo Hook, *American Journal of Human Genetics*, vol. 30, no. 19, 1978.

The risk for complications with the procedure is one-half percent above the natural complication rate for this period in pregnancy."

Standard amniocentesis is performed between the fifteenth and eighteenth weeks after the last menstrual period. Early amniocentesis is done between the twelfth and fifteenth weeks. The risks of the latter, newer procedure still are being evaluated. An ultrasound scan shows the exact location of the baby in the womb. Watching the baby's movements on the TV-like screen, the doctor carefully inserts a thin, hollow needle through the mother's abdomen into the uterus. A small amount of the clear amniotic fluid that surrounds and cushions the baby in its amniotic sac is extracted for analysis. Although this sounds painful and can be upsetting, one patient described it as "not much worse than having blood drawn."

Floating in the amniotic fluid are fetal cells such as skin cells. These cells are tissue-cultured and examined to detect genetic abnormalities and other defects. The results are available in two to three weeks. The chromosome analysis is over 99 percent accurate, and the test for neural tube defects is greater than 90 percent accurate. If the fetus is found to have a severe congenital defect, the pregnancy can be terminated.

The problem with standard amniocentesis is that, by the time the test results are completed, the fetus is eighteen to twenty-one weeks old. If the baby is found to be severely abnormal, the couple has to decide whether to have a therapeutic abortion or to raise a handicapped child. Although I don't have to make this decision or terminate the pregnancy, I have lived through the nightmare with many of my patients. By this time, the mother has felt the quickening of the baby and must go through the labor-and-delivery process to end the pregnancy. This is an emotionally traumatic experience for everyone in the family, from the grandparents to the other siblings.

Some patients who, for religious or moral reasons, would not have a therapeutic abortion still choose to have amniocentesis. If the results indicate that the baby is severely abnormal, this procedure gives the parents time to prepare to care for a handicapped infant.

Although amniocentesis cannot guarantee that the baby will be without genetic abnormalities, prenatal testing can pinpoint many problems that are of concern to families in high-risk categories. Often, to the relief of everyone, no fetal abnormality is discovered.

Chorionic-Villus Sampling

Some of the larger medical centers such as the Baylor College of Medicine offer an innovative prenatal genetic screening test called chorionic-villus sampling (CVS). Since 1982, thousands of these tests have been performed throughout the world. Women thirty-three years of age or older, or couples at risk of having a child with a chromosome abnormality or genetic disease may wish to consider CVS. Although Down's syndrome and disorders such as hemophilia or sickle-cell anemia can be diagnosed, not all abnormalities can be detected prenatally with CVS. Neural-tube defects such as spina bifida cannot be diagnosed. Fortunately, a special blood test called the "Maternal Serum AFP test" is available that is over 80 percent accurate in screening neural-tube defects.

The advantage of chorionic-villus sampling over amniocentesis is that CVS is performed earlier in pregnancy than is amniocentesis, usually between the tenth and twelfth weeks, rather than between the fifteenth and eighteenth weeks. Results following CVS are available in about two weeks, although some special studies may take longer. If the fetus is found to have a serious genetic defect and the parents feel incapable of caring for a child with a severe handicap, CVS often gives them the option of choosing a first trimester abortion.

In CVS, a sample of the chorionic villi (the fingerlike projections of the outermost fetal membrane) is harvested and the cells are analyzed (see fig. 8.2). After the position of the baby in the womb is located with ultrasound, a thin, hollow needle is passed either through the vagina and cervix or through the abdomen. A small amount of chorionic tissue is aspirated through the needle into a syringe. These cells, which develop from the fertilized egg, have the same genetic makeup as the fetus. Although CVS sounds painful, most of my patients report that the procedure is only slightly uncomfortable.

Of utmost importance is the safety of the mother and the fetus. In the past, the rate of fetal loss following chorionic-villus sampling ran as high as 5 to 10 percent. Consequently doctors used to suggest this test only if the fetus was at great risk of a genetic defect. Although CVS is still a relatively new technique, today, in highly skilled hands, the risk of miscarriage has been sharply reduced to about one-half to 1 percent.

Unfortunately, there have been reports of an increase in limb abnormalities in babies whose mothers have had a CVS procedure. Say experts at Baylor's Kleberg Center: "Although it is uncertain whether there is an increased risk of limb abnormalities following CVS, we believe it is important for our patients to understand that the absolute risk may

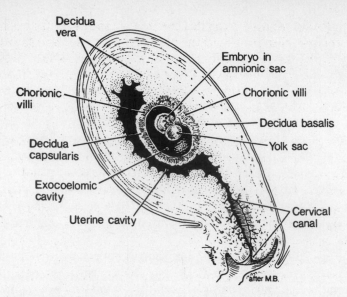

Decidua
vera

Embryo in
amnionic sac

Chorionic
villi

Chorionic villi

Decidua basalis

Decidua
capsularis

Yolk sac

Exocoelomic
cavity

Uterine cavity

Cervical
canal

after M.B.

FIGURE 8.2. Early pregnancy. Note the chorionic villi. (Reproduced, with permission, from J. A. Pritchard, P. C. MacDonald, and N. F. Gant, Williams Obstetrics, 17th ed., copyright © Appleton-Century-Crofts, 1985.)

be in the order of one in three thousand births." The expertise of the operator is vital.

The Role of Endometriosis and Adenomyosis

Forty-three percent of patients diagnosed as having endometriosis also have had a miscarriage. The incidence of spontaneous abortion among other infertile women is approximately 13 percent. One study found that conservative surgery for endometriosis reduced the abortion rate to 20 percent. Although doctors cannot prove that endometriosis causes abortion, our experience is that, if we treat this disease, a higher percentage of patients carry their babies to term.

Exactly how endometriosis causes miscarriage is not known. Doctors think, however, that it is related to hormonal imbalances (primarily luteal-phase defects) and to the prostaglandin activity often associated with endometriosis. You will recall that the prostaglandins are fatty acids that cause smooth muscles such as the uterus to contract. Patients with mild endometriosis have a higher incidence of miscarriage than those with severe cases, partly because women with severe untreated endometriosis seldom get pregnant. In addition, as the disease progresses, the endometrial cells burn out and produce smaller amounts of prostaglandins.

Patients hear that pregnancy helps women with endometriosis. This is only true, however, after a woman has carried a baby to term—after she has been exposed to placental progesterone over a long period of time. During the first two or three months of pregnancy, endometriosis often gets worse. The increased estrogen stimulation of pregnancy can cause the nodules of endometriosis to grow, making the uterus irritable. Before such a patient miscarries, she may experience cramping and bleeding, but sometimes she has no warning at all.

A condition related to endometriosis called "adenomyosis," which we discussed earlier, is also associated with spontaneous abortion. Formerly referred to as "internal endometriosis," adenomyosis occurs when some of the glands and cells of the endometrium are found *within* the muscle *wall* of the uterus (see fig. 2.20). This condition, which probably is more common than once thought, can make the womb irritable.

Although adenomyosis often can be treated successfully before pregnancy with a GnRH agonist (this drug is discussed in detail in chapter 2), the disease is extremely difficult to diagnose, even with an X-ray followed by a laparoscopy. Sometimes doctors have trouble deciding whether a patient has adenomyosis or benign fibroid tumors. Both make the uterus look knotty. The clues pointing to adenomyosis are a relatively large, tender, knotty uterus with symptoms of extremely heavy menses and clotting, cramping, backache, and bleeding between periods. Often a patient is laparoscoped because she has symptoms of endometriosis. But when the doctor looks at the pelvis, the endometriosis is mild. The cause of the symptoms and of some miscarriages is the adenomyosis inside the uterine wall.

Hormonal Causes: Luteal-Phase Defects

Doctors think that luteal-phase defects are a common hormonal cause of spontaneous abortion. If the corpus luteum, which forms in the ovary after ovulation, produces an inadequate amount of the female sex hormone progesterone, the patient is said to have a luteal-phase defect. As you now know, without sufficient progesterone at the proper time in the menstrual cycle, the uterine lining will be underdeveloped and the fertilized egg cannot implant itself.

Sometimes the developing embryo implants itself in the endometrium, and the corpus luteum suddenly stops making enough progesterone. Since during approximately the first eight weeks of pregnancy the embryo is dependent upon the corpus luteum for this hormone, its function is vital. When the corpus luteum fails early in pregnancy, the uterine lining will degenerate, and miscarriage will follow. Robbed of its crucial food supply, the embryo will die. A few days later, it will be expelled from the body. After about the first two months of pregnancy, the placenta takes over progesterone production. A crucial point, this is when some pregnancies are lost. After about the third or fourth month, the doctor looks for other causes of pregnancy loss, such as enlarging fibroids and worsening endometriosis. (See chapter 2 for further information on the diagnosis of luteal-phase defects.)

Doctors think that luteal-phase problems are associated with endometriosis and with aberrations in the secretion of the pituitary sex hormones FSH and sometimes LH, which stimulate the ovaries into action. When these hormones are out of balance, the ovaries malfunction. The problem also may lie with the cells that make up the follicle. Ovulatory stimulants such as Clomid and Pergonal sometimes help. Once the woman conceives, progesterone suppositories are given.

Malformations of the Uterus

Congenital

THE UNICORNUATE UTERUS

Some women are born with uterine anomalies. This simply means that the womb is misshapen in one of a variety of ways (see fig. 8.3). Although many women with a malformed uterus carry babies to term, some have recurrent pregnancy loss. In fact, a uterine anomaly is found in 10 to 15 percent of women who have repeated miscarriages. Unlike the normal pear-shaped uterus that stretches as the baby grows, a misshapen womb often cannot accommodate a developing fetus or provide it with adequate nutrients.

Some women who have uterine anomalies are born with a "half-uterus." Since it looks rather like a unicorn, or as if it has a single horn,

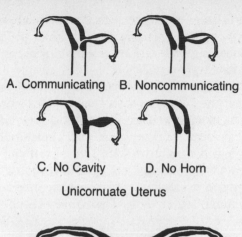

A. Communicating   B. Noncommunicating

C. No Cavity   D. No Horn

Unicornuate Uterus

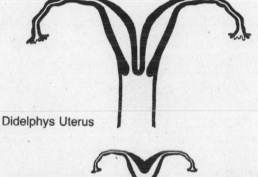

Didelphys Uterus

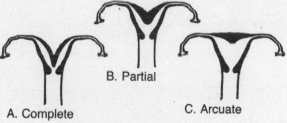

B. Partial

A. Complete   C. Arcuate

Bicornuate Uterus

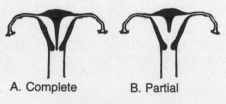

A. Complete   B. Partial

Septate Uterus

FIGURE 8.3. *Uterine anomalies. (From V. C. Buttram,* Surgical Treatment of the Infertile Female, *Baltimore: Williams & Wilkins Co., 1985.)*

this malformation is called a "unicornuate uterus." It is diagnosed with an HSG X-ray (hysterosalpingogram). These patients usually don't have much trouble conceiving and seldom require major uterine surgery. Some, however, have retrograde flow that is probably a function of a small cervical diameter. These patients can develop endometriosis. When this happens, they often do have trouble getting pregnant.

The major problem with the unicornuate uterus is that it is associated with an increased incidence of miscarriage and premature delivery. The cervix is smaller and generally weaker than normal and must not be traumatized. Many times gynecologists have to reinforce such a cervix with a purse-string suture called a "cervical cerclage," or a "stitch" such as the McDonald stitch (see fig. 8.4). This literally keeps the baby from

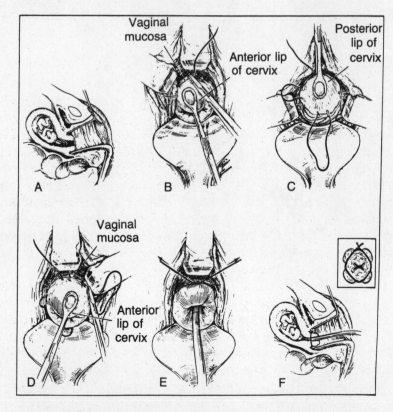

FIGURE 8.4. McDonald stitch for an incompetent cervix. (Reproduced, with permission, from J. A. Pritchard, P. C. MacDonald, and N. F. Gant, Williams Obstetrics, 17th ed., copyright © Appleton-Century-Crofts, 1985.)

falling out of the womb. Whether putting a stitch around an incompetent (weak) cervix is absolutely scientific or not, doctors feel that the procedure has saved many babies. (This obviously isn't an area that lends itself to scientific double-blind studies, in which some women receive a stitch while others do not, with neither the doctors nor the patients knowing who received treatment.)

Although management of these patients has to be highly individualized, in general they should avoid constipation, intercourse, and heavy exercise. They sometimes have to stay in bed, depending on the amount of uterine activity, dilation of the cervix, and bleeding. With care, I have had patients with a "half-uterus" deliver eight-pound babies.

Pregnant women with a unicornuate uterus have a higher than normal incidence of cesarean sections. They tend to have breech births, in which the baby's feet, not the head, are delivered first. Since the uterus is small, the baby cannot move around; once it gets in one position, it stays there.

THE SEPTATE UTERUS

Some women are born with another kind of anomaly, in which the uterus is either partially or completely divided by a wall known as a "septum" (see fig. 8.3). Called a "septate uterus," this malformation, which is the most common non-drug-related uterine anomaly, is associated with an 80-to-90-percent incidence of pregnancy loss. As with the unicornuate uterus, the septate uterus is diagnosed with an HSG X-ray. Fortunately, a septum is one problem that usually can be treated successfully, often with only minor surgery. Once the septum is removed, the incidence of spontaneous abortion approaches that among the general population. In one study, 88 percent of patients who conceived after removal of a septate uterus delivered a viable infant.

Like patients with a unicornuate uterus, women with a uterine septum have no difficulty conceiving if they are free of other reproductive disorders. Unfortunately, however, the septate uterus also is associated with an increased risk of endometriosis and adhesions, either of which can interfere with conception. It is my impression that patients with anomalies also have an increased incidence of ovulation problems.

How does a uterine septum cause pregnancy loss? Doctors suspect that the fertilized egg often implants itself on the septum. Since the septum has a poor blood supply and thus an inadequate endometrium, the embryo probably aborts because it is undernourished. These patients also tend to have decreased uterine capacity and a weakened cervix.

Since both are associated with premature delivery, careful monitoring is imperative during pregnancy.

If patients with a septate uterus do manage to carry a baby to term, they sometimes have complications during labor. Fragments of the placenta can be retained in the uterus instead of being expelled from the body. When this happens, a D&C (dilatation and curettage) is necessary to scrape the retained tissue from the womb.

In the past, a patient with a uterine septum often had the choice of continuing to miscarry or of having the septum removed during a major operation called "metroplasty." After one spontaneous abortion, doctors often suggested correcting the problem. Since the incidence of miscarriage is high with a septum, we hesitated to withhold treatment until a patient had lost three babies. The hope was that we could prevent further miscarriages.

Nowadays a patient with a thin uterine septum, and sometimes even with a thick one, can have it removed under general anesthesia without undergoing major abdominal surgery. An endoscopic instrument called a "hysteroscope" is inserted through the dilated opening of the cervix. A fiber-optic light bundle attached to the hysteroscope allows the doctor to look inside the uterine cavity at the septum. The surgeon can remove the dividing wall with miniature scissors or with a laser, either of which can be passed through the operating channel of the 'scope. Since the septum has a poor blood supply, blood loss is minimal. Other problems, such as adhesions inside the uterine cavity, some fibroid tumors (those on a pedicle or stalk), polyps, and scars, also can often be treated with the 'scope.

Although the septum usually can be removed with minor surgery through the 'scope, in rare cases, especially if the septum extends all the way to the cervix, a major abdominal operation may be necessary (see fig. 8.5). During this procedure, one incision is made in the abdomen and another in the uterus. The septum is then removed with the laser. About the only time I do metroplasty with the abdomen open is if I have to perform major surgery for other reasons, such as endometriosis or large fibroid tumors.

THE BICORNUATE UTERUS

Some patients are born with a womb that looks rather like a heart on the inside and often also on the outside (see fig. 8.3). Called a "bicornuate uterus," this anomaly is associated with an incidence of miscarriage that is approximately twice that of the general population,

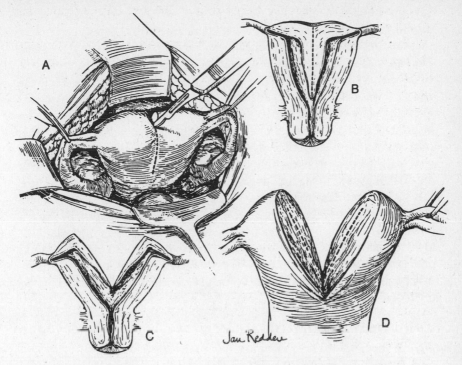

FIGURE 8.5. Major surgery to remove a uterine septum (dividing wall). (From V. C. Buttram, Surgical Treatment of the Infertile Female, Baltimore: Williams & Wilkins Co., 1985.)

or about 35 percent. Since the blood supply to the baby is usually better with this anomaly than with a septate uterus, patients with a bicornuate uterus have a lower rate of spontaneous abortion.

Patients with a bicornuate uterus, like women with the other anomalies just discussed, don't have difficulty conceiving if they are free of other reproductive disorders. Unfortunately, as we have seen, endometriosis is about three or four times more common in patients with anomalies than in patients with a normal uterus. Like the unicornuate uterus and the septate uterus, the bicornuate uterus also increases the incidence of complications during labor, especially the risk of retained placental fragments.

Before Dr. Veasy C. Buttram, Jr., classified uterine anomalies in the early 1970s, many patients with a uterine septum were diagnosed as having a bicornuate uterus. In fact, the septate uterus and the bicornuate uterus are still sometimes lumped together under the term "double uterus." Few doctors saw enough anomalies to know which patients needed repair. Although the HSG X-ray is the best tool for diagnosing a "double uterus," it wasn't until the advent of the laparoscope that doctors could make the distinction between the septate uterus and the bicornuate uterus without opening the abdomen.

Today we can not only diagnose a "double uterus" with an HSG X-ray, but we can also determine the classification with the laparoscope. Precise diagnosis is extremely important, because the septate and the bicornuate uterus are treated differently. Repair of the bicornuate uterus requires a major operation (see fig. 8.6). Since a high percentage of women with this problem can carry babies, I let these patients show me that they are going to have trouble before offering surgery. Once the patient has miscarried, she has shown that she is fertile, and her uterus is easier to repair because it has been stretched. After the uterus is cut, subsequent births must be delivered by cesarean section. Following unification of a bicornuate uterus, about 75 to 80 percent of the patients are able to have a baby. Even when uterine surgery is unnecessary, putting a stitch around the cervix may help the patient carry to term or near term.

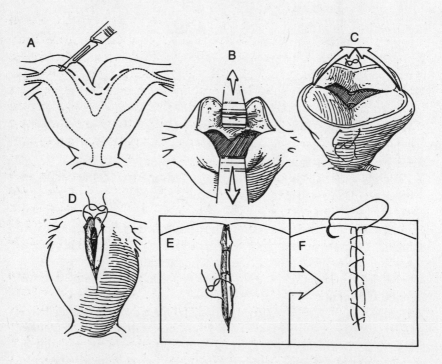

FIGURE 8.6. Unification of a bicornuate uterus. (From V. C. Buttram, Surgical Treatment of the Infertile Female, Baltimore: Williams & Wilkins Co., 1985.)

Acquired

ADHESIONS INSIDE THE UTERUS

Sometimes women form adhesions inside the uterus after a D&C, especially if it is performed immediately after delivery of a baby or after a therapeutic or spontaneous abortion. Other operations that carry a slight risk of postoperative adhesions within the uterus are metroplasty, to repair a malformed uterus, and myomectomy, to remove fibroids inside the uterine cavity. Called "Asherman's syndrome," adhesions within the cavity can cause infertility and spontaneous abortion.

Should a woman be afraid to have a D&C, especially after pregnancy? Perhaps! Sometimes a D&C is life-saving—there may be no other way to stop bleeding inside the uterus or to remove placental fragments. But, as with any other surgical procedure, a D&C should be performed only when absolutely indicated. If it has to be done, it should be performed as gently as possible. If vigorous scraping of the uterus is necessary to stop bleeding, the patient usually should be given hormones to rebuild the endometrium.

The way to diagnose Asherman's syndrome is first to suspect it. If a patient who has had uterine surgery ovulates but fails to menstruate, the first test the doctor does is an hCG pregnancy test. If the results are negative—two times in a row—progesterone is prescribed to make her have a period. If the woman doesn't have withdrawal bleeding after administration of progesterone, then estrogen followed by progesterone is given. If she still has no period, I do an HSG X-ray of the uterus and fallopian tubes. If necessary, I look inside the uterus with the hysteroscope.

Nobody knows why Asherman's causes spontaneous abortion. And nobody knows why intrauterine adhesions seem to be associated with infertility. Doctors think, however, that the condition limits the capacity of the uterus. I also feel that the adhesions reduce the amount of endometrium available to the growing fetus, thus decreasing its food supply.

Asherman's syndrome can be not only diagnosed but also treated through the cervix with the hysteroscope. After the adhesions are cut, an IUD or some other space-occupying material is inserted into the uterine cavity. Hormone therapy (estrogen and progesterone) is given to rebuild the endometrium. Following successful treatment in which all of the adhesions are removed, over 85 percent of patients are able to carry a baby to term. This figure approaches that among the general population.

FIBROIDS

Leiomyomas, which are often called "fibroids," are muscular tumors commonly found in the uterus (see fig. 8.7). Although they are benign—and often insignificant—they occasionally prevent conception; should pregnancy occur, they sometimes cause spontaneous abortion.

Hormonally dependent, some leiomyomas grow on the outside of the uterus, some within the uterine wall, and others within the cavity (see fig. 2.14). If fibroids block the entrances to both fallopian tubes inside the uterus, the sperm obviously cannot reach the egg. Not only does the fibroid take up precious space within the uterus, the endometrium

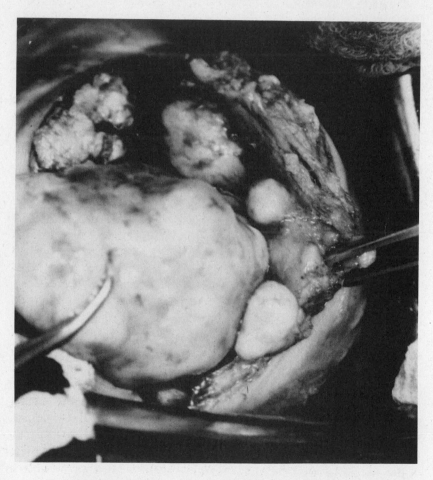

FIGURE 8.7. Photograph of the surgical removal of fibroid tumors in a twenty-six-year-old patient. She later carried a baby to term.

covering the fibroid is stretched and thus abnormal. If the embryo manages to implant itself over a fibroid, miscarriage is likely, because the food supply will be inadequate. In addition, the endometrium around the fibroid may be locally inflamed. This creates an unfriendly nesting place for the embryo. Large fibroids especially can cause the uterus to be so irritable that the fetus is expelled. Leiomyomas also appear to cause the veins of the uterus to empty poorly, so that the uterus becomes congested with blood. This makes the womb still more irritable, sometimes leading to abortion.

Even fibroid tumors that are small and insignificant before pregnancy can cause miscarriage or premature labor, because they often expand under the increased stimulation of estrogen and progesterone present during pregnancy. This was the cause of Alice's miscarriage. Two fibroids inside the uterine wall that were small before conception had grown large enough during her pregnancy to cause her to abort. Eighteen months after the fibroids were removed, she conceived again. This time Alice was able to carry her baby to term.

Pedunculated leiomyomas, those on a stalklike pedicle, are often successfully treated with the hysteroscope through the vagina. Unfortunately, this instrument cannot be used to remove all fibroids inside the uterus. In the case of some leiomyomas in the cavity, we just shave off the top, but the results aren't as good as when the whole fibroid is removed. Large fibroids and those that are in the uterine wall have to be removed surgically during a myomectomy, a major procedure.

It is sometimes difficult to decide whether a fibroid is going to cause trouble—many are insignificant. Doctors want to remove fibroids that appear to be causing infertility or miscarriage, but they must avoid performing unnecessary operations. Although the location and size of the fibroid are important, nobody knows exactly how to define a "significant" fibroid. We do know, however, that if leiomyomas are allowed to become too large the fertility rate drops after surgical removal. So, for best results, there is a critical time to do the myomectomy. This appears to be before the fibroid becomes larger than a ten-to-twelve-week pregnancy. It is more difficult to achieve good results after the muscle tumor approaches the size of an eighteen-to-twenty-week fetus.

Dr. Buttram has reported on the success of myomectomy in reducing miscarriage. He reviewed 1,941 cases of surgical removal of fibroids and reported that "spontaneous abortion was reduced from 41 percent preoperatively to 19 percent postmyomectomy, a figure approaching the 10 percent rate reported in the general population." In general, once a cut is made two-thirds through the uterus to remove a fibroid, delivery of a subsequent pregnancy requires a cesarean section.

Incompetent Cervix

Sometimes a woman miscarries during the second or early-third trimester of pregnancy because her cervix is too weak to support the increasing weight of her baby. This patient is said to have an "incompetent cervix." Without help, she may be unable to carry a baby to term. This condition can be congenital; sometimes it is associated with a "double uterus." In some cases, the cervix has been weakened by a previous trauma, such as a D&C. Unlike early spontaneous abortion, during which the body often expels the embryo because it has died, in late pregnancy loss the baby is aborted and then dies. Since the cervix is weak, it painlessly dilates, and the fetal membranes fall into the vagina. As the membranes rupture, the fetus dies because it is too immature to survive on its own.

Many patients with an incompetent cervix can carry a baby to term with the aid of cervical cerclage, a procedure whereby a purse-string stitch is put around the cervix to prevent it from dilating (to keep the cervix closed). Doctors use several cerclage techniques to support a pregnancy, the simplest of which is the McDonald suture (see fig. 8.4). This stitch may be removed near term so that the baby can be delivered vaginally. Patients with an extremely weak or scarred cervix may need a more permanent type of cerclage called the "Shirodkar procedure." This technique requires extensive resection of the cervix and should be done between pregnancies. Usually when I put in a Shirodkar stitch, I recommend a C-section. Every time this stitch is removed, more scar tissue forms, making the stitch difficult to replace.

The old school of medical thinking says that a woman should go through two and even three pregnancy losses before having cervical cerclage. In my opinion, this is outrageous. Once a woman has lost a baby because of cervical incompetence, she is likely to lose the next one the same way. The more trauma to the cervix from pregnancy loss or from any kind of manipulation, the weaker the cervix becomes. Doctors used to worry about securing a "blighted ovum," but ultrasound has rendered this possibility passé. Nowadays, we never secure a pregnancy that cannot be seen with ultrasound.

Any patient with a McDonald or Shirodkar stitch must be carefully watched. If signs of miscarriage develop after the cervical stitch is in place, the fetal tissue sometimes can be aspirated through the small opening left in the cervix. If the fetus is too large to be removed through the cervix, the stitch must be removed immediately. Although a patient may have minor contractions throughout the pregnancy, the forceful contractions of labor can amputate the cervix. The pressure of strong uterine contractions can cause the uterus or cervix to rupture, causing infection!

Infections

If a woman has an intrauterine infection, she may have difficulty getting pregnant, or, if she does conceive, she may abort. A host of infections are thought to be associated with pregnancy wastage. I see patients with streptococci, chlamydia, and mycoplasma infections who miscarry. Although the exact role of both of the latter is controversial, when I find an infection I treat it. The bacteria are not supposed to be there, and it seems illogical to refuse to treat an infection just because statisticians have failed to prove that it causes miscarriage.

Even flu viruses are thought to cause spontaneous abortions. When a flu epidemic spreads through the population, two or three weeks later there is an increased incidence of spontaneous abortions. No reason for that increase has been determined, but perhaps the high fever, which can cause uterine irritability, is the culprit. Or perhaps the virus invades the placenta.

Occasionally the body fails to expel a fetus that has died. This is called a "missed abortion." Either labor must be induced or a D&C performed to clean out the uterus. Any tissue fragments left in the womb can lead to a dangerous infection.

Other Risk Factors

Many other risk factors are thought to cause pregnancy wastage. Diabetes (especially if uncontrolled), thyroid disease, abnormalities of the immune system such as systemic lupus erythematosus (SLE), cardiovascular disease, ABO blood-group incompatibility between parents, cigarette smoking, and drug and alcohol abuse are associated with miscarriage. Even toxic substances in the environment can cause fetal loss. Women who work around anesthesia in hospitals, for example, are known to have a high incidence of spontaneous abortion.

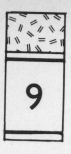

9

Breakthroughs in Assisted Reproductive Technology (ART)

ROBERT R. FRANKLIN, M.D.,
GEORGE M. GRUNERT, M.D., AND
DOROTHY KAY BROCKMAN

"Test-Tube" Babies: *In-Vitro* Fertilization (IVF)

Cuddling our six-month-old infant in her arms, my wife, Twyla, gently stroked our baby's downy curls. While our beautiful tow-headed Suzy contentedly nursed, Twyla drifted to sleep, and her wooden rocking chair slowed to a stop. Twenty minutes passed. Awakened by our baby's unnatural stillness, Twyla looked down at our tiny child. Suzy lay motionless—she had stopped breathing.

Screaming for help, Twyla ran down the stairs with lifeless Suzy in her arms. Her pink lips had turned gray. "Did she swallow anything," I cried, placing her facedown and patting her back to clear her airways.

"No," said Twyla, frantically trying to dial 911. I turned my daughter on her back on the kitchen table, gently tilted her little head backward, and blew small, cheek-sized puffs of air into Suzy's mouth and nose. Counting, I rhythmically pushed on her tiny chest.

Color immediately returned to Suzy's cheeks, and she opened her dark blue eyes. "Thank God," I wept as I held my beloved baby to my chest. Cardiopulmonary resuscitation (CPR) had brought my Suzy back to life—even if only for a while.

The hospital was ten minutes away. Suzy's pediatrician rushed through the emergency room door right behind the ambulance. After examining our baby, Dr. Jackson said, "We will have to wait for our test results before we can try to explain why Suzy stopped breathing. On preliminary investigation, I see no signs of meningitis or obvious disease. She is breathing fine now, and her heart sounds OK. Unfortunately, sometimes we just don't know why this happens. It may never happen again, or it could reoccur tonight. We need to watch her in intensive care for a few days. We'll place a cardiorespiratory monitor on her to warn the nurses if she stops breathing again."

Three sleepless nights later, Twyla and I returned to our small frame house with our little one. Although Suzy seemed less active than most babies her age, the doctors found nothing wrong with her.

Even though Suzy's monitor tracked her every breath and heartbeat, fear clouded my wife's every waking moment. Twyla almost never let our baby out of her sight. Feeling a crushing sense of responsibility, my wife checked on Suzy every twenty minutes, day and night. Twyla was not going to let our baby die. My wife refused to leave our little girl with a sitter or even the child's grandparents. Since Twyla would not set foot outside our house—for any reason—I did all the shopping. All Twyla asked from life was to keep our precious little baby alive. But fate had other plans.

Late one afternoon while Twyla was washing her hair, the sound of Suzy's alarm ripped our lives apart. Our child had stopped breathing again. Twyla ran into the bedroom and started applying CPR, refusing to give up for forty-five minutes.

When I came home that evening, the second I opened the back door, fear shot through my body. Enshrouded in darkness our fifty-year-old house sat totally silent. I flew to the top of the stairs, my heart churning in my throat. As I stared helplessly into my daughter's nursery, I found Twyla motionless in the rocking chair clinging to Suzy's tiny body. The doctors could find no cause for our infant's sudden death.

Twyla and I were completely unprepared for the tragedy that had befallen us. We were unable to fathom God's purpose for our Suzy. The afternoon of the funeral, Twyla walked out of the cemetery, got into our car alone, and drove to the office of the obstetrician who had delivered Suzy. My wife told her doctor that she wanted to be sterilized—saying that she hated being a mother and that she never wanted another baby. The doctor had no knowledge of Suzy's death.

Without telling anyone about her drastic plans, the following week Twyla had her tubes tied. When I found out, I was stunned. All the buried anger smoldering deep inside me exploded to the surface. Unable to speak, I hurled my fist through the wall and stormed out of my home, leaving all my belongings.

Six months passed. The black hole called my heart kept us apart.

Then one Saturday morning as I was driving to a convenience store,

I caught a glimpse of Twyla's frail frame getting into her car. I had missed her so. At last, tears poured down my cheeks. I felt totally out of control, but somehow my ten-year-old car found its way to our home. When Twyla pulled into the gravel driveway, I was sitting on the leaf-covered porch waiting for her.

Two years passed. With time and many hours of intensive counseling, we started to hope again. When Twyla told me that she wanted reversal surgery, I was overjoyed. Perhaps we dreamed that we could somehow regain a part of our lost Suzy. A friend, who was an infertility patient, recommended Dr. Franklin. She said that he would understand the hell we had endured. Since our baby had died, we decided to get genetic counseling. Although analysis of our genes failed to pinpoint any unusual problems, I wondered if an ill-fated roll of the genetic dice had caused my darling little girl's death.

After Dr. Franklin studied Twyla's medical records, he said: "The doctor that did your tubal ligation surgically removed part of the ampulla, the portion of each fallopian tube where fertilization often occurs. Repair requires a major operation. Although the overall pregnancy rate following reversal surgery is almost 60 percent, the rate after repair of the ampulla is around 40 percent. Before considering any surgery, we should do an HSG X-ray to see if the tubes also are blocked near the uterus, which sometimes happens after sterilization. Even though you have conceived before, we will need to evaluate your current ovulatory pattern and Gene's sperm count and check for any infections."

After Dr. Franklin read Twyla's HSG X-ray, he looked grim. He told her that both of her fallopian tubes appeared blocked—not only at the site of sterilization, but also where each enters the uterus. In other words, both tubes were probably blocked from scarring in at least two places, decreasing the odds that the sperm could reach the egg after a reversal operation. He said that our postsurgical chances for pregnancy probably were marginal.

Dr. Franklin told Twyla that she was a good candidate for in-vitro fertilization (IVF) or "test-tube" fertilization, a procedure in which conception occurs outside the body, completely bypassing the fallopian tubes. He said that about two hundred of his patients had gotten pregnant with IVF.

Said Dr. Franklin: "An expensive, high-tech procedure, IVF is stressful for most couples, even though the only surgery required to remove the eggs from the ovaries is a relatively minor procedure. The pregnancy rate is about 20 percent per cycle at some clinics, but, according to the latest American Society for Reproductive Medicine figures, the live-birth rate is now approximately 17 percent per attempt across the country."

Since our insurance paid for reversal surgery, but not IVF, Twyla decided to have her tubes repaired, even though Dr. Franklin had told us that the odds were against us.

As the years passed after her operation, Twyla, still childless and now thirty-five years old, became more and more depressed. Haunted by bitter loneliness, Twyla decided to learn more about "test-tube" fertilization. She contacted IVF expert Dr. George M. Grunert, director of the Assisted Reproductive Technology Program at the Woman's Hospital of Texas.

Dr. Grunert told us that IVF, one of the Assisted Reproductive Technologies (ART), begins with superovulation, a process of hormonally stimulating the ovaries with fertility drugs to produce more than one egg during the IVF menstrual cycle. "Pregnancy rates," he said, "seem to improve if multiple eggs are removed from the ovaries, fertilized, and the resulting embryos returned to the uterus. The success rates depend on many factors. The causes of infertility, the woman's age, the ovarian response to stimulation (the quality of the eggs and the embryos), the ability of the sperm to fertilize eggs, and the experience of the IVF team are primary considerations. The IVF pregnancy rate starts falling as the woman's age reaches the mid-thirties, dropping significantly at age forty. In couples such as you with no male factor where the woman is under forty years old, the IVF pregnancy rate is about 25 percent per cycle at most good programs, with some centers running over 30 percent."

I had plenty of reservations about putting Twyla through IVF. I just couldn't bear to have her disappointed again. Furthermore, superovulation requires daily hormone injections for about a week or two. Although we had almost saved enough money for one attempt at test-tube fertilization, the thought of my delicate Twyla becoming a human dart board made me extremely uneasy. My wife, however, was determined to try all that reproductive medicine had to offer. She feared that time was against us. Her hope was that if we attempted IVF and were lucky—we might end up with a baby.

Harvesting the Eggs and Transferring the Embryo

The birth of the world's first "test-tube" baby, Louise Brown, almost twenty years ago launched a new era in reproductive medicine—an age yielding powerful new knowledge, stunning scientific advances, and endless controversy. Pioneered in England by Drs. Steptoe and Edwards, IVF offers hope to childless couples who formerly couldn't be helped. By moving the miracle of fertilization outside of the mother's body, IVF has allowed many infertile couples to start their families. To date, over one hundred thousand *in-vitro* babies have been born—all of whom have been conceived in a test tube or laboratory dish.

Most of these infants were born to women with blocked oviducts, endometriosis, pelvic adhesions, antisperm antibodies, or poor cervical mucus. Recent remarkable breakthroughs have brought about the *in-vitro* conception of children by men who formerly were labeled "sterile" because their semen yielded immotile sperm, few sperm, or no sperm. Striking advancements in genetic testing of the fertilized egg in the "test tube" have allowed known carriers of some devastating heritable diseases to attempt pregnancy with less fear. In today's brave new world, a child can have as many as five parents—a biological mother and father, an adoptive mother and father, and an unrelated birth mother—and a menopausal grandmother can give birth to her own grandchildren.

How is this breakthrough technology, which has altered the definition of parenthood forever, possible? How are multiple eggs brought to fertilizable maturity when nature normally fully ripens only one each menstrual cycle? How are such eggs removed from deep in an infertile woman's body so that they can be fertilized in a laboratory dish? How can genetic testing of the resulting embryos help known carriers of some devastating diseases? How is an embryo returned to its mother so that it can implant itself in her womb?

To answer these questions, let's follow Twyla and her IVF doctor through the *in-vitro* fertilization and embryo transfer process. Picture this scenario: Draped with sterile sheets, Twyla is about to undergo an egg-recovery method called "transvaginal ultrasound-guided oocyte (egg) retrieval." During this fifteen-minute procedure, an attempt will be made to harvest Twyla's eggs from her ovaries through a hollow needle that is passed through the vagina (see fig. 9.1). Twyla has been given an IV sedative. No incision is necessary, but if Twyla becomes uncomfortable she can ask to have a general anesthesia.

Twyla's doctor begins by gently placing an ultrasound transducer (scanner), which bounces sound waves off internal organs, in the vagina. Super-sharp images of the inside of the abdomen immediately appear on the black-and-white TV screen. Since Twyla has taken fertility drugs, six bubblelike follicles can be seen on the surface of her ovaries. Some of the bulging follicles may contain an egg. Attached to the top of the scanner is the needle. Asking Twyla how she is doing, the *in-vitro* specialist passes the needle through the vaginal wall. Even though this sounds painful, Twyla doesn't seem to mind. A computer has calculated a path for the needle to follow through the abdomen and has drawn a line on the screen to an ovary. Although sleepy, Twyla is able to watch

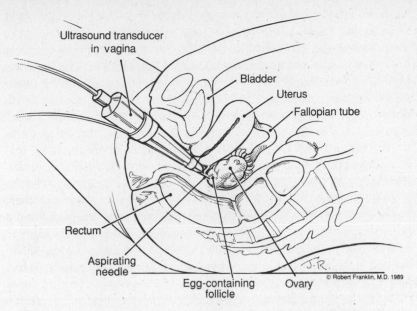

FIGURE 9.1. *Transvaginal ultrasound-guided oocyte (egg) retrieval. Eggs are harvested via a hollow needle passed through the vaginal wall. The needle is attached to the ultrasound scanner. (Research for drawing courtesy of Dr. G. Grunert and ADR Ultrasound, a division of Advanced Technology Laboratories.)*

the needle enter one of the grape-sized follicles. By applying suction to the needle, her doctor aspirates the potentially egg-harboring follicular fluid. Seventy-five percent of the time, hidden in this blood-streaked liquid is the cherished egg.

Wasting no time, a nurse rushes the precious fluid to the nearby Embryo Culture Laboratory. Here the biologist checks to see if the egg, which is no bigger than a speck, is floating in the liquid. With the aid of a microscope, Twyla's egg is quickly located, and its maturity and shape are carefully evaluated. The egg is kept in a clear plastic petri (laboratory) dish containing a special culture solution made of the patient's blood serum and other ingredients. Depending on its maturity, the egg will be preincubated from four to twenty-four hours before it is exposed to the sperm.

Meanwhile, during the same operation, Twyla's doctor has harvested five more eggs from their follicles. They have been uniformly ripened by using a combination of medications, first to put the woman's hormonal system in a rest state, and then to stimulate her ovaries with fertility drugs. As we will explain in detail later, unless the patient's ovaries are suppressed before she is given fertility drugs the eggs generally will not be at similar stages of development for retrieval.

But the eggs are only half the story. Before they were gathered, Twyla's husband was asked to produce the sperm for a semen analysis. Men say that this can be an anxiety-producing request. To take pressure off the husband, we offer him the opportunity to obtain a specimen the day before the eggs are harvested. We don't want to harvest a dozen eggs and have the laboratory tell us that they can't find any living sperm.

Back to our story. Earlier, when the semen arrived in the laboratory, it was allowed to liquefy. The sperm then were "washed" to remove the abnormally shaped sperm and those that weren't moving. The concentrated sperm also were capacitated, which, as you now know, is a biochemical process by which the enzyme inhibitor is stripped from the sperm head. Unless capacitated, the sperm cannot penetrate the relatively thick membrane surrounding the egg. In fact, before doctors learned to mimic the female reproductive tract's ability to capacitate sperm, IVF was impossible.

With the sperm and the eggs collected, *in-vitro* fertilization can now be attempted. Twenty-five thousand to fifty thousand of Gene's best-swimming sperm are mixed with each of Twyla's eggs in a plastic petri dish. (Although *in-vitro* literally means "in glass" as opposed to *in-vivo*, or "in the body," today plastic dishes are used.) When there is doubt about the ability of the sperm to fertilize an egg, the sperm concentration can be increased. Sometimes the sperm are such poor swimmers, or they are so few in number, that fertilization is only possible if a single otherwise normal-appearing sperm is injected directly into the cytoplasm of the egg. Called intracytoplasmic sperm injection (ICSI), this technically difficult microinjection technique, which was discussed in detail in chapter 6, is a major step forward in the treatment of male infertility. You will recall that ICSI results in fertilization of approximately 50 percent of the eggs injected, with conception rates varying widely, depending on the quality of the eggs and sperm. With some couples all of the eggs fertilize while with other patients none do.

Despite a vigorous effort by Gene's sperm, the first egg exposed is never penetrated. The next five, however, do fertilize, becoming pre-embryos! (Pre-embryos are the results of conception from day 1 until the nervous system starts to form, at approximately fourteen days.) Generally 70 to 80 percent of mature eggs will fertilize *in vitro*.

After fertilization, the pre-embryos are put in a temperature-controlled incubator, where they are allowed to grow at 98.6 degrees for forty-eight to seventy-two hours. As each pre-embryo divides, the biologist carefully studies its appearance and notes its rate of cleavage (cell division). Some programs take the pre-embryo's picture—couples have been known to call these photos their first "baby" pictures—but we prefer not to expose the dividing cells to light.

Although we are unable to screen an embryo for all inherited diseases, we now can look for a specific genetic disease such as Tay-Sachs, Duchenne muscular dystrophy, cystic fibrosis, or fragile X syndrome. The latter is a leading cause of mental retardation in the United States. During a delicate IVF process called BABI, short for preimplantation blastomere biopsy, a molecular geneticist carefully removes two cells from the eight-celled fertilized egg. By analyzing the DNA of these cells, doctors get a picture of the pre-embryo's genetic makeup. If Twyla's and Gene's earlier chromosome analysis had indicated that they were carriers of a disease that can be diagnosed with BABI, we could have identified the unaffected pre-embryos. At this time, the couple could have chosen to transfer the healthy embryos to Twyla's uterus. In the future, doctors hope to do routine chromosome analysis of pre-embryos to detect major genetic abnormalities such as Down's syndrome.

It is now time to proceed to the next IVF step—the implantation procedure. Once again, we need "Mom's" help. With Gene by her side, the embryos are transferred to Twyla's uterus one to three days after fertilization. She is awake during this short process, which she later says reminds her of a pelvic exam. At this time, the couple's dividing eight-celled pre-embryos are gently placed in the patient's womb. The *in-vitro* specialist uses a narrow plastic catheter (tube) that is gently passed through the cervix. Afterward, when some of the excitement is over, Twyla remains in bed and falls asleep for about two hours. Although some IVF programs send the woman home right after the transfer, Twyla's doctor wants her to rest for a while.

A crucial point: Implantation is when most IVF failures occur. If the lining of the uterus is either underdeveloped or past its prime for that cycle, none of the pre-embryos floating in Twyla's womb will implant itself. On the other hand, if the endometrial nest is in perfect readiness, one or more pre-embryos may burrow their way into the lining of the uterus. If any attach, Twyla at last will be pregnant.

We have had over four hundred IVF pregnancies at our ART clinic. To these families—who have brought home a "test-tube" baby—*in-vitro* fertilization is a miracle of modern technology, the long-awaited answer to their endless prayers.

In recent years, the ultrasound-guided retrieval method described above has replaced laparoscopy as the procedure of choice for gathering eggs. About the only time we still use the 'scope to retrieve eggs is when the patient needs a laparoscopy for other reasons, such as in the diagnosis and treatment of endometriosis or pelvic adhesions. In general, ultrasound-guided retrieval offers tremendous advantages over laparoscopy as an egg-recovery method. Vaginal retrieval is easier on the patient, involves less risk, and is cheaper. Eggs inaccessible with laparoscopy often can be recovered with ultrasound. If, for instance, the pelvic organs are covered with sheets of adhesions, ultrasound can "see" right through them (see fig. 2.3). The complication rate with vaginal retrieval is less than with laparoscopy. Nevertheless, even with ultrasound there is a slight risk that the needle might hit other pelvic structures such as the intestines, the bladder, or blood vessels.

When there is a reason to use the laparoscope to recover eggs, the patient usually is given general anesthesia. The 'scope is inserted through a half-inch incision near the navel. When the doctor looks through the 'scope at the ovaries, he or she usually sees several nearly ripe follicles. If adhesions or endometriosis is found, both conditions often can be treated at this time with the laser. Once the ovary is accessible it must be stabilized with tiny grasping forceps passed through a second puncture site. To retrieve the egg, a narrow, hollow needle is inserted, either through the laparoscope or through a third puncture site in the abdomen. Suction is applied to the needle to remove the fluid from each follicle. Next the eggs are examined and fertilized, and the resulting pre-embryos are incubated. Forty-eight to seventy-two hours later, the pre-embryos are transferred to the infertile woman, using the same method described on the previous page.

IVF Success Rates

What determines whether assisted reproductive technologies such as *in-vitro* fertilization and embryo transfer are successful for couples such as Twyla and Gene? In general, IVF pregnancy rates depend on the age of the patient, the cause of infertility, the ovarian response to stimulation (the quality of the eggs and the embryos), the ability of the sperm to fertilize eggs, and the experience of the ART team.

At first glance, ART statistics can be confusing. One way to understand IVF success rates, for example, is to consider results in 1,000 patients under age forty whose husbands have normal sperm function. If all of them start an IVF cycle at our clinic, we will recover eggs from approximately 950. Some eggs won't fertilize, hence about 900 women will undergo embryo transfer. Of these, about 300 patients will get pregnant. They must be carefully monitored because 50 will spontaneously abort (miscarry) and 5 or more will have an ectopic (misplaced) pregnancy in a fallopian tube. Hence, of the original 1,000 women, about

245, or 25 percent, will deliver a baby each IVF cycle. Keep in mind that these are averages; couples with poor sperm function or with a maternal age of over thirty-nine have a lower chance of pregnancy, while optimal IVF candidates may do better.

The averages for the country, which include older couples and those with male factor infertility, are lower than those stated above. According to a 1992 nationwide study published in the December 1994 issue of *Fertility and Sterility*, the rate of deliveries per retrieval for IVF cycles was 16.8 percent; for GIFT cycles, 26.3 percent; for ZIFT cycles, 22.8 percent; and for combined cycles using IVF and one of the tubal transfer techniques, 27.9 percent. Frozen embryo transfers produced 13.9 percent deliveries per procedure.

Although ART teams are judged by such success rates, what the couple really wants is a baby in their arms. In other words, the ART statistic that counts is the "take-home-baby rate." With this in mind, the husband and wife should thoroughly evaluate the ART program under consideration. If they are contemplating "test-tube" fertilization, they should ask a prospective center exactly how many IVF births—not pregnancies—it has produced. The husband and wife should make certain that they aren't quoted another center's statistics. In the past, the American Society for Reproductive Medicine (ASRM) found that programs that do more than eighty cycles a year are more successful than centers with a low patient volume. In fact, some IVF programs in the U.S. have yet to produce a successful pregnancy.

An ART program should meet the guidelines of the American Society for Reproductive Medicine. Says the association's Ethics Committee: "After reports surfaced that some clinics were misstating or exaggerating success rates, congressional hearings were held and legislation enacted to address this problem. The Fertility Clinic Success Rate and Certification Act of 1992 requires that every assisted reproductive program report its rate of live births 'per number of stimulation procedures attempted' and 'per number of successful egg retrieval procedures' to the Centers for Disease Control or its designee." Every laboratory must now pass inspection by the College of American Pathologists.

The scientific knowledge necessary to make *in-vitro* work is mind-boggling. Many programs employ a team of medical specialists including a reproductive endocrinologist, an embryologist, a gynecologist skilled in laparoscopy and ultrasound aspiration, an andrologist, nurses, and laboratory technicians. Sometimes one person fills several of these functions. With hard-core commitment, these specialists research ways to overcome the most difficult cases of infertility. They supervise hormone therapy, monitor the growth of follicles with ultrasound and hormone tests, harvest eggs, and transfer embryos. All of these drugs and tests make IVF physically exhausting and expensive for the patient, although, as we discuss in detail later, sometimes expenses are at least partially covered by medical insurance.

Surrounded by so much attention, the couple often feel that IVF is the grand finale of infertility treatments. If, after all this effort, reproductive medicine fails to produce a viable infant, the couple once again go home to an empty nursery. A difficult time, this is when their doctor should listen to the couple and try to help them consider their final options.

When we have to tell a couple that they have a negative hCG pregnancy test, they look at us as if they have been hit by a truck. To help them through their disappointment, we point out that even though the wife didn't get pregnant, they have gained important new information. The husband and wife may have learned, for example, that the woman can ovulate on fertility drugs, that her eggs can be fertilized by her husband's sperm, and that the couple can produce healthy-appearing pre-embryos. Just knowing this can be reassuring to a patient and her husband and can help direct the couple's future medical therapy.

If, on the other hand, no eggs fertilize (an IVF outcome made rare by microinjection of the egg), this information also is extremely valuable. Some couple's eggs do fertilize, but none of them implant. When these patients request genetic testing of their nontransferred pre-embryos, we often learn that the majority are chromosomally abnormal. This may be the major reason pre-embryos fail to attach to the uterine lining. As you know, such genetic aberrations also often lead to spontaneous abortion.

Unfortunate IVF results can tell the couple that their options are either to stop trying to get pregnant or to consider using artificial insemination by donor or donor eggs. But, even though the couple learn a great deal about their chances of having a baby, sometimes they are so devastated when IVF fails that they need the help of a specially trained infertility counselor.

Fortunately, the last few years have brought astonishing new advances that have enabled more IVF patients to become pregnant. Today *in-vitro* fertilization is no longer an experimental procedure; it is standard medical practice. Although much remains to be discovered, doctors have gained valuable new insight into the intricate reproductive process by monitoring ovulation induction and by observing fertilization in the laboratory. As you now know, the use of fertility drugs, which make more eggs available for fertilization, has improved the pregnancy rate. As Twyla's case shows, the new egg-retrieval methods, which permit eggs to be gathered under IV sedative, have made IVF easier on the patient. With experience, more precise timing of egg recovery has evolved. The relatively new practice of freezing and storing extra human pre-embryos can ease the patient's physical burden. This technology permits transfer attempts during several cycles without the need for additional courses of fertility drugs or further invasive procedures to harvest more eggs. (We will discuss cryopreservation of pre-embryos in detail later.)

Although at first glance *in-vitro* pregnancy rates seem low, they are put in perspective when compared with those found in nature. Natural reproduction is *not* an efficient process. For a young couple having regular intercourse with no fertility problem, 90 percent of the time an embryo will be created every menstrual cycle. During this same time, however, the pregnancy rate is only about 15 to 25 percent. In other words, many fertilized eggs fail to attach themselves to the uterine lining. This means that in nature about 17 to 18 percent of human embryos implant. So although the IVF implantation rate (currently about 15 percent) is low, it is catching up with Mother Nature. Considering the number of fertilized eggs that fail to implant in fertile couples, it isn't surprising that implantation is the weak link in infertile IVF patients. Amazingly enough, for some causes of infertility, pregnancy rates at the more experienced IVF centers exceed natural pregnancy rates for fertile couples. This is no small accomplishment, considering that IVF doctors attempt to overcome the most stubborn infertility cases.

Although IVF has a high miscarriage rate, many spontaneous conceptions also end in miscarriage. Doctors estimate that about 50 percent of all pregnancies are aborted. As stated earlier, many of these miscarriages occur before the woman even knows that she has conceived. Among clinically proven pregnancies, the incidence of spontaneous abortion runs about 10 to 15 percent. Since pregnancies are diagnosed sooner during the IVF cycle, early miscarriages may be discovered that normally would go unnoticed. If one looks at pregnancies beyond eight weeks, the abortion rate with IVF is about the same as with spontaneous pregnancies.

Who Might Benefit?

Generally a patient is considered a candidate for IVF only after all other, conventional infertility therapies have failed. Considering all the facts, the couple with the help of their doctors have to decide whether IVF is the appropriate technology to solve their particular infertility problems—that no other procedure would be more successful or less expensive.

In the past, *in-vitro* programs primarily accepted women with missing or damaged fallopian tubes. Such a patient often has had both oviducts blocked as the result of previous pelvic infections or an irreversible tubal-ligation (tubal-sterilization) procedure. Depending on the location and extent of the blockage, laparoscopic repair of the tubes or tubal micro-surgery often is the first-line treatment. If the tubes aren't operable, if they reocclude, or if after several years no pregnancy occurs, IVF still offers some hope. In fact, sometimes women over age thirty-five, who are concerned that the age of their eggs is becoming a significant fertility factor, try IVF before tubal surgery.

Nowadays *in-vitro* programs also are accepting patients with endo-metriosis, pelvic adhesions, cervical factors, immunological infertility, unexplained infertility, as well as wives of men with low sperm counts. Couples who are known carriers of genetic diseases that can be diag-nosed by preimplantation blastomere analysis also are candidates for IVF. Some endometriosis patients have such severe adhesions that tra-ditional surgery cannot restore fertility. In the worst cases, the pelvis is covered with sheets of scar tissue, and the organs cannot be identified (see fig 2.3). In these patients, the eggs have little chance of reaching the tubes. With ultrasound guidance, however, the doctor can retrieve the eggs and fertilize them in a petri dish. A few women have repeated ectopic pregnancies because of interruptions in the little avenues that line the inside of the oviducts. These patients also are best treated with IVF, because it totally bypasses the fallopian tubes.

IVF has helped some husbands with subfertile sperm father children. Since the sperm are directly incubated with the egg in a dish, they don't have to swim through the female reproductive tract. Doctors think that "washing" the sperm to remove those of poor quality, along with the acidic semen and the sperm autoantibodies, has led to many IVF preg-nancies. Adding more concentrated sperm to the egg *in vitro* increases pregnancy rates. IVF also may allow pregnancy in some women with hostile or inadequate cervical mucus. Since the cervix is bypassed, the sperm don't have to maneuver through the mucus to reach the egg.

Unfortunately, in the past IVF results using sperm with poor mor-phology (shape and structure) haven't been good. The total number, concentration, and motility of sperm hasn't been as important as their morphology. Although shape is more critical than motility, if there's no motility, there's no sperm function and thus no fertilization. A poorly shaped sperm is seldom a good swimmer. And, of course, if the sperm aren't strong swimmers, they have a difficult time penetrating the egg—even when placed right next to it "in glass." The exciting news is that ICSI or microinjection of a sperm into the center of an egg may help overcome problems of sperm number, motility, and shape. Nowadays if a sperm has normal-appearing genetic material, it doesn't have to be an Olympic swimmer to initiate conception.

Why do doctors sometimes recommend *in-vitro* fertilization to patients with immunological infertility, a problem in which the wife's or sometimes the husband's system attacks the sperm as foreign invaders? (These patients have antisperm antibodies that decrease sperm motility, which leads to agglutination or clumping.) By bypassing the female genital tract, IVF reduces sperm exposure to the woman's immune system. In these patients, doctors obviously don't use the woman's blood serum in the IVF culture medium. In theory, IVF also should help men who produce autoantibodies (antibodies against their own sperm). In these men, some autoantibodies are found in the semen itself. Although "washing" the sperm before mixing them with the eggs should reduce the number of these antibodies, in the past success with IVF in patients with autoantibodies was limited. Hence, IVF without micromanipulation of the egg wasn't very helpful in treating the patient who had developed antisperm antibodies after a vasectomy. Nowadays, however, by injecting the sperm directly into the egg, doctors are able to help more couples with autoantibody problems.

Since immunologic infertility is a nebulous problem—some *fertile* women carry sperm antibodies   experts are often slow to recommend IVF to these patients. But if a patient has immunological infertility, and no other apparent problems can be found, we think she should be told that IVF is available.

Since IVF is expensive, time-consuming, and exhausting, it should be offered only to infertility patients with a fighting chance of taking home a baby. It is easy to understand why the patient must be healthy, without a contraindication to pregnancy, and why both partners should be free of infections. The woman must have a normal uterus, and her ovaries must be responsive to stimulation with fertility drugs. If we cannot retrieve eggs, we cannot do IVF, that is unless the couple want to consider donor eggs. In addition, the patient's husband's sperm must be able to fertilize eggs, unless donor sperm is used.

Ethically, the doctor has two key questions to consider: Does IVF make sense for this particular couple? Does it have a reasonable chance of succeeding in a reasonable period of time? Since we know that the pregnancy rate starts to decline after the fourth IVF cycle, we think that it is reasonable to counsel people to stop after that. (Keep in mind that not only does an IVF cycle consist of hormone stimulation, egg recovery, and embryo transfer, it includes transfers of all frozen embryos produced during that cycle.) There is an exception to the above four-cycle rule. As you know, in the past IVF failed many of our patients with some difficult sperm problems. But nowadays, by adding ICSI to a fifth IVF attempt, we finally are helping a few of these couples have a baby.

The upper age limit of the wife used to be thirty-five years, but now many IVF programs accept patients into their late forties. There is, of course, an increased risk of chromosomal abnormalities related to age. For this reason, pre-implantation or prenatal genetic counseling can be helpful. In addition, there is a higher incidence of miscarriage. Although the IVF pregnancy rate is almost the same at age forty-five as it is at forty, the miscarriage rate increases from 35 percent at forty years of age to 60 percent at forty-five. In other words, some older women might get pregnant with IVF, but many of them won't end up with a baby. Doctors think this is caused by the effect of the aging process on the eggs rather than on the endometrial nest.

More and more older women are having babies with IVF. In France, for example, a sixty-five-year-old woman became pregnant using donor eggs. In South Africa, a woman in her late forties gave birth to her own twin granddaughters—her daughter's and son-in-law's babies. In other words, the daughter's eggs were removed and fertilized in a laboratory dish with the son-in-law's sperm; then the resulting pre-embryos were placed in Grandma's uterus. So the endometrium of an older woman can support a pregnancy. In this case, the daughter had had a hysterectomy, but she still had healthy ovaries. To have a family she, in essence, "borrowed" her mother's womb.

Superovulation: Hormonally Stimulating the Ovaries

ART doctors give fertility drugs to fool Mother Nature into maturing more than one egg. Called superovulation, this process of stimulating the ovaries increases the chances that multiple eggs will be fertilized and returned to the uterus. Using controlled ovarian hyperstimulation (COH), doctors stimulate the ovaries to recruit multiple egg-harboring follicles rather than letting one dominate. The pregnancy rate with IVF appears to be directly proportional to the number of eggs recovered and fertilized. And, up to a point, the more eggs transferred, the greater the likelihood of pregnancy. If two fertilized eggs are placed in the uterus, the chances of pregnancy more than double. The best chance for success occurs if three or four pre-embryos are transferred per IVF cycle.

The extra maturing follicles make the whole reproductive mechanism more efficient. Not only are more eggs available for fertilization (all exposed to sperm usually don't fertilize), the additional estrogen produced by the extra follicles makes the endometrium lush for implantation. Transferring more than four pre-embryos, however, fails to improve pregnancy rates while increasing the risk of multiple births and the accompanying complications.

What medications does the doctor prescribe to stimulate the ovaries? Depending on the patient, various combinations of fertility drugs such as clomiphene citrate (Clomid or Serophene), human menopausal gonadotropin (Pergonal), or pure follicle-stimulating hormone (FSH) (Metrodin) are used to increase the number of eggs ripened each cycle. Simply put, clomiphene works indirectly by making the pituitary (the master gland) release FSH and LH. Metrodin is FSH; Pergonal is FSH and LH. By selectively using these drugs, which are made in the laboratory instead of in the patient's head, doctors can override the ovaries' normal limitations of maturing only one egg at a time.

The exact medications the endocrinologist chooses depend on the individual patient's hormonal system. The doctor must constantly reevaluate the ovarian reaction to drug stimulation in order to pick the most effective medications.* Expertise in this area is the key to the success of an IVF program! In the initial cycle, 95 percent of our patients respond well enough to proceed to surgery. Sometimes, however, cycles have to be discontinued because the patient fails to respond. Of these women, approximately 70 percent will ripen follicles in a later cycle.

As the follicles ripen under hormonal stimulation, their progress is monitored with ultrasound imaging. Follicles of different sizes usually can be seen on the TV-like screen, indicating that the eggs are at varying stages of development. As mentioned earlier, to make the follicles reach maturity at about the same time, we prescribe a GnRH agonist to keep the pituitary gland from recruiting eggs. With the ovaries at rest, the IVF specialist uses fertility drugs to bring multiple high-quality eggs to maturity at the same time.

Based on recent evidence, we feel that resting the ovaries before stimulating them with fertility drugs gives a better pregnancy rate. One of the most successful stimulation regimens starts by completely suppressing the ovaries with one of the GnRH agonists a week before menstruation. Once the ovaries are in a rest state, which usually takes two to three weeks, we begin stimulating them with either Metrodin or

---

*Unconfirmed preliminary studies have reported a slight increase in the incidence of ovarian cancer following the use of ovulation induction drugs.

Pergonal. Clomid won't work because with a GnRH agonist the pituitary gland isn't playing a role. The advantage is that all of the stimulation is coming from the drug store. Not only do we get more ripe eggs, but also the cancellation rate, which usually is 30 to 40 percent per cycle, drops to about 10 percent. Consequently, more patients get to the operating room for egg retrieval. For some patients this ovarian stimulation regimen, along with other changes, has increased the IVF pregnancy rate between 15 and 25 percent per transfer to between 30 and 40 percent per transfer.

Since the follicles secrete increasing amounts of estrogen into the bloodstream as they grow, daily blood tests for estrogen help doctors track growth of the follicles. Once these tests, along with ultrasound imaging of the ovaries, indicate that the follicles are almost ripe, maturation of the egg is triggered with a shot of hCG (human chorionic gonadotropin). Proper timing of this injection is crucial! The doctor schedules egg retrieval thirty-four to thirty-six hours later. If the IVF specialist waited forty-four to forty-eight hours after administration of hCG, the patient would already have ovulated on her own. The goal in IVF cycles is to retrieve the eggs when they are mature enough to finish ripening outside of the ovary but before ovulation.

In spontaneous cycles, luteinizing hormone (LH) is released by the pituitary. This causes maturation of the eggs and, later, ovulation. In COH cycles, hCG mimics the action of LH. If the pituitary releases LH spontaneously, before hCG is given, ovulation can occur before surgery, resulting in cancellation of the IVF cycle. When a GnRH agonist is used, spontaneous LH production and premature ovulation are prevented.

Sometimes more eggs are recovered than should be fertilized and transferred at one time. When this is the case, the couple has three ethically acceptable options. The first is to fertilize only some of the eggs and discard the rest. The second option is to donate the extra eggs to an infertility patient who cannot recover eggs. The third choice is to fertilize all of them. If the couple ends up with more embryos than should be transferred to the wife's womb, they can freeze the others for implantation during a subsequent cycle. Whichever option the couple chooses, they must decide the fate of any extra fertilized eggs before beginning IVF.

Natural Cycle IVF

IVF is sometimes performed for patients under thirty-five years of age during spontaneous cycles without the use of fertility drugs. "Test-tube" fertilization during a natural cycle is simpler and cheaper than during a hormonally stimulated cycle. Egg retrieval is quicker, and concerns about multiple births are reduced, although twins are possible. Requiring less medication and monitoring, natural cycle IVF is easier and less stressful on the patient. Nevertheless, sonograms and blood tests are needed to follow the development of the egg.

During an unstimulated cycle the egg is retrieved vaginally right after the LH surge. Doctors often trigger egg maturation with an injection of hCG, harvesting the egg about 34 hours later. If the egg fertilizes, the pre-embryo is placed in the uterus. With only one follicle producing progesterone, levels of this critical pregnancy-supporting hormone are lower than during stimulated cycles. For this reason, hCG, or rarely progesterone, shots may be necessary to maintain the early pregnancy.

Unfortunately, pregnancy rates are low with natural cycle *in-vitro* fertilization. In an unstimulated cycle, even if the patient ovulates and menstruates regularly, the stress of IVF can throw her reproductive clock off balance, making the timing of the egg retrieval more difficult. In women over thirty-five, even though we often recover an egg after spontaneous ovulation, the pregnancy rate is poor. After this age, we find an increasing number of abnormal eggs.

Monitoring the Pregnancy

IVF patients say that the two weeks following the embryo transfer until the hCG pregnancy test seem like an eternity. Twyla experienced a rainbow of emotions, ranging from hopeful anticipation and exhilaration to apprehension and depression. She said that all her grief over the loss of her daughter Suzy and her disappointment over being unable to have another baby haunted her nights of waiting.

Like most IVF patients, Twyla "felt pregnant," but her defense mechanisms had convinced her that she wasn't. She kept reminding herself that her IVF doctor had said she could try again. But since her medical insurance didn't pay for *in-vitro* fertilization, she and Gene wouldn't be able to afford a second IVF attempt for several years. Although IVF coverage is offered by law in some states, many employers don't purchase such coverage. In Texas, IVF, which treats infertility alone, often isn't paid for by insurance, unless the couple have specific coverage for it. As mentioned earlier, medical expenses for the evaluation and treatment of diseases such as endometriosis are generally covered. For Twyla and Gene, it seemed as though one attempt at *in-vitro* fertilization would be the couple's only chance to have a baby before she turned forty years old.

The night before Twyla was to have her pregnancy test, the couple slept one hour. First thing in the morning, Twyla rushed to the laboratory to have blood drawn. That afternoon, with her heart pounding in her chest, she picked up the phone to dial her doctor. The nurse on the other end of the line instantly recognized the couple's name. Her voice sounded excited as she said: "Twyla, I have great news for you. Your hCG test was positive. I think that you are pregnant!"

Even though IVF has left many couples without a baby, the joy it brought to Twyla and her husband made all the effort focused on this million-dollar technology worthwhile. When we heard Twyla's good news, we were thrilled. We had believed that she had been an excellent IVF candidate. Nothing had been wrong with her reproductive system except that her fallopian tubes had been damaged.

Now that Twyla was pregnant, her progress had to be carefully followed by her obstetrician. Although IVF bypasses the fallopian tubes, there is a 1.2 percent chance that, following transfer, IVF-conceived embryos will implant themselves in the oviducts rather than in the uterus. These ectopic pregnancies are dangerous and either must be treated medically with a drug called methotrexate (MTX) or removed surgically before the tube ruptures. Since ectopic gestations are the leading cause of maternal death, we recommend early ultrasound monitoring not only for pregnant IVF patients but for all high-risk pregnancies. If an out-of-place pregnancy is diagnosed soon enough, drug rather than surgical therapy may be possible. The doctor also has to be aware that in every two hundred IVF pregnancies one patient will have simultaneous tubal and uterine gestations.

Ultrasound imaging allows us to see if the pregnancy is in the uterus by about two and one-half to three weeks after the embryo transfer. If there are multiple pregnancies, we can identify all of them by about three weeks. It is important to follow these patients with ultrasound until they are out of risk for spontaneous abortion. Once we can see that the baby is moving and can monitor its heartbeat, the chance of miscarriage with a single pregnancy is low.

Pregnant IVF patients have a high incidence of multiple births. When three or four pre-embryos are transferred, the multiple-pregnancy rate is approximately 25 percent. Fortunately, the vast majority of these are twins.

Prospective IVF parents can be reassured that the risk of their full-term baby's having a birth defect is no greater than if it had been conceived following intercourse. The collaborative registry of IVF babies shows that the incidence of birth defects is the same as would be expected with spontaneous pregnancies in patients in the same age range. In other words, there have been a number of IVF children born with birth defects, but the incidence is no higher than in the general population and apparently isn't related to IVF.

There is an unconfirmed study from Australia, adjusted for multiple pregnancies, indicating a higher risk to IVF patients of prematurity and fetal distress in labor. Doctors don't know whether such problems are caused by the IVF process or by the high incidence of pelvic disease in IVF patients. With the Australian medical system, the patient goes to an IVF center for egg retrieval and transfer, but returns to a general practitioner for obstetrical care. It obviously is important for IVF patients to plan to deliver in an area that has excellent facilities for obstetrical and natal care. All ART patients should choose an obstetrician who feels comfortable with treating high-risk pregnancies.

Superovulation and Intrauterine Insemination (IUI)

One of the first ART procedures doctors recommend for carefully selected couples is superovulation combined with intrauterine insemination (IUI). For this to work, the woman must have at least one ovary capable of responding to fertility drugs, and its corresponding oviduct must be open. During IUI, large numbers of washed motile sperm are deposited inside the uterus via a syringe or a narrow tube. By boosting sperm and egg density, doctors hope to increase the chances that the sperm and eggs will meet in the fallopian tubes.

Superovulation combined with IUI is more economical and easier on the patient than IVF. Hence, before proceeding to "test-tube" fertilization, we recommend fertility drugs followed by IUI for every couple with open tubes and normal sperm function. This ART procedure can increase the odds of conception in couples with a small chance of having a baby in any given menstrual cycle. Our goal is to give people a better chance at pregnancy in a shorter period of time.

GIFT: Putting the Eggs and Sperm
Directly into the Tubes

Some infertile patients with intact fallopian tubes have conceived with the help of GIFT, an acronym for "gamete intrafallopian transfer." Pioneered by Dr. Ricardo H. Asch, GIFT is a procedure in which the gametes (the technical name for eggs or sperm) are placed directly in the fallopian tubes. As you now know, during the GIFT process, the eggs are harvested from stimulated ovaries via laparoscopy with the woman under general anesthesia. The eggs are placed in a catheter,

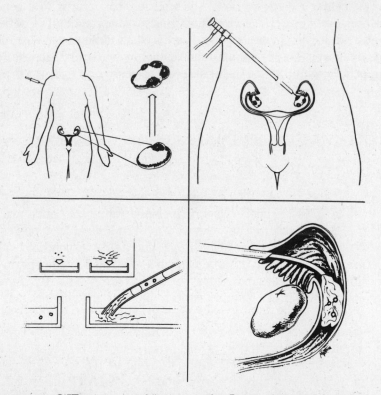

FIGURE 9.2. GIFT: gamete intrafallopian transfer. Eggs are harvested from the ovaries by laparoscopy, placed in a catheter, and, together with the husband's sperm, immediately injected directly into the outer end of the fallopian tubes. (From R. H. Asch, J. P. Balmaced, L. R. Ellsworth, et al., "Gamete Intrafallopian Transfer [GIFT]: A New Treatment for Infertility," International Journal of Fertility, vol. 30, p. 41, 1985 [fig. 1, p. 43].)

and, together with the husband's sperm, immediately injected through the 'scope into the outer end of each fallopian tube (see fig. 9.2). Many centers now place four eggs and one hundred thousand sperm in each tube when GIFT is done without IVF.

Keep in mind that GIFT only works for couples with normal fallopian tubes, normal eggs, and normal sperm. But if all of these reproductive processes are working, patients often get better results with superovulation and intrauterine insemination—a process that, as mentioned earlier, doesn't require laparoscopy. With both GIFT and IUI the sperm get into the oviducts. In our experience, if couples fail to conceive with superovulation combined with IUI—which is cheaper and easier on the woman than the laparoscopic procedure—they seldom get pregnant with GIFT. In fact, in unsuccessful IUI patients our pregnancy rate with GIFT has been low—only 4 percent.

So in our experience, IVF has been more successful than GIFT, in part because we recommend superovulation and IUI for all women with open oviducts. Some nationwide studies, however, have reported little difference between the two procedures. Here again statistics are confusing because often GIFT is performed at the time of initial laparoscopy without preliminary evaluation and without first trying IUI. According to the Society for Assisted Reproductive Technology, the National IVF-ET Registry in the U.S. reported a clinical pregnancy rate of 33.9 percent for GIFT compared to 19.1 percent for IVF. Obviously, the screening process used to select GIFT candidates affects such figures.

Since our GIFT pregnancy rates have been disappointing and since GIFT requires a 'scope, we rarely use this technology anymore. Nevertheless, for older patients or for couples with religious or moral objections to IVF, GIFT may be an alternative. Some patients prefer GIFT over IVF because the former more nearly mimics natural conception; the eggs and sperm—which are separated by an air bubble in the catheter—come together in the woman's fallopian tubes rather than in a laboratory dish (see fig. 9.2). If fertilized, the dividing pre-embryo travels through the oviduct and implants itself in the lining of the uterus, just as it would following spontaneous conception.

GIFT is sometimes offered to couples if a laparoscopy is indicated for other reasons. If, for example, a patient hasn't conceived after a year following surgery for endometriosis, a second-look laparoscopy may be necessary to see if the condition has returned. If the woman can produce enough extra eggs with the aid of fertility drugs and if she has normal fallopian tubes, we sometimes perform GIFT and IVF together during the same menstrual cycle. We put two or three eggs in the oviducts with the sperm via the 'scope. Some of the remaining eggs can be fertilized *in vitro*. Depending on the couple's wishes, several of the resulting pre-embryos are transferred to the patient's uterus, and the rest are frozen. In addition to receiving the diagnostic and therapeutic benefits of the 'scope, the woman is exposed to pregnancy in two ways: through her tubes and her uterus. The couple also learns whether their eggs are fertilizing.

A complication of GIFT is that approximately 4 percent of embryos conceived following this procedure implant themselves in the oviducts instead of in the womb. For this reason, expecting GIFT patients must be followed carefully with ultrasound during early pregnancy.

ZIFT: Putting the Fertilized Eggs Directly into the Tubes

One of the latest "high-tech" treatments for infertility, ZIFT (an acronym for "zygote intrafallopian transfer"), is a combination of GIFT and IVF. As with other assisted reproductive technologies, the woman takes fertility drugs to stimulate her ovaries to produce multiple eggs. During the ZIFT procedure, mature eggs are fertilized in a dish and the resulting pre-embryos are placed in the fallopian tubes via the laparoscope. Since the pre-embryos must travel through an oviduct before implanting naturally in the uterus, at least one tubal canal must be healthy.

Our pregnancy rate per cycle with ZIFT is 35 to 40 percent per transfer, which is higher than with IVF. But here again patient selection influences success rates. If only one or two eggs fertilize, rather than perform a laparoscopy, we transfer the embryos to the uterus instead of the tube. Hence, the ZIFT pregnancy rate is higher than the IVF rate not only because of the transfer method, but also because we only do ZIFT if we have three or four good quality embryos. Like GIFT, ZIFT seems to work better than IVF in women over forty years of age. In addition, ZIFT, as mentioned earlier, is helpful for couples with primary male infertility, especially if the woman's reproductive system appears normal. Always of concern to doctors is the increased risk of misplaced pregnancies following this procedure. In our experience, the ectopic pregnancy rate has been 1.5 percent.

Freezing Human Embryos: Cryopreservation

A baby boy who began life as eight cells frozen at minus 300 degrees was reported in "good health" Thursday by the doctor [Dr. Richard P. Marrs] who introduced the parents to the technology. Wednesday's birth was the first in the U.S. and the fourth in the world from a frozen embryo.
Houston Chronicle, June 6, 1986

Human embryos now can be frozen in a cryoprotectant (a special protective solution) and stored at -196 degrees centigrade in liquid nitrogen—and about two-thirds will survive freezing and thawing. Sometimes referred to as "souls on ice" by the lay press, cryopreserved pre-embryos that resume cell division and appear viable after thawing can be transferred to the uterus of either the biological or an adopting mother. The viable pregnancy rate per frozen embryo transfer is only about 10 to 15 percent, depending on the number and quality of embryos. If four embryos are frozen, thawed, and transferred to a patient, the chances of pregnancy are about 20 percent. Millions of calves have started their lives "on ice" with no apparent increase in birth defects.

The attempted implantation can be performed during a spontaneous (unstimulated) menstrual cycle three to four days after the LH surge. An alternative plan is to monitor the patient with ultrasound and to transfer the thawed pre-embryos one to two days after ovulation.

Profound ethical questions surround the storing of human pre-embryos, not the least of which is: When does the soul enter the body? Although this question is best left to theologians, doctors must decide what they personally feel is morally right. If a procedure might help our patient and if it conforms with our moral standards, we tell the patient that it is available. If the procedure is also acceptable to the couple, we either do it or refer them to another specialist. Keeping this in mind, we think that physicians must be careful not to overstep professional boundaries by trying to impose their morality on their patients. What is right for one couple might not be right for another.

To help set up guidelines for physicians, the Ethics Committee of the American Fertility Society (1986–87) has stated: "The preembryo doesn't have differentiated organs, much less the developed brain, nervous system and capacity of sentience that legal subjects ordinarily have. Indeed, the preembryo is not yet individual, because twinning and mosaicism [the development of human cells with differing genetic makeup] can still occur. Thus, it is not surprising that the law does not recognize the preembryo as a legal subject."

The committee, made up of attorneys, medical doctors, biologists, theologians, and ethicists, adds that "it seems prudent at this time not to maintain human preembryos for research beyond the 14th day of postfertilization development. Although this limitation is somewhat arbitrary as to specific time, it recognizes that beyond this time, the definitive embryo and placenta may be structurally discriminated, individuality seems assured, and anatomic differentiation of the embryonic corpus begins."

Allowing conception and birth to be separated by years, cryopreservation of pre-embryos has set the stage for many expensive legal battles. For example, if the couple divorces, who has custody of their frozen embryos? What inheritance rights do pre-embryos implanted and born after the father's death have? Not only do laws vary depending on the state, but trial court decisions may be rejected by higher state courts.

There reportedly have been four pregnancies using mature human eggs that were frozen and thawed. Two of these patients miscarried and two delivered. The technical problems are considerable because the human egg is extremely fragile.

Theoretically, doctors might even take cryopreservation of eggs one step further. Why not freeze the entire ovary? Studies in animals are currently under way. When a young woman has to have her ovaries removed for medical reasons, it would ease her concerns about sterility if at least part of an ovary could be preserved by freezing. If the eggs could be ripened outside the body in a special culture medium, she still would have the potential to have children. This is becoming more science than fiction. Although storing human ovaries is currently impossible, two Australian pregnancies have been reported in which oocytes were recovered from a sedated patient's unstimulated ovaries, stimulated to maturity in the laboratory, and fertilized in a "test-tube." After conception the pre-embryos were transferred to the patients. This may hold promise for the future.

Donor Eggs: Hope for Women Without Eggs

A few women are born with no egg-containing follicles. Other patients experience menopause prematurely or have their ovaries destroyed by disease, chemotherapy, or radiation. Still others are afraid of passing on a crippling genetic abnormality to their children. Some patients have little hope of establishing an IVF pregnancy with their own eggs because of maternal age. A number of these women have relied on donor eggs in order to give birth.

If a patient without eggs has a normal uterus, a donor's eggs can be fertilized in a laboratory dish with the sperm of the infertile woman's husband. The resulting embryos can then be transferred to the uterus of the patient without any eggs. Obviously the menstrual cycles of the donor and the recipient must be synchronized so that the latter's endometrium is at the right stage of development to accept and support a pregnancy at the time of implantation. The age of the donor greatly affects the success rate: If she is thirty years old and the recipient is forty, pregnancy occurs 40 percent of the time; if the donor is forty and the recipient is thirty, the pregnancy rate is only 10 percent.

Sources of donor eggs usually are relatives and close friends. With ultrasound-guided recovery of eggs, we now can gather eggs from well-meaning relatives with minimal risk, cost, and discomfort. Sometimes a sister, for instance, will undergo ovarian stimulation and egg retrieval to help her infertile sibling. The sister's eggs are aspirated via a hollow needle through the vagina and then fertilized in a laboratory dish with the sperm of her brother-in-law. The resulting embryos are transferred to the hormonally prepared endometrial nest of the infertile woman. Some clinics have donor eggs available from compensated, anonymous donors.

The reservations surrounding the use of donor eggs are discussed in chapter 17 of *Ethical Considerations of Assisted Reproductive Technologies*, dated November 1994. The Ethics Committee of the American Society for Reproductive Medicine considers all the pros and cons of this and the other ART procedures in this publication. It can be ordered from the ASRM, 2131 Magnolia Avenue, Suite 201, Birmingham, AL 35282-9990. In addition to ethical concerns, legal issues must be addressed. State laws vary. Hence, we always recommend that an infertile couple seek expert legal advice before attempting pregnancy with a donor egg.

The Host Uterus: Hope for Women Without a Uterus?

Some of our patients cannot have children because they continually abort. Others were born with no uterus or have had a hysterectomy at an early age. Still other women have medical contraindications to pregnancy, but are healthy enough to be parents. Nowadays such patients have the potential to become parents of biologically related children—as long as they have at least part of a functioning ovary.

Using IVF techniques, it is possible for a sister or a caring friend to carry the "infertile" couple's baby. The eggs of the woman without a uterus can be gathered under ultrasonic guidance. Her husband's sperm can be added to the eggs in a petri dish. If the eggs fertilize, they can be transferred to the uterus of the woman who has promised to carry the "infertile" couple's offspring. The child will be genetically related to the couple, not to the surrogate carrier—that is, unless the carrier is the biological mother's sister. Then, of course, the birth mother would be the baby's aunt!

The advantages of this arrangement are that the couple can have a genetically related baby and the carrier can give the gift of life. But there also are disadvantages. If the carrier bonds to the baby and refuses to give it to the couple—who in this case are its parents—a custody battle could follow. Once again state laws vary. The woman the infertile couple ask to carry their biological child must be a very trusted person indeed.

There are other concerns about using a host uterus. For example, could a woman be pressured into carrying her infertile sister's baby, especially since the infertile couple may have no other way of having a genetically related child? Is there a possibility that the baby carried by another woman might *not* belong to the infertile couple?

According to the Ethics Committee of the American Society for Reproductive Medicine: "It is possible that a surrogate might inadvertently become pregnant with her own partner, rather than with the transferred embryo. So that the contracting couple can avoid rearing the wrong child, human leukocyte antigen typing can be done to establish that they are the actual genetic parents of the child born to the gestational surrogate." The ASRM Ethics Committee discusses its reservations concerning the use of gestational surrogate mothers in chapter 24 of *Ethical Considerations of Assisted Reproductive Technologies* (see page 247).

Perhaps the greatest ethical dilemma surrounding all of the new reproductive technologies is deciding when to stop using them in attempting to help a patient become pregnant. If the woman has no ovaries, we can get eggs from someone else. If a patient has no uterus, we can borrow someone else's womb. If the husband's sperm won't fertilize his wife's egg, we can use donor sperm. Where do you stop? We think that physicians—with the help of their patients—have to accept the responsibility of setting some reasonable guidelines as to when to give up.

After all, infertility isn't a communicable or fatal disease. It may make people wish they were dead, and it may keep people from being created, but nobody has ever died from not getting pregnant. A few women have died, unfortunately, during the surgery to treat infertility. It is extremely rare, but it has happened. We feel that it is the doctor's responsibility to remind patients that the treatment of infertility is a 101 percent elective procedure. The sheriff isn't going to throw you in jail because you haven't produced an offspring.

Microscopic and Laser Surgery

Looking at the surgical field through a microscope and suturing with fibers finer than a human hair, doctors strive to improve the results of fertility surgery (see fig. 9.3). With dazzling light scalpels called lasers, microsurgeons can destroy disease while tissue only a few cells away from the laser's cutting beam remains undamaged. This pinpoint accuracy, which has reduced surgical trauma and bleeding, has revolutionized infertility surgery.

The "bloodless" carbon-dioxide (CO_2) laser, the one most commonly used in gynecological surgery, is never dull and always sterile. A powerful concentration of energy, laser light, unlike sunlight, is focused in one direction at one wavelength. Guided by a colored red laser, the CO_2 laser's invisible beam can be defocused to coagulate tissue and refocused to cut it. The laser can vaporize endometriosis and repair fallopian tubes damaged by pelvic infections and tubal sterilization procedures. Since bleeding is reduced, the operating field is easier to see. Swelling, adhesion formation, and infection are minimized. In selected cases, other lasers, such as the argon laser, the YAG laser, and KTP laser are used. Although I strongly feel that, in expert hands, the laser offers patients the best treatment, some outstanding microsurgeons think that microelectrocautery (surgery using electric current to cut and seal blood vessels) is equally effective.

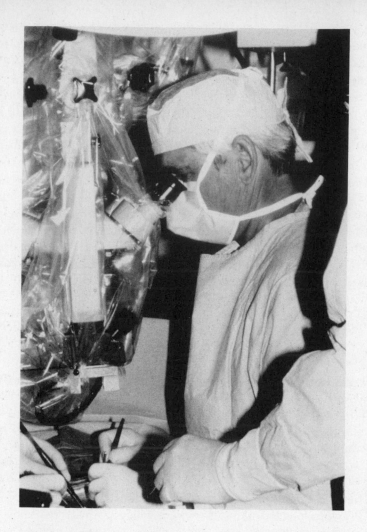

FIGURE 9.3. *Operating microscope used to perform microsurgery.*

Considering the recent stunning advances in infertility surgery and in "test-tube" fertilization, patients often ask me if they should have microsurgery to repair their damaged fallopian tubes or *in-vitro* fertilization and embryo transfer. The answer is: It depends entirely on the individual case!

Nowhere in medicine does treatment have to be more individualized than in this area. Often the choice of therapies is an extremely difficult judgment call. In general, the pregnancy rates after tubal microsurgery still are higher than with *in-vitro* fertilization. But on a case-by-case basis the success of surgery depends on the section of the tube affected and the degree of damage sustained. Even when the outsides of the tubes are damaged, if the insides are healthy, the pregnancy rate following surgery is 70 to 80 percent. If the tubes are damaged in several places, however, the pregnancy rate drops below 30 percent. If the fimbriated ends of both tubes have been destroyed by disease, the success rate is even lower.

The problem is that, even though the doctor does everything possible to prognosticate, it is difficult to predict the patient's postsurgical chances for pregnancy. The HSG X-ray, which shows how the oviducts dilate, gives some indication of tubal damage. But until the tubes are actually opened during surgery, the doctor can't accurately estimate what the patient's chances for pregnancy will be after tubal microsurgery (see chapter 3).

The disadvantage of tubal surgery is that, unless it can be done with the laparoscope, repair of the fallopian tubes requires major abdominal surgery. Unfortunately, this operation not only increases the chance of a uterine pregnancy, but it also increases the risk of an ectopic pregnancy in an oviduct. Although a pregnancy conceived with IVF can also end up in a tube after transfer, the risk is less than it is following tubal surgery.

One major advantage of microsurgical repair of the oviducts is that, if the tubal damage is "cured," the patient usually can have as many babies as she wants without further help. In other words, once repaired, the tube generally remains normal. With *in-vitro* fertilization, however, every time the patient with blocked tubes wants a child she has to go through the expensive IVF process. Even when IVF works, it may take several cycles for the embryo to implant. Nevertheless, when the potential pregnancy rate for a particular type of surgical repair approaches the rate for IVF, some patients may wish to try IVF first.

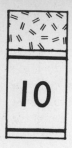

10

The Emotions of Infertility

SHERRY M. WILSON, M.S.W., AND
DOROTHY KAY BROCKMAN,
and introduced by Robert R. Franklin, M.D.

Introduction

There is no question that going through an infertility workup can be stressful. The tests and therapies designed to help infertile couples are hard work. Patients usually can tolerate focusing on trying to have a baby for only a limited time before their frustration builds to the point where they stop seeking medical help.

Although I get some of the most difficult cases, almost two-thirds of my patients deliver a baby. In fact, with the newer reproductive technologies, such as *in-vitro* fertilization and GIFT, that we covered in the previous chapter, the figure may run as high as 75 percent. Although this means nothing to the 25 to 30 percent who do not get pregnant, it does mean that the majority of patients undergoing an infertility workup have good reason to be optimistic.

Part of my job as an infertility specialist is to keep an eye on how the medical process is affecting my patient's emotional well-being. She needs to be able to open up and talk about her feelings. After all, optimal treatment includes reassurance. The doctor must try to guide her and her husband through this difficult process in a positive way. At times, every patient feels disappointed, frustrated, and sad that the baby hasn't arrived yet. When a patient shares her "baby blues" with me, I help her understand that it is normal to have brief periods of unhappiness during the infertility workup. Most patients regain their optimistic outlook when they balance their doubts about their ability to conceive with the hope offered by reproductive medicine.

For some patients, however, this is not the case. Over time, if the medical workup fails, patients can become depressed or compulsive about having a baby. If they are older, they may fear their time is running out. For them, a therapist such as Sherry Wilson can be extremely helpful. Therapy often enables a couple to confront their fears and sadness. This frees them not only to work positively toward their goal of pregnancy but also to return their attention to the other aspects of their lives.

For the minority of couples who go home without a baby, infertility is a tragedy. It is a loss—and one that is not easy to accept. When a patient leaves my care without a child in her arms after trying to conceive for years, it hurts. In fact, after working with infertile couples for almost thirty years, I still get angry and sad just thinking about the unfairness of infertility.

Even for a doctor used to dealing with infertility, the following chapter on the healing powers of grief is not easy to handle. I encourage my patients to be positive and hopeful. Sometimes, however, we have no choice but to come to grips with sadness so that the patient can continue through the infertility workup with renewed energy. When the medical workup fails, as it did in the following story about Linda and Will, the couple must accept the final diagnosis so that they can go forward with their lives. Unless they face the problem squarely, the hurt can fester deep inside them, causing untold emotional damage.

It was time for Linda and Will to come to grips with the truth: they probably would never have a baby. For seven difficult years they had tried everything medical science had to offer, including hormones to improve Will's sperm count, surgery to rid Linda's ovaries of endometriosis, and four unsuccessful attempts at *in-vitro* fertilization. Although Will's sperm fertilized many of Linda's eggs in a "test tube," none of the pre-embryos had implanted itself in her uterus.

Linda, a homemaker, was director of children's ministries at her church. She spent many hours working on educational projects for grade-school children. At first, this helped keep her mind off infertility. But as the years passed, and pregnancy seemed increasingly unlikely, working with other people's youngsters became an intolerable reminder of her own childlessness. One day, after a freckle-faced little boy threw his arms around her saying, "I love you! You remind me of my mommy!," Linda walked out of her church in tears. She didn't go back.

Linda desperately needed to talk about her growing unhappiness with someone, especially with her husband. But he was suffering from his own emotional pain and was unable to discuss his feelings with anyone. So much so that from the beginning he had adamantly insisted that they tell no one about their struggle to conceive—not even their parents or closest friends. As time passed, Will, a computer operator, became still more withdrawn, often working overtime in the evenings and all day Saturdays. This left Linda totally alone much of the time, giving her many hours to think about her inability to have a baby and her infertility workup.

Realizing that Linda was becoming increasingly depressed, I suggested that she and her husband have a visit with Sherry Wilson, a therapist who works with infertile couples. I wanted the couple to work through their feelings about infertility so that they could "come out on the other side" feeling closer to each other and good about themselves.

—Robert R. Franklin, M.D.

Stress and Infertility

Society has elaborate rituals to comfort the bereaved in death. Infertility is different. There is no funeral, no wake, no grave upon which to lay flowers. Family and friends may never even know. The infertile couple often grieves alone.

BARBARA ECK MENNING, *Infertility: Diagnosis and Management*

When a friend tells you that she has heart disease, you know that she and her family have suffered devastating emotional trauma and pain. Yet few people are aware of the overwhelming impact that the inability to have a child can have on a couple. Infertility, which strikes at the inner fiber of a person's being, can profoundly alter a couple's life by threatening their individual identities, mutual intimacy, and social interactions.

For a couple to cope with the emotional complexities of infertility, they must discern the roles that stress and grief are playing in their lives. They need to learn to balance these feelings with the hope that lies in every infertility case. To ignore the importance of handling stress and grief in a positive way can seriously jeopardize not only their medical prognosis but also their personal health and marital relationship.

External Stressors

Words are inadequate to describe the stress of infertility. As months of hoping for a baby turned into years of longing, Linda and Will were exposed to a continual barrage of stresses from the outside world.

The greatest external stressor was the medical workup. With their dream of a child at stake, it was necessary for them to expose the most personal aspects of their private lives to strangers. Although Dr. Franklin's medical team tried to be extremely sensitive to their feelings, no amount of tender loving care could completely alleviate the stress the couple felt about revealing the intimate details of their marriage. As Linda said: "We can tolerate the temperature charts, the pills, and the nuisance of all those doctors' appointments, but to have to tell people we hardly know how, when, and why we did 'it' is almost more than we can bear!"

The financial burden can be another source of stress. Infertility procedures are expensive. Linda and Will made major sacrifices to afford them. Hoping to achieve their ultimate dream, the couple postponed other goals such as plans for higher education and a home. Said Linda bitterly: "Our friends take trips to Hawaii while we take trips to the hospital."

Social situations also contributed to their stress; often those closest to the couple caused them the most heartache—usually unintended. Unfortunately, many of these stressors were intricately intertwined with the couple's life. Asked Linda: "How can I avoid Aunt Mary's questions and Mom's talk of grandchildren?"

And there was the outside world to contend with: the pregnant woman with three kids in the mall, the neighbor's baby shower, the men's locker-room jokes, and Will's cousin's pregnant teenage daughter were all reminders of the couple's pain. On the surface, the only alternatives appeared to be to "grin and bear it" or to isolate; but as I will discuss later, these were no options at all!

Internal Stressors

Internal stressors are the messages that a couple such as Linda and Will give themselves as a result of experiencing the external stressors. One of the most painful, stress-producing messages they inflicted upon themselves was: "I am a failure!" They expressed this in a variety of ways: "I am not a worthwhile woman." "I am not a real man." "I am being punished." "Without children we have no future together." "If I am not a parent, I am nothing."

These thoughts were reactions to the external stressors, but unfortunately the couple didn't understand this. Instead they mistakenly believed that the negative messages were facts about themselves. This led to more stress and an adverse effect on the marital relationship.

Said Linda: "We have spent all our money, yet we have no child. I feel I have failed Will, and he thinks he has failed me. He hurts so much, but he won't speak out. My ache is so deep that I no longer reach out. We are drifting apart. After all the pain, after all the disappointment, how will we ever become close to each other again?"

Linda and Will needed to manage their internal stressors—quickly and appropriately—or risk destroying their marriage. As we will discuss in detail, this management entailed facing the problem, experiencing and working through their grief, redirecting anger, learning crucial new communication skills, gaining a more accurate picture of themselves, and undergoing a process that therapists call "reframing."

How Infertility Can Cause Marital Stress

Although many marriages are strengthened during an infertility workup, the divorce rate is high among infertile couples, especially among those unable to share their feelings. Sexual relations, for example, can become an ordeal rather than a pleasure. As Dr. Franklin explained in the chapter on endometriosis, intercourse can be physically painful for some women with this disease. Until the husband understands his wife's pain, he may believe that she is rejecting him. Feeling hurt, the husband may pull away and focus on something other than his wife. It may be his work, a hobby, or another person. His withdrawal makes his wife feel unloved, creating a vicious cycle with no open avenues for intimacy.

Sometimes it is the husband who is unable to perform. Months of having intercourse because the woman's temperature indicates that she is ovulating can make the man feel like a sex object. When men first hear this, they grin and say: "Bring on the temperature chart. That will never happen to me." But when I see these same men after they have been struggling with infertility for a year or two, they often feel different. By this time, sex has become a test of performance that they fear they may fail. Unlike women, most men have never been treated like a sex object, and the thought is absolutely horrifying to them. In the privacy of my office, they will say: "I cannot tolerate the idea of sex. If I have to have sex on demand once more, I . . ."

When the husband becomes unable to perform on demand, he feels humiliated, ineffectual, and impotent. The fear of impotency threatens his masculinity, often becoming an obsession with him. It is normal for a man to be unable to perform occasionally; maybe he drank too much or was just exhausted. But if this happens over and over—at the "scheduled" time—it can stress the relationship.

When I see a couple "worn out" from their infertility and suspect that the marriage is suffering, I recommend a break. I say: "Let's think about a vacation from your medical workup. Put away that thermometer! Put away that temperature chart! Get back to discovering each other. Make love because you love each other. Forget about trying to have a baby for a while."

One woman replied: "But I'm thirty-seven years old. I am running out of time!"

I answered: "Let's talk about what it is going to cost both of you if you don't take a break. You are exhausted and, I sense, losing sight of each other in the process. Is the workup worth making you feel this way? Why not let up for a couple of months? You'll come back rested, renewed, and more in love. It's not worth gaining a baby if you lose each other in the process."

I believe that the major source of marital stress in infertility is the failure of couples to communicate. This certainly seemed to be a major part of Linda and Will's problem. Most couples will discuss their hopes, joys, and expectations with their partners, but far too many refuse to share their frustrations, pain, and fears. Often the motive for this is to "protect" the partner, but the end result is lack of communication, leading to feelings of isolation and rejection.

Rather than skirting the issue or ignoring it completely, Linda and Will needed to address their feelings and to share them with each other. A caring exchange of thoughts keeps unpleasant feelings from blocking each partner's desire to be supportive. Shared feelings are the foundation of emotional intimacy.

Once Linda and Will began communicating, they started seeing each other's point of view. Rather than inaccurately guessing what the other was thinking, each spouse began to learn the other's needs. This gave both partners an excellent opportunity to provide and to receive the support and nurturing so essential to coping with infertility. Rather than let infertility continue to drive them apart, they grew closer and more intimate by expressing their feelings. Their marriage grew stronger, and so did they.

Grief and Infertility

Infertility can put a couple on an emotional roller-coaster ride. One minute they are up and hopeful, and the next they are down and disappointed. Once the couple understand that this is an unfortunate but normal side effect of trying to overcome infertility, they tolerate it reasonably well, and at times even with a sense of humor. But if infertility persists, as it did for Linda and Will, the cycle may change; and the temporary "baby blues" can become more pervasive, propelling a couple into a deeper emotional state called "grief."

Ranging from unhappiness to deep, intense sorrow, grief is a cluster of emotions felt when we either anticipate or experience a loss. Most people resist facing their grief. As Linda and Will's therapist, I tried to help them see that grief is a normal, healthy bodily response not only to losing someone or something very dear but also to losing a dream. Indeed, grief is the body's natural healer of loss. As such, it must be experienced if we are to purge ourselves of the pain.

We grieve over actual losses, such as the death of a loved one or the loss of a significant relationship, a valued job, our home, or a pet. But we also grieve over the loss of our fantasies. In infertility, our dream is to have a child. It is the loss of that dream or its feared loss that pushes the infertile couple into the grieving state.

In infertility, loss is experienced two ways.

The first is through an identifiable loss such as a miscarriage, a stillborn baby, a hysterectomy, or the diagnosis of sterility. Once it is acknowledged, the infertile couple experience their feelings through grieving this loss and eventually go on with their lives.

The second way couples mourn the loss of their dream child is through anticipatory grief. This kind of grief is experienced in advance of a loss when it is feared to be inevitable. For Linda and Will, anticipatory loss began when their efforts to have a baby had been unsuccessful for a long time. The couple started to anticipate or fear that pregnancy would never happen. Their bodies sensed this fear and evoked grief to help heal their fear and pain. But since there was *not* an identified loss (as in miscarriage) or a diagnosed loss (as in hysterectomy), the couple thought that their grief was unfounded. As Linda told me: "Sometimes I think I must be crazy for feeling so unhappy and depressed." What she failed to understand was that the arrival of each menstrual period symbolized that her dream would not happen that month. As time passed, she began to worry that she would never have a child. This fear was in anticipation of a loss; hence anticipatory grief began—a process just as painful as a grief that has been identified.

One of my patients was describing anticipatory grief when she said: "I don't understand why I'm so sad all the time. All I do is cry. It's not as though I will never have kids; we just haven't been able to yet. My doctor is optimistic—why can't I be? I know that the majority of patients do get pregnant, but that doesn't seem to help. What is wrong with me?"

Regardless of whether grief is identified or anticipated, it must be experienced. It is by experiencing our feelings of grief that we help them go away. If we fail to do this, they linger, causing us more suffering. Since experiencing our grief can be a gut-wrenching process, we often try to protect ourselves from meeting sorrow head on. But by refusing to face our anguish, we get stuck in our misery, prolonging the agony— sometimes for the rest of our lives.

Once I identify a couple's emotional state as grief, I teach them the stages of grief. This helps them understand what they are feeling and why. They need to see grief as a normal healing process.

Stages of Grief

Grieving is a process, and as such it has predictable and universal stages regardless of what is being grieved. But no two people grieve in exactly the same way. Each of us has unique life experiences and coping styles that influence the way we feel. Regardless of our style of grieving, we all go through the same stages, although not in the same order, in the same way, or at the same pace. At first, almost everyone goes through the stages of shock and denial. How and when a person experiences the other stages depends entirely on previous experience with grief and other life circumstances. Consider the five most common stages of grief:

I. SHOCK AND DENIAL: "NOT ME!"

Almost every couple is stunned to discover that they have a fertility problem. As Linda told me: "We had no idea that we wouldn't be able to have a baby—no one in either of our families has ever had this problem."

Since our bodies will not tolerate shock for long, we move into denial. This stage is important because it gives the couple time—if they are willing—to accept the problem and to develop the internal and external resources needed to cope with infertility. Said one patient: "We refused to believe we had a problem. As soon as we left the doctor's office, we began discussing with close friends what the doctor had said. They gave us the comfort and support we needed before we could face another doctor. After a while, when no pregnancy occurred, we quit denying the problem and sought help. By this time, however, the diagnosis wasn't so painful to hear." Through verbalizing their shock and disbelief, the couple were able to move out of this stage of grief.

Some people will avoid telling anyone about the problem but will quickly get a second opinion. Confirmation of the original diagnosis also helps a couple pass through the denial stage. As they learn more about the problem, they no longer deny its existence.

II. ANGER: "WHY ME?"

Anger is probably the most common response to any situation in which a person feels misunderstood, unfairly treated, or abused. Infertility causes all of these insults. Infertile patients often are extremely misunderstood; infertility is grossly unfair; and the body and mind feel abused by the endless medical testing and emotional stress. Sooner or later, anger develops in response to all of these unpleasant circumstances.

The first anger an infertile couple experience is what I call the "Why me?" response. Said Will: "Why me? When so many people can and often shouldn't have a baby!" This anger is compounded after the couple do everything humanly possible but no pregnancy occurs. Sometimes the anger borders on rage.

Anger often gets directed away from "Why me?" to "Why you?" Anyone who is a reminder of the couple's infertile state becomes the target of their anger. This includes the doctors, the nurses, friends, family members, and the "pregnant world" at large.

Sometimes God is the recipient of the couple's anger. Linda felt ignored or abandoned by God, in that her prayers had not been answered. She felt that she didn't deserve her fate, because she had been devout in her faith. Will wondered if God was punishing him for some past "evil" thought or deed. He felt that, if God was so angry with him, he could be angry with God too! But this reaction made him feel even more abandoned and hopeless.

In my experience, the greatest and most harmful anger is not at God (God can take it) but at the spouse or at the self. Anger toward one's mate needs to be discussed, but unfortunately it rarely is. Instead the anger gets "acted out." Will's behavior said, "I am not happy with you," but his anger was never openly examined until he started therapy. It is not unusual for an irate spouse to become silent and withdrawn. This is when he or she may get overinvolved in work, a hobby, TV, reading— or another person. All of these indirect methods of expressing anger jeopardize the marriage. The longer the anger remains unresolved, the greater the damage to the marriage.

When the anger of infertility is directed against the self, individuals can become enraged with themselves. They are continually haunted by self-abusive thoughts such as: I'm an idiot for not seeing the doctor sooner; I'm paying for having an abortion; or, as Linda said: "I'm worthless to my mate if I can't have a baby." Such thoughts, of course, are irrational. Whatever happened in the past may have been the best solution to the problem at that time. Self-directed anger can cloud one's memory. Patients may ridicule themselves so severely that self-esteem falls, leaving only an overwhelming sense of failure.

III. BARGAINING: "IF I DO THIS, SURELY I'LL BECOME PREGNANT."

Bargaining is an agreement, usually made with God by a desperate individual, to do something good in exchange for a pregnancy. The person is attempting to gain control of a situation in which she feels totally out of control. Sadly, however, the more the individual bargains, the more out of control she feels, because the "good deed" seldom produces the desired result—a child.

As Linda said in tears: "I promised God that I'd do volunteer work, become a Sunday-school teacher, and a whole lot more. For years, I faithfully kept my part of the bargain, but I was not rewarded. I'm not pregnant; I'm exhausted. I did my part—why doesn't God do His?"

IV. DEPRESSION: "NOTHING WORKS; I FEEL HOPELESS AND HELPLESS!"

As a couple move through their infertility workup without a pregnancy, they start to feel hopeless, helpless, and desperate. Eventually they begin to believe that there are no positive options. They may see no hope.

Many couples refer to this stage as the "black hole." For some, this is a temporary period of depression brought on by the arrival of menstruation, by negative test results, or by some other setback. After a few days, the couple pull themselves out of the "hole" by looking forward to the next cycle or by turning their attention elsewhere.

As time passes, however, the depression can become overwhelming for some patients. For Linda and Will, months of pulling out of the "hole," only to be thrown in again the following month, had a wearing-down effect. Gradually the couple lost their resilience. Lacking the mental energy to develop new options, they became depressed and needed professional help to learn effective coping skills.

V. ACCEPTANCE: "WE HAVE A FERTILITY PROBLEM."

The final stage of grieving is acceptance. I believe couples reach this stage when they no longer need to protect themselves from the pain of infertility. For Linda and Will, this was when they could finally openly say: "Yes, we have a fertility problem and it hurts—it hurts a lot."

Acceptance does not mean that the heartache is gone but, rather, that it is managed—and managed in a way that is healthy for them as individuals and as a couple. In the acceptance stage one can say: "Yes, infertility hurts. I desperately wanted a baby. But I can live with the pain. It doesn't control me—I can cope with it." This is acceptance; this is resolution.

Secondary Infertility: Stress and Grief

The feelings of couples struggling with secondary infertility (the inability to have more than one child) are often slighted. Since they have a child, people tend to think that these patients feel only mild disappointment or frustration. This simply is not so! Not every couple wants more than one child, but for those who do, secondary infertility causes the same stress-and-grief reaction as primary infertility. Some women with secondary infertility may suffer less from a feeling of failure because they have proved to themselves that they can conceive. In my experience, however, they are in the minority. Most of these patients also seem to feel a sense of failure. They grieve as deeply as the woman who never gives birth, because they too feel the loss of their dream.

One of my patients with secondary infertility described her sadness this way: "I love my child—but I dreamed of having four children. It hurts to think I'll only have one, yet I can't talk about this pain. If I do, everyone says that I'm not grateful for the one I have. Believe me, I am—but what do I do when my heart aches for the others I will never have?"

Therapy for secondary infertility is exactly the same as for primary infertility. It involves managing stress in a productive manner and learning positive coping skills. If a pregnancy does not occur for a long time, the focus needs to be on handling anticipatory grief. This helps the couple as they work their way through the medical infertility procedures.

If the final diagnosis indicates the probability of no more biological children, I guide the couple through their grieving process. We re-examine their fantasy of more children. Eventually they are able to say goodbye to their dream of two children, a white house with a picket fence, and a Ford station wagon. Only when they grieve their loss will they be able to go on to new dreams.

Special Issues in Infertility

Identity Problems and Feelings of Failure

Even today, despite all the career options available to women, society still places a premium on a woman's role as a mother. Although Linda was successful in other areas, she was continually bombarded with the idea that she must be a mother. Ignoring her significant accomplishments, she measured her self-worth by her ability to have a child.

Much of our identity centers on the roles we assume. When an infertile woman thinks that her main purpose in life is to be a mother, she will have an enormous problem dealing with her childlessness. Even though she may be extremely successful in her other roles as a businesswoman, church worker, wife, lover, homemaker, and friend, she may feel like a "nobody" without children. For this woman, the inability to have a child is more than a medical diagnosis; it is a judgment sentencing her to hell. Said Linda: "If I can't have children, I have no value to my husband or myself. I am worthless."

Although I see more women overtly struggling with these self-defeating feelings than men, it would be unfair to say that the problem is only a female-related issue. Men also can feel a tremendous sense of failure if pregnancy is difficult to achieve, especially if the medical problem lies with them.

Even so, a man's emotional reaction to infertility is usually different from a woman's. There are exceptions, but a man's feelings of failure are not as overtly encompassing—infertility is not an "all-or-nothing" situation to him. To cope with his feelings of disappointment, he tends to lose himself in other endeavors. Whereas an infertile woman's sense of failure may paralyze her emotionally, a man's feelings often drive him compulsively to work harder in the other areas of his life.

Feelings of Isolation

In a world that values parenthood, infertile couples feel alone and different; Linda and Will were often the only couple at the picnic or the family reunion without children. Eventually they began to feel as if they did not belong in this parent-oriented society; they felt abandoned and isolated.

Isolation, a feeling brought on by a reaction to a specific stimulus or situation, can be either healthy or unhealthy, depending on when and why the couple withdraw. When used as a nurturing retreat until a person is better able to cope, isolation is healthy. I frequently tell my patients: "Don't go to that baby shower or party if you cannot handle it at this time. Be good to yourself! Nurture yourself until you can work through this period and feel stronger."

Sometimes, however, the couple isolate themselves indefinitely in order to hide from the pain of infertility. Like Will, they may be unable to share their problem even with those closest to them. Therapy helped him see that this was unhealthy. He said: "I have been living in an emotional closet because I haven't wanted anyone to know that we can't have a baby. I just couldn't face all of those prying questions."

Linda and Will had separated themselves from those who loved them. They had been unable to work through the pain and break out of the isolation without therapy. By hiding their struggle with infertility, they had set themselves up for annoying statements such as: "When are you going to start your family?" Or "Is something wrong with you two?" Continuing to isolate without support led to depression.

Unsuccessful Coping Mechanisms

Most people are guided by the following set of worthwhile values:

1. Dreams are accomplished through hard work.
2. Do right and life will treat you right.
3. There is justice in this world.

These ideals say that, if we work hard enough and do right by our fellow man, we will get our just rewards. Although such values may hold true in many aspects of our lives, they do not help us cope with infertility.

Most childless couples work hard, doing everything they can to have a baby, but sometimes their dream still does not come true. Justice does not prevail. There is no just reason, there is no sane reason why the woman cannot get pregnant. When Linda asked me, "Why should this happen to me?," I could not come up with one logical reason. It just happens.

The important values that governed the rest of Linda and Will's lives were not helping them deal with their childlessness. In order to survive their infertility experience, they had to learn new coping skills. This wasn't easy, but eventually they did it.

Unresolved Past Experiences

Until handled, unresolved feelings about crises from the past can resurface at any time, causing anguish and pain. In infertility, I see several such unsettled life experiences reappearing again and again. They are feelings associated with the person's childhood, with a previous parenting experience, or with an unwanted pregnancy. These ghosts from the past—which lie dormant, waiting to reappear as anger, rage, depression, or other emotions—can drive the knife of infertility deeper.

A previous abortion that has not been resolved can be one of the most painful memories that an infertile patient has to face. She often will need therapy to help her examine and resolve her feelings about this issue. A therapist will try to determine whether such a patient sees her infertility as a punishment. If so, she needs to reconsider the circumstances surrounding the abortion. It is important for her to resolve her guilt so that she can avoid carrying it into another pregnancy, thus averting possible serious emotional conflict for herself, her husband, and her future baby.

The woman needs to understand that abortion is a loss and must be grieved in order to heal the pain. Often the first feeling after an unwanted pregnancy is terminated is relief. But even though the abortion seemed the right choice for the woman at a particular time in her life, she usually regrets that things couldn't have been different. I have never talked with a woman who didn't have some buried pain after an abortion. Sometimes it surfaces months or years later. She may see a stranger's toddler and think: My baby would be that age, or: My baby would have huge blue eyes like that little girl. Ignoring the sadness does not make it go away—the hurt is just shoved back. There is a fantasy child.

Every pregnancy is unique, with its own set of issues and emotions. These need to be understood and experienced before another pregnancy is created. Once a past abortion is grieved, the woman is free to attempt a new pregnancy. If she conceives, her joy doesn't have to be shared with the sadness of an unhappy or unresolved past experience.

Abortion can greatly affect how a woman feels about herself. The negative messages she gives herself because of a past abortion need to be examined. Once these feelings are resolved, she can enter into a new pregnancy feeling good about herself and her ability to be a mother.

Special Problems of the Husband

Although men generally react differently to emotional crises than women, this doesn't mean that men don't hurt or that infertility doesn't bother them. How unfair such assumptions are to men.

Men care! Men hurt! Men cry! But, unlike women, men don't always get the opportunity to show their emotions in public. Sometimes they won't take the chance even in private. Just because a man doesn't cry, stay home from work, or hate all pregnant women doesn't mean that he is insensitive. Men tend to grieve silently and alone. They usually don't let their emotions surface, nor do they seek comfort and support as easily as women do. Not because men don't need it, but because they have been taught that "it is not OK."

Unlike many infertile women, who see themselves mainly in the role of mother, men tend to base their identity on other roles in addition to that of parent. Nevertheless, if the medical problem is within his body, a man's sense of masculinity can be deeply affected. A woman who is unable to bear children is still considered extremely feminine. A man, however, too often feels unmasculine if he cannot initiate a pregnancy. This view of masculinity is changing—and it certainly should be—but it is still a powerful force in the mind of today's male.

To resolve the pain of infertility, the male needs to be willing to discuss his feelings regarding his sense of masculinity. For Will, this was so frightening that he suffered in silence for years, denying the impact of infertility rather than asking for help. Until he gained a clearer understanding of the true definition of masculinity, his self-esteem and marriage suffered.

A man's feelings concerning his sexuality are closely tied to his sense of masculinity. When sex is constantly "demanded" rather than "desired," most men sooner or later experience temporary impotence. This can be embarrassing, humiliating, and painful unless both partners understand that it is often a side effect of the infertility workup. The husband needs to be able to discuss his feelings openly with an understanding wife. Otherwise it is too easy for the husband to start doubting or questioning his sexuality. When this happens, his self-esteem drops, often creating emotional problems. This leads some men to feel the need to "prove" their sexuality and masculinity in ways that are potentially harmful to the marriage.

Therapy can help a man see his masculinity, sexuality, and infertility in the right perspective. When Will finally looked at the way he had been taught from childhood to handle emotions, he decided to make changes that brought him comfort, support, and a sense of freedom. Therapy helped him develop a sense of intimacy with Linda that he could never have had as long as the "old" messages ruled his life. Said Will during therapy: "This is the first time in my life that I have been able to talk about my feelings. It is the greatest feeling in the world. I'm so free! Finally, I can say what I'm thinking; I can ask for what I need. Infertility still hurts, but it doesn't have the same power over me. I feel better about myself and closer to Linda."

Bizarre Reasons for Seeking an Infertility Workup

Several patients have come to Dr. Franklin seeking an infertility workup while trying to *avoid* pregnancy! Psychologists think a woman does this to punish her husband. Her anger toward him often stems from some mental or physical injury inflicted by a male during her childhood.

When no reason for "infertility" can be found, the woman blames her childlessness on her husband, using it as a sword to wound him psychologically. Becoming compulsive about sexual relations, she insists on intercourse in the middle of her cycle while secretly taking birth-control pills. Her goal is not only to make her husband feel guilty for being unable to father a child, but also eventually to make him impotent. If the doctor fails to perceive what is happening, the husband can be devastated.

As unbelievable as this is, it does happen, and the infertility specialist has to be aware of the signs that point to the problem. How a husband and wife treat each other often gives important clues as to whether they really want a baby.

Sometimes it is the husband who has the psychological problems. A few men let their wives go through major surgery and, when the woman's chances of pregnancy are increased, ask for a divorce. Some of these men never intended to father a child—their reason for paying for an expensive infertility workup was to punish their wives!

Coping with Infertility

Much More Than Their Reproductive Process

When a couple are infertile, it is because their reproductive process is failing, not because they are failures. Their totality is infinitely more than one biological process within their bodies. I try to move a couple away from the false feeling that there is something wrong with either of them as a human being or as a total person. What is wrong is a physical process. But in order for them to accept this, they have to develop a correct sense of themselves—they must realize that they are far more than just their ability to conceive.

When I draw a pie and cut it into wedges, a couple can see that their reproductive process represents only one slice of their lives. Think of the pie as the person's whole being and of procreation as only one slice. When infertility dominates the couple's lives, they sometimes think that, since the reproductive wedge is failing, all the other slices are insignificant. There is no denying that procreation is extremely important, but their totality goes far beyond their ability to reproduce. If couples are to cope with infertility, they must get it into perspective.

Positive Stress Management

Positive stress management does not entail punching some busybody in the nose—even though it may be tempting. Nor does it mean working constantly, eating excessively, swallowing pills, or gulping alcohol.

To cope well with infertility, a couple must learn to manage their stress in a positive way, and they must allow themselves to grieve. This is much harder than it sounds.

There are three ways to manage stress successfully.

First, exercise. This has a wonderful tension-reducing effect. Physical exercise, which helps us shed the outer layer of stress, rejuvenates the body, giving us more energy to deal with our problems. But exercise alone is not enough.

Second, try to alter the external stressors that are causing the problem. This generally means talking more rather than less with close friends and family in order to receive the kind of support required.

Sometimes a couple may need to avoid a particular family gathering or supper club until they feel stronger. They might decide to read more, to attend workshops, or to become involved in an infertility support group such as Resolve, Inc. Whatever form of stress management they use, the infertile couple can and should face the external stressors and manipulate them to their benefit. When they feel more in control of what they can regulate—their own actions—their stress will be reduced. (This also may mean that couples might choose to stop their medical workup temporarily, in order to get the stress under control. This is *not* failing; this is taking care of themselves and constitutes positive stress management.)

Finally, when the external stressors cannot be changed—and many of them cannot—the meaning we give them must be changed. For Linda and Will, this entailed taking a hard look at infertility and altering the internal messages they had about the situation. Since they were unable to change the problem, they had to alter the significance they gave it in order to reduce their stress. This was done through a process called "reframing."

Reframing is changing a thought or a belief from a negative to a positive or at least to a more acceptable form. In order to reframe, we must discover the origins of our negative messages, even though this can be painful. We have to be open to suggestions, to consider other points of view, and to explore new options.

Changing the recurrent message "I am a failure" to "The infertility workup is failing, but I am not" is an example of reframing. For people who have difficulty doing this, a professional can help identify the negative messages and reframe them so that infertility can be seen more positively.

When the medical infertility workup continues for many months with no success, a good therapist can help the couple stay positively focused. This can go a long way toward reducing stress. Once tension is minimized, as Dr. Franklin discusses later in this book, the chances for conception increase!

Grief: A Step Toward Recovery

Although a couple will feel better when stress is handled positively, its management does not rid them of their need to grieve. Coping with loss means that the couple have to grieve periodically—a process most of us tend to avoid if at all possible.

A childless couple needs to realize that grief—the body's natural healer of an emotional loss—will help them take an important step toward recovery. Our bodies heal naturally from a wound by sending in the blood: the red cells, the white cells, and the platelets. We heal emotionally by slowly letting ourselves feel our sorrow.

Grieving is our right, but to be successful, it has to be experienced openly, unashamedly, and without guilt. It must be worked through in its totality—every feeling of every stage needs expression. It must not be hidden deep inside the heart. To allow ourselves to feel only part of our sorrow is like taking only half the medicine. Recovery takes twice as long if it happens at all.

For grieving to be successful, it must be shared with another person. This is the key to healing. If we are unable to share our unhappiness, all our emotions and negative messages stay bottled up within us, causing more pain than the situation demands. When we are not able to communicate our feelings, we become cut off from those we need the most. Alone and paralyzed by the pain, we stagnate in our misery, unable to focus on all the marvelous options that life has to offer.

With whom do we share our grief? With our partner first. As I told Linda and Will: "You wouldn't dream of excluding your mate from your joy. Neither should your spouse miss the sorrow."

It is in communicating our vulnerability and our pain that we lay the building blocks of intimacy. When both partners share their grief, they tend to go through infertility together, usually growing closer and becoming more intimate. Even sorrow can help a couple grow when it is shared within the marriage. It is not that the hurt will disappear, but that the bond of understanding and affection deepens. As we learn to understand each other's pain, we can pass through each crisis in a positive way—no matter what the outcome.

The problem is that often each spouse suffers through the pain of infertility alone. When a husband and wife feel isolated from each other, they can drift apart. Sadly, many couples fail to share their pain with each other because they get stuck with: It is his problem; it is her problem; it is my problem. As one infertility patient said: "I told everybody that I had major surgery for endometriosis. I could sense that my husband didn't want people to think that he had a problem. I could handle it. He couldn't. After all, it wasn't my fault."

I helped this woman understand that infertility is a "we" problem, not a "his" or "her" problem. The therapist needs to move the couple away from concentrating on whether the physical problem is with the male or female. A couple are like a lock and key. They fit together. Whether there is something wrong with the fallopian tubes, the ovaries, or the sperm count, reproduction is their process.

Unfortunately, some people refuse to allow themselves to grieve. They cannot share their pain. When Will first started therapy, he said: "I don't want to think about it. I just want it behind me so I can go on." For years he had tried to ignore it, refusing to face his unhappiness. But the ache continued to burn deep within him, making him emotionally fragile. This was *not* resolving grief—this was getting *stuck* in grief.

Whereas at one time he could handle large problems, eventually little ones upset him. His hurt became rechanneled into anger to the point where he was increasingly withdrawn and occasionally verbally abusive toward Linda.

Conditioned to express feelings from childhood, Linda wanted to share her grief with Will, but he was unable to listen. Like many men, he had been conditioned to be "strong and silent," like John Wayne. Henry Ford summed up this approach when he said: "Don't complain; don't explain." This may work for men in business or poker—but it can hurt a marriage struggling with infertility. Silence not only blocks marital intimacy but also denies the male the relief he needs from his pain.

Therapy helped Linda and Will face infertility together by letting them look at their coping styles as individuals and as a couple. As I began to understand each spouse's grieving style, I worked to bring them closer together, so that they could make allowances for their differences. In time, Linda began to understand that her husband also had grief, but that he had been conditioned to deal with it differently. In time, Will was able to share some of his pain with Linda. Together they began to realize that the way feelings were handled in their childhood families was not working in their marriage—that they needed to develop new ways of handling problems that would work for both of them.

By the time Linda and Will finished therapy, they understood that an extremely complex problem such as infertility requires not only careful fine tuning of the bodily processes but also positive stress management and a continual fine tuning of the grieving process.

Developing Communication Skills

EXPRESSING

Good communication skills are absolutely essential in order to cope with infertility. It was the responsibility of Linda and Will to let people know how they wanted to be treated. I tell my patients that communication is more than just talking—parrots can do that. On the other hand, it's also more than staying quiet—the dead do that! Instead good communication involves two processes: expressing and listening.

To express ourselves clearly, we have to give a "whole" message. In their book *Messages: The Communications Skills Book*, Matthew McKay, Martha Davis, and Patrick Fanning define a whole message as one that includes four important parts. These are: what we observe, what we think, what we feel, and what we need. All of these pieces of the message must be included for effective communication.

According to these authors, if we fail to include every part of the message, we confuse our listeners. They will sense that something is missing, but won't know what. When listeners are confused and unable to respond appropriately, speakers fail to get their needs met.

Infertile couples often communicate what the problem is and what they think about it, but they don't always let their listeners know the other important parts of the message—what they feel and what they need. Consider the incomplete message that Linda gave Will every month: "I started my period today. I don't think I'll ever get pregnant!" This message included what Linda observed and what she thought about it, but not what she felt or needed.

Now consider the complete message: "I started my period today. I don't think I'll ever get pregnant! I feel miserable and hopeless." Going to her husband, she continues: "I just need to be held close and told that everything will be OK."

In the second example, Linda is much more likely to be understood and comforted, because she communicated the entire message. She didn't wait to see if her husband could read her mind. Instead she told him what she needed, and she got it.

In the first example, Will couldn't be certain what to do to help his wife. The response to incomplete communication often is to say nothing rather than risk doing the wrong thing. By not effectively communicating her needs, Linda was left with her pain.

An infertile couple need to pick their listeners carefully; to be helpful, listeners must be interested and caring. Not every relationship or encounter requires a whole message. The mailman and grocery clerk obviously didn't need to know about Linda's infertility problem, nor did they require complete messages. The more important the problem and the more significant the relationship, the greater the need to use whole messages when expressing oneself.

LISTENING

Listening, according to the authors of *Messages*, is not just keeping your mouth shut and your ears open. Listening, whether to your spouse or to a friend, is a commitment and a compliment. The commitment involves carefully trying to understand what the speaker is saying. This means temporarily putting aside your own thoughts, feelings, and needs in order to see the situation from the speaker's point of view. This kind of listening is a compliment to your speaker because it says: "I care about you and I want to understand your view of the problem as much as my own."

Once Linda and Will started really listening to each other in an open, caring manner and each started delivering whole messages in the same way, both began to have their needs met. This also helped their relationships with caring friends and relatives.

Redirecting Anger

Anger is an important part of grieving. For Linda and Will to cope with infertility, they needed to express their anger. First they had to pinpoint what was making them so unhappy. Occasionally their displeasure was directed at medical professionals, other times at friends, family members, or co-workers. Each situation needed to be examined carefully so that the anger could be understood and appropriately resolved. Although infertile couples often have good reasons to be angry with people, most of their anger is really at the problem of infertility. Recognizing this, however, can be difficult for couples. It is much easier to be upset with the doctor or a pregnant teenager than to be angry with something as abstract as an infertility problem. I tried to help Linda and Will interpret their anger so that they could redirect it away from the person to the problem. Once they were able to do this, they began to find peace and resolution, because they could express their feelings.

One infertile man came to see me because he was extremely angry with his brother and an adoption agency. He said: "I saw my kid brother and his pregnant wife today. When he said, 'Hi, how are you?,' I felt like saying, 'Go to hell. . . . I don't want to talk with you.' "

I helped this patient realize that he was angry at the problem (his infertility), not at his brother. After trying to father a child for four years, my patient was hurt because at age thirty-three he had not succeeded in doing what his brother had done at age nineteen. Therapy helped him understand the source of his anger. Eventually he was able to say to his little brother: "I have shut you out of my life. I've shunned you and I've ignored you. And it wasn't anything you did. I'm sorry. I miss you and the great times we used to have together."

When this same patient and his wife were going through adoption proceedings, he came to see me one day and said: "I don't know what is wrong with me. When the social worker left my house, I was livid. I hate her, but I don't know why, because she told us that she liked us. Everything went perfectly. I know that we are in. Why am I so angry?"

I said, "What are you having to do?"

"I am having to pass approval to get a child, when most people just have one anytime they want . . . and sometimes when they don't."

I asked: "Are you really angry at the social worker or at the situation?"

He paused, looked at the floor, and said: "You're right. I'm angry at the problem, not at the person."

This patient had succeeded in redirecting his anger away from the person back to where it belonged—at the problem. By doing so, he felt better about himself and his relationships with other people.

When Infertility Becomes an Obsession

Sometimes the slice of life called "baby" takes over a couple's thoughts to the exclusion of everything else. This happens for several reasons, depending on the person's history and on the powerful messages he or she carries from childhood—the "tapes" that say, for example: "I must be a mother. Whatever I set out to do I must accomplish, no matter what!"

If the woman fails to get pregnant, ultimately one of three things happens: The couple adopt a child; they pursue a purposeful life without children; or they become obsessed with trying to have a baby.

The purpose of a compulsion or an obsession is to avoid feeling. What the infertile person is shunning is the fear that she may never conceive: And then what? What does that say about me? How does that affect our life together? These questions evoke so much dread for some people that they become compulsive about infertility.

Stuck in grief, these patients need to share the problem with a professional counselor. Sharing grief and being obsessive are not the same thing. When grief is shared, there is knowledge, support, and insight, so that the couple are able to move forward. When patients become obsessive about infertility, they talk—but they fail to listen or to grow. They refuse to reframe in order to tolerate the negatives of the experience.

I try to help couples look at the reasons for their obsession. These are usually found by looking at the origins of their internal stressors, which I discussed earlier. They are obsessive about conceiving because they don't want to face their fear of what it means to each of them as a person if they cannot have a child. They need to examine their negative internal messages so that they can put them in the proper perspective.

To help infertile Linda and Will see their lives more clearly, I said: "Yes, infertility hurts. How do you live with this?" Then I asked them to draw the slice of the pie of life that was called "grief" or "baby." I asked: "Is it consuming your life?" When they saw the huge chunk of their being that their sadness represented—that they had lost the other aspects of their lives—they began to understand why they were compulsive about trying to have a baby. Facing and letting go of an obsession is hard work—but absolutely essential if a couple are to endure successfully and even grow from the infertility experience.

If the Medical Workup Fails

When the best medical minds tell you that you probably will never become pregnant, you are stunned by the vast loss: you cannot have a baby. You think to yourself: All those years that we worried about protecting against pregnancy. This cannot be happening.

Before you can go forward with your life, you must resolve the past. You have the right to say goodbye to a dream—to what Barbara Eck Menning calls "the loss of a potential."

Without therapy, it is sometimes difficult to find the positives in the infertility process. It seems like such a bleak, bitter experience. Even time cannot totally dissolve the lump in our throats. But when couples walk down the long, hard road of infertility arm in arm, they can think back on their pain and say: My God, that was a difficult time; we never got our baby and it hurts—even now. But with the love of those who cared, as we faced our grief together, we uncovered the powerful current of courage flowing deep within us; and with a deeper insight and commitment, we grew stronger.

As one childless woman said: "We looked our loss straight in the eye, we saw our agony reflected in each other's glance, and for a fleeting instant—a forever memory—we were one."

Goodbye is never easy. It is uncomfortable. We do not like it, but sometimes we have to say it.

"Grief closes the door behind us so that we can open the one ahead."

Linda and Will eventually decided to apply for adoption. Today they have new dreams. With a three-month-old daughter in their arms and a freckle-faced boy in training pants, the couple are too busy to think about a less happy time.

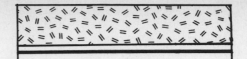

Part IV

Alternative Solutions

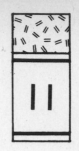

Artificial Insemination by Donor (AID)

LARRY I. LIPSHULTZ, M.D., AND
DOROTHY KAY BROCKMAN

> *The couple is ready for [artificial] insemination only if*
> *they view the child not as a product of AID, but as a*
> *product of their marriage.*
>
> LORI ANDREWS, *New Conceptions*

Many couples whose infertility is caused by a male factor that cannot be cured have turned to artificial insemination by donor (AID) to start their families. During a simple procedure, which usually takes place in a doctor's office, the wife of the infertile man is inseminated with sperm from an anonymous donor. Using a syringe, the doctor, his assistant, or the woman's husband places the sperm into the wife's vagina and cervical canal. If she becomes pregnant, the husband in essence "adopts" the donor's sperm. Other, less common indications for AID are Rh blood-type incompatibility, in which the mother makes antibodies capable of destroying fetal blood cells; proven genetic errors in the husband; a recessive gene for a genetic disease such as Tay-Sachs; or possibly immunological infertility in which the wife makes antibodies against her husband's sperm.

Since the wife often has no known fertility problems and the donor's semen has been screened for fertility potential, the success rate of AID equals the pregnancy rate of the fertile population. Approximately 70 to 80 percent of couples using AID conceive, and about 75 percent of them do so during the first six cycles.

279

The Emotional Impact of AID

The majority of couples who have a baby with the help of AID are happy with their families. In fact, most couples decide to have more than one child this way. Nevertheless, before proceeding with AID, all medical avenues should be investigated, and both the husband and wife should be convinced that artificial insemination is the best solution to their infertility. It is important that each family member has confidence that the other enthusiastically supports the decision to use donor sperm; neither partner should feel pressured to agree to the AID process just to please the other. In some cases, the religious background of an individual may affect his or her attitude toward AID. The Catholic Church opposes it, although people of many religious faiths often make this decision for themselves. If the couple are unable to communicate their feelings, professional counseling may help them bring their expectations and anxieties about AID out in the open. Although deciding to use AID can be an emotionally charged issue for a couple to face, once they finally decide to use donor sperm most people appear to cope with the AID process quite well.

Couples who spend months making this decision are best prepared for the emotional impact of the AID process. They have a much lower divorce rate than the national average. Although the divorce rate among infertile couples is high, the marriage of a couple who use AID has already been tested and often grows stronger. Such couples realize that their relationship is built on much more than whether both parties contribute the genetic material for a baby. Thoughtful consideration of the true meaning of parenthood has enabled many infertile men to see that, in the long run, caring for and loving a child is what builds the bond of love between a father and his son or daughter.

Donor Selection

Couples considering AID have many questions concerning the screening and selection of the donor. It is important that they have confidence in their doctor, and that they have an opportunity to discuss the AID process with him in detail. Couples are often most concerned about the donor's health and intelligence. Frequent questions are: How do you know that the donor is fertile? Has he been tested for sexually transmitted diseases such as AIDS (acquired immune-deficiency syndrome), gonorrhea, syphilis, herpes, hepatitis B, and chlamydia? Has the donor been screened for genetic diseases? Do his physical characteristics resemble the husband's? What is his educational background? Will his identity be kept anonymous? How many AID children has he fathered? Whose name will be put on the father's line on the birth certificate?

In order for a man to donate sperm, his semen analysis must indicate that his sperm have a good chance of initiating a pregnancy. Generally a semen specimen of at least fifty million sperm per cubic centimeter and a motility of 70 to 80 percent with good forward progression meets the AID requirements. By using semen that meets these criteria, we can ensure that more than 95 percent of selected donors will initiate a pregnancy.

Medical students, residents, and other doctors have traditionally been chosen as sperm donors because they tend to be of above-average intelligence, reliable, and available. My nurse and I interview each potential donor to try to determine if he is stable. His identity remains anonymous.

Why do men donate sperm? Usually it is because they need the money that is paid per specimen. Many are going through medical school and are on a tight budget. Some of them may contribute because they want to help someone else.

When a potential donor responds to an appeal to give sperm, he is asked to fill out a historical-information sheet. He describes his hobbies, interests, and background. The donor's medical history, which is reported by him, and his physical examination are of utmost importance. He is questioned about his family health history and is asked to answer a genetic questionnaire. Any known hereditary illness will disqualify him as a donor. Our AID program includes genetic testing (karyotyping) of the donor, because one person in 150 carries a chromosomal abnormality. Karyotyping won't pick up every genetic disease, but such testing does identify a possible donor's risk of passing on some of the major ones. Not all AID programs do this type of testing, because it is expensive; many rely on the donors' medical history to eliminate men with genetic diseases.

If the potential donor's medical history qualifies him to donate sperm, semen analysis and laboratory testing is done. It is crucial to screen him for AIDS. But even though we test each donor every three months for AIDS antibodies, we cannot guarantee that an inseminated woman won't get the disease. It takes at least three months from an infected person's date of exposure to the virus before he will test positive. Symptoms may not appear for years. Fearing the spread of this deadly disease to the woman, her husband, and the unborn baby, the American Society for Reproductive Medicine now strongly recommends that only frozen sperm be used for insemination, and only after a six-month quarantine period has been satisfied. Freezing doesn't kill the virus and won't eliminate the risk of AIDS, but time for additional testing may help reduce the risk. Since thawed sperm are less fertile than fresh, however, conception may take longer—perhaps up to nine months, instead of two to six months with fresh semen.

We also carefully test potential donors for gonorrhea, herpes, mycoplasma, chlamydia, syphilis, and hepatitis B. If the donor is Jewish, he should be tested for Tay-Sachs disease; if black, for sickle-cell anemia. To ensure that the mother and fetus will have Rh blood-type compatibility, the donor's blood type is obtained.

Since most fathers want their child to look as much like themselves as possible, the physical characteristics of the donor and the husband should be matched. We are very particular about this, and also about matching blood types. Since the mother gets pregnant, carries the baby, and delivers it, many couples don't tell anyone how their baby was conceived. Sometimes the child, who may mimic his or her "adopting" dad's mannerisms and speech patterns, actually resembles him. But even though careful matching of race, height, hair color, and eye color is done, the child might not look like the father.

Timing of Insemination

The timing of artificial insemination is crucial if the woman is to become pregnant. Since the sperm can live in the female reproductive tract for at least forty-eight hours and up to seventy-two hours in a good environment, usually only two inseminations are scheduled around ovulation. The basal-body-temperature chart and one of the ovulation kits that measure LH are used to determine the day of ovulation. If there is a problem with timing, ultrasound will indicate whether there is a mature follicle, and also when the egg is released. Generally the insemination is done the day after the LH surge, and possibly again the next day. The process, however, is individualized to each woman's particular ovulatory pattern. We try to do at least two inseminations per cycle, although three inseminations with a day between each pair would be ideal. If the woman normally has an irregular ovulatory pattern, or if the stress of the AID process causes lack of ovulation, she can be regulated with fertility drugs. Clomiphene citrate (Clomid or Serophene) or a combination of Pergonal and hCG often will cause her to ovulate on a predictable schedule. If clomiphene is given, the patient must be carefully monitored, because the drug can have a negative effect on the cervical mucus.

Sperm Mixing

Some AID programs mix the donor's sperm with the husband's, on the slight chance that the husband's sperm may fertilize the egg. Mixing sperm, however, might lower the chances of conception, because antibodies in the husband's semen may attack the donor's sperm. Even though some doctors report that mixing sperm doesn't decrease the pregnancy rate, I don't physically mix the donor's and husband's sperm. Instead couples may wish to have intercourse on the evening of each insemination day. This avoids the antibody problem, and in a few reported cases the baby has turned out to be the husband's.

Although we don't encourage it, some couples ask to have the semen processed for sex selection to increase the odds of having either a boy or a girl. This involves a fairly new and expensive technique, and its efficacy has yet to be clearly proved.

AID Techniques

Artificial insemination can be performed in several ways. During the cervicovaginal method, most of the semen is placed in the vagina and a small amount is put in the cervical canal. More often, however, insemination is done using the intracervical method, a technique in which a small amount of the semen is placed into the opening of the cervix with a syringe. A cervical cup containing the rest of the sperm is placed over the cervix for four or five hours. Since the cup keeps the sperm from falling back into the vagina, all of the semen remains in contact with the cervical mucus and is protected from the acidic vaginal environment. With a third insemination method, intrauterine insemination, the physician puts the semen directly into the uterus with a small catheter. Although this approach places the sperm closer to the egg than the other insemination procedures, implanting the semen in the uterus carries additional risks: it can cause infection and uterine cramping. If more than 0.3 percent of a milliliter of semen is placed in the uterus, the semen can be expelled. We have to process semen specially before placing it directly in the uterus to remove the seminal components that cause uterine cramping. Considering the added risks, intrauterine insemination usually is reserved for women with poor or hostile cervical mucus that prevents the sperm from entering the uterus, or for patients with unexplained infertility. In all cases, the doctor and nurse must do everything possible to make the woman comfortable and to help her relax.

Semen Preservation

Mixed with a cryoprotective agent such as glycerol and/or a protein-rich buffer, semen can be frozen in liquid nitrogen for three to ten years and sometimes longer. Years of experience with frozen semen of both cattle and humans indicates that freezing doesn't damage the genetic material of the sperm. In a study of the use of frozen human semen, Dr. J. K. Sherman reported a congenital abnormality rate of 1 percent of AID pregnancies, and a spontaneous-abortion rate under 10 percent. This means that the incidence of birth defects and spontaneous abortions with donor insemination was less in this study than in the general population. The pregnancy rates, which are lower with frozen sperm than with fresh semen, occur because freezing can decrease sperm motility. Conception rates with thawed semen are 50 to 60 percent, as opposed to 70 to 80 percent with fresh semen.

The use of frozen semen offers many advantages to couples with male infertility. Because semen from one donor is frozen in multiple strawlike containers, the couple can have several children by the same donor, and the siblings will be more likely to resemble one another. Frozen semen, most of which is stored in the nation's sixteen major frozen-sperm banks, can be screened for diseases. Adequate testing of fresh semen is difficult, and freezing gives the laboratory more time to study the specimen. By using frozen sperm, the donor can be retested for the AIDS virus three to six months after he donates the sperm, but before the semen is used for insemination.

Legal Issues

Infertile couples considering artificial insemination by donor often have many questions about the legal status of an AID child. It is important for both husband and wife to sign a form, in the presence of a notary or an attorney, consenting to the insemination. Although it is advisable to consult a lawyer who is expert in the laws of your state, in most states the husband is considered the legal father. Courts in the United States have protected children fathered by donor sperm, saying that such offspring have a right to support by the husband, who consented to having his wife artificially inseminated.

Some husbands choose to adopt a child conceived by donor sperm to protect the child's inheritance. Others, not wishing to make the pregnancy a matter of public record, decide that adoption is unnecessary. Says Dr. William W. Beck, Jr., M.D., in *Infertility in the Male*, edited by Larry I. Lipshultz and Stuart S. Howards: "The legitimacy issue in AID has sporadically found its way into the courts because of divorce proceedings that involve child support and/or inheritance. Happily this is rare, thanks to the solidarity of AID couples. With the national divorce rate approaching 40 percent, less than 1 percent of AID couples experience irreconcilable marital problems. On occasion, however, a husband has left and rejected responsibility for the AID child, claiming that it was not his child. Court rulings in the United States have generally supported the AID child. The highest ruling was made by the Supreme Court of California in 1968, and stated that there is no question about the legitimacy of an AID child providing that there has been voluntary involvement and an informed written consent on the part of both husband and wife. Since that time, a number of states have passed statutes that legalize the insemination process and assure the legitimacy of the child conceived by AID."

Special Problems with AID

The American Fertility Society recommends that no single donor initiate more than fifteen AID pregnancies. The concern is that siblings who are unaware that they were fathered by the same donor might marry and thus unknowingly commit incest. Although the chances are slight, it could happen. In her book *New Conceptions*, Lori Andrews tells the following story: ". . . in Tel Aviv, a marriage has already occurred between two AID children fathered by the same donor. In the United States a similar marriage was stopped by a doctor who revealed to the couple their genetic link. Thus, it seems wise to put some limit on the number of donor pregnancies a man is allowed to initiate."

Another problem with some AID programs is that the donor may not be screened adequately to meet the infertile couple's requirements. Lori Andrews also says: "It is ironic that the screening of donor sperm for human AID is much less stringent than that of bull sperm in the cattle industry." Although we cannot speak for every donor insemination program, we can speak for ours. We spend a great deal of time, effort, and money screening donors and matching them to infertile couples. It is our hope that this will reduce the stress of starting a family with the aid of a donor.

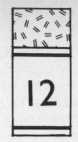

Surrogate Motherhood

Fighting a Losing Battle

It is extremely depressing to tell a teenage girl about to be married that she may never be able to have children. But Nancy's endometriosis was unusually severe. I had no option but to explain the bitter facts to her family: unless we could stop the progression of this "benign" disease, Nancy eventually would need a hysterectomy.

When I first met Nancy in 1969, she was a nineteen-year-old college sophomore. Her uncle, a pediatrician, had sent her to me because she was having monthly menstrual pain, nausea, and weakness. Although Nancy's original gynecologist had said that her worse-than-"normal" cramping was "all in her head," her uncle disagreed. He thought that she might have endometriosis.

Unfortunately, Nancy's uncle was correct—his niece's pain definitely was not "in her head." On physical examination, I could feel endometriosis on the ligaments supporting her uterus. And when I looked at her reproductive organs through an optical instrument used to view the inside of the body, I could see purplish endometrial implants all over her ovaries, the ligaments—everywhere. Nancy's prognosis wasn't good.

Immediately after Nancy learned the devastating news, she tried to break off her engagement to Mike. But he wouldn't hear of it. He was totally devoted to her and bought her a diamond ring before she left the hospital; a year later they were married.

Twenty-five years ago we lacked many of the infertility drugs and advanced laser and microsurgical techniques that we have today. Nowadays we could dry up some of the endometriosis with drugs before surgery. Back then the best nonsurgical treatment was to stop Nancy's periods temporarily with medication. I hoped at least to maintain the status quo and maybe dissolve some of the endometriosis.

After a few months of treatment, Nancy's uncle wrote me: "Nancy feels so much better and is a greatly changed young lady." But within six months after we stopped the drug, the severe cramping that had brought her to me in the first place had returned.

Meanwhile, Nancy and Mike were trying unsuccessfully to have a baby. In 1970, when she was only twenty-one years old, I put her in the hospital for conservative surgery for endometriosis (an exploratory laparotomy). I hoped to remove the disease before it became any worse and totally destroyed her ability to get pregnant. After this major operation, I remember feeling quite optimistic. At that time, I thought that she had over a 70-percent chance of conceiving.

Unfortunately, Mike also had a problem; his sperm count was below normal. He had a varicose vein of the testicle. When this was corrected surgically, his sperm production improved significantly. But, in the meantime, another year had passed, and Nancy still wasn't pregnant.

Our problems were far from solved. As discussed earlier, endometriosis patients often form adhesions that can bind the pelvic organs in rubbery bands of scar tissue. Furthermore, the very surgery designed to eradicate endometriosis can lead to additional pelvic adhesive disease. In the early 1970s, today's intricate microsurgical techniques, which partially reduce postsurgical scar-tissue formation, were unknown. At that time, the best medical science had to offer Nancy was not good enough.

In December of 1971, an X-ray of her uterus and fallopian tubes showed that both of the tubes where fertilization occurs were totally blocked. When I looked directly at Nancy's tubes and ovaries through the lighted pencil-sized laparoscope, I instantly knew why she wasn't pregnant. Not only had cobweblike adhesions covered the ends of both tubes, but thicker scar tissue had pulled the entrance to each oviduct away from its ovary. The petallike tubal ends or "fingers" were not free to whisk the egg from the surface of the ovary into the tube.

Without another major operation, Nancy's chances of having a baby were almost zero. In October 1972, this determined young patient underwent her second major surgery for infertility. Afterward her prognosis appeared better; we were delighted to see that both tubes were open once again.

But the endometriosis came back! Nancy's fallopian tubes needed to be open for conception to occur. When they were, however, the menstrual debris would back up through the oviducts onto her ovaries. Each period was like throwing gasoline on a fire. We would operate on her to remove the endometriosis, flush out her tubes with cortisone, and the implants would return. It was incredibly discouraging.

Finally, Nancy decided that she could stand the chronic menstrual pain no more. For two days a month, she was unable to get out of bed. The strain of infertility was taking its toll. She wanted a hysterectomy. But when my surgical team went in to remove her uterus, I couldn't do it. At that point, everything still looked too good. I knew how desperately she and Mike wanted children, and she was so young—only twenty-six.

When Nancy woke up, I was in trouble. To say that she was unhappy with me is an understatement. She had had three major operations and several laparoscopies. After all this surgery, she still had her uterus, the source of her endometriosis—but no baby.

She said to me: "All my life, I have succeeded in everything that I have tried. This is the one thing that I wanted to do for my husband; the one thing that other women can do so easily. I have tried and tried and tried. And I have met with constant failure."

In the end, her pain and bleeding became intolerable. I was finally forced to give her a total hysterectomy. By this time, recurrent endometriosis had destroyed both of her ovaries. She had extensive intestinal involvement, and all of her reproductive organs were covered with rubbery adhesions. We had to face the heartbreaking truth—Nancy would never give birth.

After the hysterectomy, *she* tried to make *me* feel better. She said: "I'm not sad, Dr. Franklin. For the first time, I finally feel a peace within me. I know that I have done everything that I possibly could do— everything that I am willing to do. I have no regrets. I know that you have tried incredibly hard to help me. If I had to live these past ten years over again, I would act precisely as I did.

"I love my husband," she continued. "He has stuck by me from the beginning—even before we were married. He has longed for children as much as I. But I know that it just is not going to be. And I can face this."

Nancy did face her loss—the loss of a child never born. She dealt with her grief in a positive way. Determined to get on with her life, she returned to her job helping children who needed her love—teaching handicapped preschool children.

A Glimmer of Hope

Two more years passed. Although Nancy and Mike never dreamed that they would become parents, a glimmer of hope still remained. There might be a way that the remarkable young woman could be the mother of her husband's biological child. She could turn to a surrogate-parent program for help.

This type of agency arranges for a surrogate mother to have a baby for an infertile couple. The surrogate is artificially inseminated with the husband's sperm, carries the baby to term, and allows the infertile woman to adopt the infant. The couple puts money into a trust to pay the surrogate for her services.

At first, Mike was against the idea. He feared that state laws might consider surrogate parenting baby selling. Or what if, after the birth, the surrogate mother decided to keep *his* baby? He would feel responsible for it, but he might have to share custody with a stranger and pay child support. And, worst of all, he feared that if they lost again it would break Nancy's heart.

But after two more childless years and much soul searching, they decided at least to consider this final option. The first program that they visited gave the couple an uneasy feeling. Although they would be allowed to see the mother's psychological profile and her IQ, they could not meet her. This really bothered both of them. It made them feel the situation was totally out of their control. They felt that they would be turning over the most important thing in their lives to a stranger. For nine months, they would not know if the surrogate mother was taking care of the tiny being that they had created. They could not live with this.

Then, one morning, while Nancy and Mike were lying in bed reading the Sunday newspaper, they saw an article on surrogate parenting by a reporter who had interviewed several agencies. The story mentioned that the agency that the couple had visited had had some serious problems. In one case, the surrogate had kept the baby. In another, the surrogate's husband turned out to be the father.

When the couple called the woman who wrote the article, she told them that she felt the most comfortable with Dr. Nina Kellogg's Surrogate Parent Program of Los Angeles. The reporter had visited several agencies and thought that Nina, a psychologist who works with infertile couples, had the best-thought-out program.

That was Thanksgiving. After many long-distance phone calls to California, the couple decided to take the plunge: Christmas vacation, they would visit Nina's agency. They felt that her program gave the surrogates more support than some of the other agencies. All of the mothers lived in California and met with the psychologist every other week, during and for a while after the pregnancy. This was extremely important to Nancy and Mike.

As Nina now says: "In a way, babies born to a surrogate mother are *team babies*. They are so *wanted*. You have a surrogate, and her husband, if she's married. You've got the couple. You have the couple's parents and the surrogate's parents. You have the other surrogates in the support group. You have me. And, of course, you have the obstetrician. All these people are concerned about the baby. Their hope, delight, and happiness "cradle" the baby in incredible love—even before it's born."

Three weeks after their phone call to Nina, right before Christmas, the couple were walking into Nina's office in Los Angeles for a holiday party. Most of the agency's surrogate mothers were there—all big and round and pregnant. Some appeared ready to deliver at any minute.

At first Nancy could not enter. She clung to the door, overwhelmed by the sight of a small room bursting with pregnant women. She would leave as soon as politely possible.

But as she and Mike were shaking hands with Nina, one of the mothers spotted Nancy's sad face. A rosy-cheeked woman who was just beginning to show, Carol (not her real name) walked up to Nancy, put an arm around her, and brought her into the party. Nancy had wondered what sort of woman would have a baby for someone else. Carol, at least, seemed much like her neighbors—just a nice married lady who wanted to earn money to stay home with her two small children.

As the couple walked toward their car, they exchanged hopeful glances. They both had a good feeling. They believed that most of the surrogate mothers were in the program for the right reasons.

Nancy and Mike decided to meet with a potential surrogate. Within a few days, the psychologist introduced them to Pat (not her real name). They met not only Pat's husband, who had had a vasectomy, but also Pat's parents, her grandparents, and one of her two daughters. Knowing the whole family meant a great deal to the couple.

As Nina now says: "As important as it was for the couple to know the surrogate, it was even more important for *her* to meet *them*. Understanding the infertile couple's story enables the surrogate to carry *their* baby for the whole nine months.

"Before she promises to have a baby for them," continues the psychologist, "I make certain that she understands that this couple cannot have a child if she keeps the baby—that she will have a power to destroy them.

"This is why the face-to-face meeting is extremely important," says Nina. "Surrogate motherhood is a relationship based on incredible trust and love. When Pat said to Mike and Nancy, 'Yes, this is your baby—it will never be my baby,' I believed that she would honor her word," says Nina.

Before long, the couple were told the good news: the second artificial insemination had taken—Pat was pregnant. Nancy and Mike were unbelievably excited. Fifteen years after Nancy's first surgery, she was going to be a mother.

Then, only two days after they learned of the conception, a tragedy occurred in Pat's family. Her sister died of cancer.

Perhaps it was because Pat had lost her only sister, or maybe it was the depth of Nancy's gratitude, but an unbelievable bond grew between the two women. To Nancy, Pat was the most unselfish person she had ever known. How could Nancy fail to love this woman—the woman who was willing to hand her her dream? To Pat, Nancy was a friend of deep spiritual faith and understanding in her time of grief—a woman who had fought valiantly with infertility and lost. Pat's reward was in giving.

Pat did everything she knew to assure the couple that she was caring for the new life inside her. Writing Nancy and Mike almost every week, she sent them a tape recording of the fetal heartbeat; she mailed them a picture of the ultrasound; she told them of the baby's first kick.

Nancy and Mike had a little book with wonderful colored pictures that told of the monthly stages of the development of their baby. Each month they would think about how it was growing; each picture showed one miracle occurring after another. Nancy felt just as if she were having the baby. She did not feel that she was missing anything.

"You see," says Nina, "although the baby obviously isn't in the adoptive mom's body, in a sense she goes through the pregnancy with the surrogate. Often, the infertile woman even helps the surrogate pick out maternity clothes. The whole process is so healing for the childless couple, but especially for the woman. Finally, she can look at a pregnant woman with hopeful expectancy instead of pain."

As Nancy said: "Mothers are always telling me about the birth of their babies. Well, I didn't miss out either. I was there for my baby's birth; I was the one who cut the umbilical cord."

The birth of Nancy and Mike's baby was the happiest event that ever happened. In almost thirty years of practice, I have never known such a thrilled couple. Nancy sat beside Pat's bed holding her hand during the entire labor and delivery. She rubbed her back, winced from her pain, and wept with incredible joy as a tiny sandy-haired girl was placed in her arms. The bond of love was forever.

As the new parents left the hospital with their sleeping baby cuddled on Nancy's shoulder, a nurse rolled Pat to the door to say goodbye. The couple would never forget the sad look on the surrogate mother's face—Nancy was extremely worried about her friend.

Trying to reassure Nancy, Pat said that she wasn't sad because she was giving up her baby. "I have always considered the baby yours," said Pat. "My tears are because I have to say goodbye to you."

Facing the Legal Mire

Nancy and Mike returned home terrified that the legal system would take their baby away from them. They had known from the beginning that surrogate parenting is encumbered with endless legal problems. When they went to court for the custody hearing, they took Mike's mother along with them; they felt that the judge would not deprive a biological grandmother of her grandbaby. If he did, they were prepared to leave the country.

The outcome depended on how the judge viewed the law. If he saw it as buying a baby, they were in trouble. If Pat had wanted to keep the child, she probably could have. In some states even the surrogate's husband, whether he has had a vasectomy or not, may have rights to the child. But Pat had reassured them that, if the court gave their daughter to her, she would immediately hand the baby right back to them.

Fortunately, this time the legal system worked! The judge indeed was wise—Nancy was allowed to adopt her husband's infant.

The psychologist and lawyers advised the couple to sever the tie with the surrogate mother. They wanted the newly formed family to be as normal as possible. The professionals are aware of the adoptive mother's tremendous feelings of gratitude toward the surrogate. As attorney Lori Andrews says in her excellent book *New Conceptions*, the infertile couple should "not feel obligated to 'share' the child with her in any way. . . ." This is one of the reasons some surrogate programs, unlike Nina's, refuse to allow the infertile couple to meet the surrogate.

Nancy, however, wanted to keep in touch with Pat. She told me: "I ached when I said goodbye to Pat—we had a living bond between us." Nancy sent Pat flowers on the baby's first birthday; Pat sent the couple cards on Mother's Day and Father's Day; and, for a while, they exchanged letters.

Like Pat, some of the surrogate mothers I have heard of have been exceptional people. They have had a baby for someone else because they cared. These women are not unlike some of the people I know in medicine—they feel that helping others makes life worthwhile.

Most surrogate mothers have enjoyed motherhood so much that they have been willing to go through pregnancy for an infertile couple. Some of them have had a childless friend or relative and have seen how devastating it is to be unable to have children. Their reward is in doing something for someone that perhaps nobody else would do.

I get some doubting looks when I say this, especially since the famous Baby M case, in which the surrogate reneged on her promise to William and Elizabeth Stern. People look on the dark side, believing that a surrogate must be a cold woman who gives up her baby for money. But in some cases the surrogate is motivated by reasons other than money. There are much easier and less risky ways of making money than having a baby for someone else.

Says psychologist Nina Kellogg: "The surrogates *do* want to help the infertile couple. But I'm not sure that most of them would do it without the money. Many people still think that women should do everything for free. Just because the surrogate wants to be paid for a twenty-four-hour-a-day job doesn't mean that she lacks altruistic motives as well."

Continues Nina: "The money Pat received enabled her to stay home with her three children. Her overall income from the escrow account was approximately ten thousand dollars. It was received in installments, with the last half paid after the custody settlement." The surrogate mother's payment was about $1.50 per hour, well below the minimum wage.

The couple's total expenses, however, were over twenty-five thousand dollars. Besides paying the surrogate, Mike and Nancy had to pay for medical expenses, insurance, airfare, and lodging, not to mention the cost of the agency and three lawyers. In 1994, the total expenses of a couple in similar circumstances could exceed forty thousand dollars.

Although Pat brought incredible joy into my patient's life, surrogate motherhood has never been the solution for every infertile couple. As the Baby M case shows, occasionally the surrogate arrangement ends in a legal battle. In this case, the bitter dispute began when surrogate mother Marybeth Whitehead Gould, who contracted to have a baby for William and Elizabeth Stern, changed her mind after childbirth and sought to keep the baby. In 1988, the New Jersey Supreme Court granted the Sterns custody but Marybeth, who has remarried and had another baby, has liberal visitation rights. The judges felt that the Sterns—William is the child's father by artificial insemination—"promise a secure home."

Although the court did not award the surrogate mother final custody, the judges viewed surrogacy as baby selling, a practice long condemned by the law. Said the court: "While we recognize the depth of the yearning of infertile couples to have their own children, we find the payment of money to a 'surrogate' mother illegal, perhaps criminal and potentially degrading to women." The court ruled that surrogacy is legal as long as the mother is not paid, providing she is allowed to change her mind after the birth.

The Baby M case and other surrogacy custody battles have cast a long shadow over surrogate motherhood. For years doctors have worried that their patients might be hurt rather than helped by turning to another woman for a baby. If a physician has negative moral feelings about surrogate parenting, he cannot mention this option. Even if properly handled, surrogacy has the potential to be an emotional minefield.

Some experts believe that the legal uncertainties surrounding surrogate motherhood point to a critical need for legislation. At present, uniform procedural guidelines are nonexistent because the United States government has skirted the issue. As of 1992, only sixteen states had passed laws regarding surrogacy. These vary. Laws range, for example, from banning surrogacy contracts outright, to prohibiting payment to a surrogate, to disallowing compensation to her but permitting the infertile couple to cover her expenses. Some states prohibit payment to an intermediary.

Of utmost concern to the infertile couple, the surrogate, and the baby is the question: Who are the legal parents of the child? Some states such as Arizona, North Dakota, and Utah recognize the surrogate and her husband as the legal parents. The laws of other states such as Arkansas, Florida, New Hampshire, and Virginia recognize the intended parents as the legal parents of the child, though the latter three give the surrogate a grace period to change her mind. Expert legal advice is obviously extremely important.

California has the most comprehensive surrogacy law. Says legal expert Lori B. Andrews in an article in *California Lawyer*, October 1992: "California's new surrogacy law is designed to regulate traditional and gestational surrogacy (a gestational surrogate carries the couple's biological child), as well as egg donation. The statute allows compensation of up to 15,000 dollars to the surrogate for her services, in addition to payment of medical expenses and legal fees connected with the formation and enforcement of the contract. Surrogates must be at least 21 years old, must have previously borne at least one child, and must have separate counsel. . . ." Both the intended parents and the surrogate must have life insurance, and the surrogate also must have health insurance.

Psychological counseling for both the infertile couple and the surrogate also is mandated. At birth, the intended parents get custody of the child, regardless of the state of its health.

The issue of *gestational* surrogacy was recently addressed by the courts in California. In 1990, after entering into such an agreement with Mark and Crispina Calvert, Anna Johnson decided against relinquishing the baby to the couple even though they were its biological parents. She petitioned the Orange County Superior Court maintaining that, "although not genetically related to the child, she was its mother because of the biological contributions she had made during gestation." The court ruled that the couple who provided the embryo were the parents based on their genetic tie to the baby and on the contract between the parties. A precedent was set when, in May of 1993, the California Supreme Court upheld this decision, saying that the surrogate was a facilitator providing a service to the infertile couple.

The Ethics Committee of the American Society for Reproductive Medicine (ASRM) discusses many of the potential problems surrounding surrogacy in *Ethical Considerations of Assisted Reproductive Technologies, Fertility and Sterility*, Supplement 1, November 1994. After mentioning the lack of research on the subject the committee says that it has "serious ethical reservations about surrogacy that cannot be fully resolved until appropriate data are available for assessment of the risks and possible benefits of this alternative." Some members "judged that surrogacy could not be ethically recommended. Others concluded that it could be cautiously recommended while research on the key issues continued." For more detailed information on this subject contact ASRM, 2131 Magnolia Avenue, Suite 201, Birmingham, AL 35282-9990.

My goal over the years has been to know as much as possible about all the ways that an infertile couple might go about starting a family, whether it be medical therapy, surgery, adoption, or surrogate motherhood. As I get to know a patient and her husband, I begin to understand their wishes. Eventually I can sense how much they can stand, emotionally, physically, and financially. Although it isn't done consciously, I'm sure that I do guide my patients. I want them to have all the facts. But in the end, only they can choose what is right for them.

If Nancy had been born ten years later, perhaps we could have won her battle against infertility. Nowadays, if we treat endometriosis early enough, we are sometimes able to stop the progression of this mysterious disease while it is still in its milder stages. No longer should a teenage girl with severe cramping be told that her pain is "all in her head." Today more physicians finally are paying attention to this complaint. After operating on between two and three hundred patients annually for many years, I know the suffering that this "benign" disease can cause. Prevention has got to be the better way.

Helping an infertile couple have a child is unbelievably rewarding. This is one of the reasons I love my work, and perhaps the reason some women become surrogate mothers. When an infertility team does a really good job for a patient, it sometimes is able to help her when nobody else could. To me this is incredibly exciting.

After all, what could be a happier sight than an infertility patient turned into a proud mother? Even though medicine failed to help Nancy, she didn't miss this joy. Her prayers for a child with whom to share her love were answered. I know: the last time Nancy came to my office, a busy blue-eyed toddler with long black lashes just like her daddy's played happily at my patient's side.

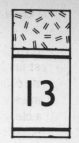

13

The Challenge of Adoption

You can adopt if you want to! You can find a child
you can love for life. To maneuver through the adop-
tion system successfully, you must be knowledgeable
and tenacious.

JACQUELINE HORNOR PLUMEZ, *Successful Adoption*

Many infertile couples have turned to adoption as a rewarding alternative way of starting a family. All of us know of a home brightened by an adopted child. Over the years, I have observed the special delight adoptive parents feel toward their children. These couples often tell me about their sons and daughters with a special unselfish pride. The love in their eyes is unmistakable. As one proud father of two teenage boys, one adopted and one not, told me: "Whether the child is adopted or biologically related, love returns in small unspoken ways as a glance, a hug, and a tear."

The current numerical imbalance between healthy white babies needing homes and white couples desiring to adopt has made adoption not for the faint of heart. For nearly two decades, prospective parents have had to pursue their goal with unwavering determination. Some struggle through the adoption maze for years before a baby finally is placed in their arms. Many of my patients have turned to outstanding private adoption agencies such as The Gladney Center in Fort Worth, Texas. (There are other excellent agencies, but Gladney, a comprehensive maternity home and child-placing agency, is the one with which I am most familiar. It can serve as a model for couples looking for an agency.) Some couples have adopted without the invaluable support and protection of an established agency, often through an intermediary such as a lawyer or a clergyman. Other couples have found their children in foreign countries, while some patients have welcomed handicapped or abandoned children into their homes.

Many of my patients have found great joy in adoption, despite its challenges. Armed with an understanding of the adoption process, these resolute couples have overcome obstacles that most people never face. Once bonded to their new arrival, they have committed themselves "for better or for worse" to parenthood—an irrevocable entrustment filled with all the joys and sorrows of a lifetime of caring.

Facing the Facts

A "shortage" of healthy white infants for adoption exists in this country, but abortion is only part of the reason. Since abortion became legal, the number of unplanned births has actually increased. Nowadays the majority of unwed mothers who deliver their babies decide to parent. Many are pressured by family members or by the biological father to keep their children.

Experts estimate that at least one hundred couples or single adults are seeking to adopt each available healthy white baby. Says Michael McMahon, president of The Gladney Center: "The interest in white infants continues to be intense. The wait to adopt such a baby from a state-licensed agency in the U.S. varies over time and depends on many factors."

Some authorities say that prospective parents hoping for a boy have more opportunities to adopt, because adoptive couples prefer girls by a ratio of three to one. Although many families will ask for a specific sex, they are often flexible. For couples capable of accepting the responsibilities of caring for an older child or one with emotional, mental, or physical handicaps, the wait to start a family is usually shorter.

There is a great need for African-American families desiring to adopt a black infant, and for interracial couples to adopt a multiethnic child. White couples hoping for an African-American baby, however, will find that some agencies, especially those in the South, discourage interracial adoptions. According to the National Council For Adoption, the National Association of Black Social Workers has come out against white couples adopting black babies, saying that transracial adoption amounts to "cultural genocide." Says Gladney's president: "There is great need for adoptive couples in our biracial and African-American programs. If at all possible, we try to keep African-American children in African-American families. But absent an African-American home, we think that every child deserves a family to love it. As of 1994, federal legislation protects children from being held in the system if caring families are available to adopt them."

There also is a need for couples to adopt Native American and Hispanic babies. Couples wishing to adopt a Native American child must comply with the Indian Child-Welfare Act of 1978. Each tribe can interpret this act differently. If the child is part Native American and the intermediary fails to comply with this law, the adoption can be set aside.

Since the number of white couples longing to adopt far exceeds the number of healthy white infants, prospective parents must be determined in their efforts to find their child, and knowledgeable about adoption sources. Adoption agencies can be discouraging. Not wishing to keep long waiting lists, a few are sometimes forced to tell callers: "We are not accepting applications at this time."

One agency in Texas (not Gladney) used to open its waiting list only one day a year. Infertile couples would camp out on the agency's door step with coolers and lawn chairs to get in line. The agency would accept applications from the first hundred people in line and then close the list for a year. Quite clearly, the adoption process can be unbelievably frustrating—but this doesn't mean that it is impossible.

Couples who finally find a child haven't let such disheartening situations, statements, or statistics cause them to forsake their pursuit of a baby. They have met the challenge of adoption by becoming informed and by being persistent! They have read books by adoption experts, kept in touch with adoption agencies, and put their names on the waiting lists of several reputable agencies. As one adoption attorney says: "Agencies sometimes cannot take applications one month but will the next. If an agency isn't accepting applications, ask why not. Then ask when the agency will be taking them again. Call back or visit in person at a later date. Some small agencies may have their positions filled for the foreseeable future, but this usually isn't the rule for all agencies."

Private and Public Agencies

The number of public and private adoption agencies in the United States changes constantly. Public agencies, run by state and local governments, still do the most placements. These agencies place many children of minority race or with special needs.

Many adoptions of healthy, native-born white infants are handled by the nation's private agencies. These agencies are licensed by the state but aren't government-funded, although some may receive grant money. Many church groups sponsor adoption agencies, some of which welcome nonmembers. In recent years, numerous religiously affiliated agencies have been founded.

Adoption in the United States is under the regulation of each state, although federal law is becoming increasingly important. Adoption laws vary tremendously from state to state and change frequently, so it is difficult to make general statements concerning adoption throughout the country. Furthermore, interpretation of these laws is complicated. Hence couples should not attempt to decipher technical legal language relative to adoption without the assistance of a reputable attorney knowledgeable about adoption or family law. As one well-respected adoption attorney said: "It is crucial for couples to put themselves in the right legal hands."

For further up-to-date information about state-by-state adoption regulations, see *Law of Adoption*, edited by Hollinger, published by Matthew Bender & Co., 1995.

The Gladney Center

Gladney places almost as many babies as ever, because of its outstanding service to pregnant women. The private adoption agency serves prospective parents from the United States and throughout the world. Unfortunately, the agency cannot serve everyone who turns to it for help. Gladney has almost four thousand inquiries annually from families wanting to adopt. In 1994, Gladney placed 246 infants.

When a pregnant woman first comes to Gladney, she finds a pleasant place to stay and caring counselors. The home carefully looks after her, providing prenatal care and educational and career development programs. The campus is open. Since her peers help provide support and control, the young woman must be able to function in a group. The home is not equipped to serve women who are mentally retarded, psychotic, or addicted to drugs.

Says a Gladney representative: "In 1994, we served approximately four hundred birth mothers. Of the young women who remained with the home until after delivery, most placed their babies for adoption. Of the 40 percent admitted to residency who left before delivery, most planned to parent. The average length of stay is about four months, but a few girls only remain a couple of days and decide that adoption isn't for them."

What determines how long a couple wait for a Gladney baby? One factor is the couple's religion. Some girls have strong feelings about the religious preference of the couple adopting their offspring. The agency makes every attempt to honor these and other preferences, as long as they don't unduly delay placement of the child. Suppose, for example, that a birth mother tells the agency: "I want my baby to go to a couple belonging to the Greek Orthodox Church. They must live in a city with a population of fewer than a hundred thousand people. The father must have a college degree, and the mother must work only in the home." The agency may not be willing to accept a child with the promise that all of these placement requests will be honored. It cannot accept a baby for placement and put it on the shelf for six months until an adoptive couple come along who meet all of these specifications.

The prospective parents may also state preferences that must be considered. Says former Gladney Executive Director Eleanor Tuck: "In general, the couple's wishes aren't difficult to meet, but a few have such a long list that matching is slowed. Gladney tries to give some preference to those who have been waiting the longest. In addition, if the couple want to adopt a second child, the agency attempts to match the new baby to the first child."

Some couples worry that their personal income might be too low for them to be considered for adoption. Says the agency: "We aren't as interested in family income as we are in how well the family manages money. We look for a good, stable marriage and for a couple who are prepared for the baby. If the mother works outside the home, the couple will need a well-thought-out plan for child care." Unlike Gladney, some agencies may want the adoptive mother to set aside her career for a while.

People over forty-five years old may find it difficult to adopt a newborn. This is the reason I bring up the subject of adoption to couples with a poor fertility prognosis who are in their late twenties or early thirties. Since it may take a while to adopt, some of them decide to put their names on an agency waiting list. The birth mothers are more in control of the selection of adoptive parents than ever before. Hence, many agencies are having an increasingly difficult time assisting older couples. Although at first this idea sounds unfair, older couples should not give up without inquiring further. Couples over forty or forty-five years old should look for an agency that doesn't adhere to a strict age rule. In addition, they should determine if the age limit applies to one or both parents, and whether it applies to adopting a first or a second child. Couples wishing to adopt an older child will find that many agencies place such children with older couples. So don't become discouraged before asking questions.

A couple usually take the first step toward adoption by making a phone inquiry to the agency. When contacting The Gladney Center, the couple must meet Gladney's basic requirements concerning emotional and physical health, soundness of marriage, and financial stability. Gladney will work with couples who already have biological children, particularly in the minority or international adoption programs. As discussed in detail later under independent adoption, Gladney's relatively new "designated" adoption program, which combines the best of private and agency adoption, may help some couples with secondary infertility add to their families. With Gladney's "agency-assisted" program, which serves young women with unplanned pregnancies, the prospective couple must provide a statement from their physician verifying their infertility.

Gladney draws from its pool of prospective adoptive parents to find homes for its babies. The agency always has a substantial number of families approved for adoption who are waiting for a baby. In the agency-assisted program, each birth mother selects the adoptive parents for her baby from this pre-approved list.

Once a couple are invited to orientation, they are asked to complete an application. Autobiographical in nature, the long questionnaire forces the couple to face many soul-searching questions. Sometimes a husband and wife haven't communicated to each other their true feelings about adoption. After they look at their motives for wanting to adopt, some couples weed themselves out of the adoption process.

After the orientation, if the couple still wish to adopt, they visit with a caseworker, first in her office and then in the couple's home. Says a Gladney representative: "During these meetings, we attempt to build a relationship of trust with the couple. Sometimes they are nervous and anxious at this time, but, from Gladney's perspective, we want these meetings to be positive. The more we know about a couple, the better we can help them with adoptive planning."

Once the prospective parents are approved, the wait for a child can take anywhere from two weeks to two years, depending on the Gladney adoption program the couple chooses. Says Gladney's president: "In the assisted adoption program, it takes about sixteen months for a couple to get a child. In the designated adoption program, the average time after approval is between six and nine months. In the international program, we have infants and toddlers waiting for adoption right now."

Ordinarily Texas law requires a six-month period of supervision, to protect the child and the adoptive parents and to provide reassurances to the birth mother that the family is adjusting to the new arrival. When all goes well, the adoption is finalized, and legal responsibility for the child is transferred from the agency to the adoptive parents. If the adoptive parents have other children, the adopted child has the same legal status as the couple's biological children.

Gladney's Triangle of Love

One reason for Gladney's success is that the agency builds adoption around what it calls the "triangle of love" formed by the birth parents, the infant, and the adoptive parents. The key member of this triangle is the young birth mother, often a teenager. Says former Gladney director Ruby Lee Piester, currently with the National Council For Adoption: "The girl is where we like to focus. When you protect the girl, you protect the others involved, the babies and the adopting parents."

The home tries to help every young woman plan for the future. By focusing on her assets, she improves her self-esteem. The agency also wants her to become aware of adoption procedures and rights. In addition, Gladney tries to help her prepare emotionally for the adoption process. For support, each pregnant woman has a specially trained counselor to call on any time of the day or night.

Says Piester: "The birth parents often need help in making the appropriate decisions for their child and for themselves. These young people also need an atmosphere in which to make these decisions that safeguards their right to make them *totally* without pressure."

Gladney also wants the biological parents to talk with parents who have adopted children of various ages. Birth parents need to see firsthand that adoptive parents have concern and respect for biological parents. Such visits enable the young woman to develop a trust that the adopting couple will nurture and love the child from infancy to adulthood.

At Gladney, every young mother is encouraged to hold and visit with her baby after the birth. This gives the girl the opportunity to satisfy her curiosity about her infant and, at the same time, helps her put the emotional birthing experience into perspective. According to Gladney, most birth mothers who plan adoption are eager for their child to be placed in the adoptive home as soon as possible, although some young women aren't ready for several weeks. The birth mother will have the opportunity to reaffirm the placement decision before a judge of a state district court.

Gladney also looks after its adoptive parents. The agency answers the questions couples have about adoption before and after placement. Agencies such as Gladney offer couples individual postadoption services, including counseling on such subjects as when to discuss adoption with the child.

Once the baby is placed with the couple, Gladney remains available for support. As mentioned earlier, Texas law ordinarily requires a six-month supervision period after placement before the prospective adoptive parents may complete the adoption; the length of time varies among states. The adoptive parents are usually extremely anxious for this time to pass. Says the agency's former director: "At Gladney this is a supportive period, when the agency is available to counsel the couple. The agency is not spying on them—it is there to help. It is possible that some problem may come to light that could call for Gladney to take action. For instance, if the stress of a baby becomes more than a couple's marriage can handle, and it seldom does, Gladney will take the baby back under its wing."

How Letters Help

Letters written by each member of the "triangle of love"—the birth mother, the adoptive parents, and an adopted adult—show the thoughtful care of all concerned. In an article written for *The Wall Street Journal*, family psychiatrist Dr. Alfred A. Messer says: "These handwritten letters provide tangible evidence of love and concern. They can be brought out and read whenever feelings of guilt or uncertainty arise in either the child or the parents. By removing some of the child's uncertainty about his origins, a letter from his birth mother helps diminish his feelings of rejection and abandonment and provides the basis for a healthier self-esteem."

When a birth mother relinquishes custody of her baby, she sometimes feels guilt. Says a Gladney representative: "She not only feels remorseful about getting pregnant, but she also feels guilty because of what she calls 'pushing her responsibility on someone else.' " An unsigned letter from the adoptive parents showing their appreciation and concern helps the biological mother see that her child is the answer to an infertile couple's prayers. The letter reassures her that the baby will be raised in a loving home.

A birth mother wrote the following poignant letter telling of the love she felt for her child:

My dearest baby girl,

I am writing this so that you will understand my feelings at this trying time. You see, I gave birth to you seven days ago and a mere two days have passed since I released you for adoption. I want you to know how great my love is for you. It is a deep and unselfish love that only mothers feel for their children. As I held you close to me I told you why I gave you up, but I know you didn't hear me. So, I feel I have to try and reach you through a letter.

I am eighteen years old and too young to be a good mother. I could give you love and my prayers. But I want you to have so much more, my darling. I want you to have teddy bears and sweet lullabies from music boxes. When you get older I want you to have a piano and a pony and a puppy, like my parents gave me. I want you, my sweet child, to have pretty dresses and, yes, blue jeans with signs of wear from happy play-days in your own big yard. There is so much I want for you, all the good things I had and even more. I can't give you these now, and I probably wouldn't be able to tear myself away from you long enough to finish college in order to give you them later. But most important of all, I want you to have a Daddy like my very own. My life wouldn't be complete without my father. I needed him to spank me when I was young and I needed him to show me how to ride my bike. I need him now to ease the pain of growing up the hard way. I need my father for love.

I can't give you your daddy, sweetheart. He's young, too, and we aren't married. He isn't ready to be a good father. I'm not prepared to be a good mother. That's why I feel like I'm giving you the greatest gift of all, by loving you so much to give you brand new parents. They are waiting for you, and have been waiting for just the right woman to have just the right baby. Well, I am that woman, and now you are the precious child they need and love.

I have no regrets over my decision. It took strength and love to make it. But I know it's right because the good Lord gave me that strength and instilled in me an unselfish love for you. That's why I must ask you to remember me as a young woman who had a child when she wasn't ready for one. Remember that I loved you enough to give you a new and happy life.

Please, darling, don't look for me. It would hurt me terribly if we were to meet in the future. I love you and I have decided on adoption because of that love. I can't explain why this was to be our destiny, only God knows the answer. But it is our destiny and I must learn to live with it. So must you. In 20 years I will probably have married a wonderful man and I will have my career in medicine. You will be a young adult and a total stranger to me. I know that sounds harsh, but my memory of you will be the tiny, sweet newborn that I called my little Cherry. I want to remember you just like that. I couldn't give you an "identity" if you were to find me. You already are a beautiful individual and you need no more than to be yourself.

I am going to close with my favorite passage from *The Prophet* by Kahlil Gibran. I hope you will read it and know the truth and depth of my love.

". . . your children are not your children. They are the sons and daughters of Life's longing for itself. They come through you, but not from you, and though they are with you, yet they belong not to you. You may give them your love but not your thoughts. For they have their own thoughts. You may house their bodies but not their souls, for their souls dwell in the house of tomorrow, which you cannot visit, not even in your dreams. You may strive to be like them, but seek not to make them like you. For life goes not backward nor tarries with yesterday.

"You are the bows from which your children as living arrows are sent forth.

"The archer sees the mark upon the path of the infinite, and He bends you with His might that His arrows may go swift and far.

"Let your bending in the archer's hand be your gladness;

"For even as he loves the arrow that flies, so He loves also the bow that is stable."

I love you,
Mother

The Alleged Father

Some young men keep in touch with their pregnant girlfriends, but most do not. It is not uncommon for alleged fathers of the baby (called "F.O.B.s" by more than one Gladney girl) to say that the baby might be theirs, but that it also could belong to many other fellows. This, of course, is extremely hurtful for the girl. She feels rejected by her boyfriend, and occasionally also by her family, in her time of need.

Says Eleanor Tuck, Gladney's former director: "Even though the father doesn't have to publicly admit that the baby is his, he has his feelings about the pregnancy. Unless he comes forward, he receives little help."

Although often painful for the unwed girl, it is important to try to find the putative father. His medical records are needed for the child's sake, and his social history helps the adoption agency match an adoptive couple to his baby.

In years past, the putative father often was ignored. During the past twenty years, however, his interests have been addressed. The U.S. Supreme Court, through decisions such as *Stanley* v. *Illinois*, has set forth guidelines governing paternal rights. Ordinarily fathers must be given an opportunity to claim their parental rights. Before an adoption, it is essential for his rights to be severed. For the adoption to be legally secure, the agency must satisfy the law's requirements with respect to the biological father of the baby.

His right of notice to participate in legal proceedings concerning the child and his signing requirements vary from state to state. A couple must never assume that, just because a birth mother desires to place her child for adoption, the "unwed" birth father is without rights or recourse with respect to the child. Many states treat the alleged father no differently than if he were married to the child's mother. It is imperative to inquire as to the identity, marital status, location, and attitudes of the birth father before any placement plans are finalized. The adoptive couple should be leery of a claim that the biological father's identity is unknown. The relinquishing birth mother usually knows who the father is. Sometimes her motive for denying knowledge of his identity is to prevent him from asserting his legal rights. If his rights aren't addressed, later the birth mother can say: "Oh! The baby's father and I have made up. We are married now. So we, of course, want our baby back. You realize, don't you, that you didn't give the father notice!"

An attorney familiar with the laws in your state should be able to interpret them with respect to the father's interests and in light of federal constitutional requirements. In Texas, if the father cannot be located, the Family Code of Texas stipulates the procedures required to terminate his rights.

What will the child learn of his background?

"At the time of placement," answers Gladney, "the adoptive couple is given nonidentifying information about the birth parents. Physical characteristics, personality traits, educational achievement, and goals may be among the items that are shared with the adoptive couple. This information is then passed on to the child at appropriate times by the adoptive parents. If the adoptive parents misplace these data or never disclose them, an adult adoptee, having reached the age of eighteen years, has the right to obtain this nonidentifying type of information from the agency or from the court that granted the adoption." Today, the adoptive parents and the birth mother often want to meet, although they usually exchange first names only. This greater openness has helped couples and birth mothers feel more comfortable with each other. The adoptive couple may have an easier time explaining the adoption story to their child when they use the birth mother's real first name.

What provisions are made to protect the identity of the members of the adoptive triangle?

In every adoption, the birth parents and adoptive parents determine how much identifying information is shared with one another. Says Gladney: "Since both couples have greater control over what information is shared, all parties to the adoption develop respect for each other's privacy and individual desires.

"In the state of Texas," continues the home, "adoption records may be sealed; sealed adoption records cannot be opened without a court order. In 1983, Texas passed a mutual-consent voluntary-adoption registry act. This act provides the means by which birth parents and adoptees, anytime after the child reaches twenty-one years of age, can arrange through an agency or the Texas Department of Protective Regulatory Services to have contact." As of April 1995, a bill was pending that could change that age to eighteen. The state registry works like this: if children wish to contact their birth mothers, the adoptees can have their names entered in a database. If the birth mother also signs the registry, a match occurs. In other words, both are willing to meet and share identifying information. This central registry is completely voluntary.

Most agencies maintain their own registries. Says Gladney's general counsel Heidi Cox, "Most private agencies provide services to help adoptees find their biological mothers. At Gladney, this service—which is based on mutual consent—is called Direct Post Adoption Contact." People who don't wish to be located may feel threatened by a registry. Since state laws vary, legal interpretation of the laws in your area can be extremely helpful.

How much does adoption cost?

In 1994, the cost to adopt a baby through The Gladney Center was between ten thousand and twenty-five thousand dollars, graduated according to ability to pay.

It cost Gladney an average of eighteen to twenty-three thousand dollars to care for each mother and baby. This included room and board, individual and group counseling, secondary education, career development and job training, excellent medical care, postadoption services, and legal services by attorneys who specialize in adoption law. The costs of processing the application, of evaluating the adoptive family, and of conducting postplacement supervision aren't included in these figures.

The National Council For Adoption says that adoption costs in 1994 ranged from zero to two thousand dollars through a public agency and from zero to twenty-five thousand dollars through a private agency. According to some experts, independent adoption generally costs between fifteen and thirty-five thousand dollars and sometimes considerably more, depending on the intermediary involved.

Children with Special Needs

> *Most children labeled "special needs" have characteristics that present too great a challenge for the average adopter. The "need" is usually that the child is school-age or of a minority heritage. Some waiting babies and children have serious handicaps.*
> JACQUELINE HORNOR PLUMEZ, *Successful Adoption*

Although there usually is a long wait for a healthy white baby, prospective parents interested in a child with special needs will find thousands of children in the United States desperately in need of a home. These children range in age from preschool through the teens, with the older ones less likely to be placed.

Many special-needs children are handicapped—either mentally, emotionally, or physically. Some are blind; others have heart disease, cerebral palsy, or Down's syndrome. Having been abused or neglected, some children have been removed from their homes by the court and are under the conservatorship of the Department of Protective and Regulatory Services (Texas) or other states' welfare departments. It is not uncommon for these youngsters to have a long history of moving from one home to another; some have had unsatisfactory foster care. These children may have emotional and behavioral problems—a few are hostile. Even though past relationships with biological family members may have been far from ideal, some children still may need contact with relatives. These youngsters need a very special kind of home. Sadly, even with the best of care, some of them have little hope for improvement. It is an unbelievably heartbreaking problem.

Some children waiting to be adopted are categorized as difficult to place because they are part of a sibling group or a minority race. There is an urgent need for caring families to adopt these youngsters. Others have problems that might be corrected with a great deal of understanding, guidance, and patience. Some need only the appropriate medical and surgical therapy in order to be able to run and play like normal children. All of them need love.

The actual process for adopting a special-needs child usually is simpler than for adopting a healthy white baby. It is possible for an older couple—say in their mid-forties—to adopt a younger child this way. Often, however, toddlers are part of a sibling group, and agencies try to keep brothers and sisters together.

Adoptive parents opening their hearts to handicapped and other special children need counseling, because such children often present difficult challenges. Says Mrs. Tuck: "Adoptive parents need extra counseling and support to help them deal with their child's psychological and physical problems. Even healthy teenagers can be a worry to parents, but when you add the problems of a special-needs child, you are talking about a major emotional commitment. It takes a very special family to adopt one of these children. Such people restore one's faith in human nature."

At present, federal aid is available to pay for some of the costs of caring for a special-needs child, although there is always a push to cut these grants. Medicaid coverage also may pay some of the medical expenses. As of April 1995, a five-thousand-dollar tax credit was pending before Congress to assist *all* adoptive couples. Although Texas has no specific funding for special-needs children, some states do offer assistance.

Says adoption expert Jacqueline Plumez: "Adopting one of these children is a big step and a big commitment. Parents who have done it will readily admit they often ask themselves why in the world they did such a foolish thing! But they also speak of the pride they take in their child's accomplishments, of the good feelings they get for providing the chance of a better life and of the love that grows as a homeless child is transformed into a son or daughter. . . . If you think you are up to the challenge—as one mother put it, to 'love a rose with thorns'—then special needs adoption may be for you. It has special challenges and special rewards, and rarely a dull moment."

Couples interested in further information about adopting a special-needs child should write the National Council For Adoption, 1930 17th Street N.W., Washington, D.C. 20009 ([202] 328-1200) or AASK America-Adopt a Special Kid, 2201 Broadway, Suite 702, Oakland, CA 94612 ([510] 451-1748).

International Adoptions

In recent years, more Americans have been turning to international adoption to build their families. Some established U.S. adoption agencies such as Gladney assist couples interested in foreign adoption. Prospective parents also can adopt abroad directly—without the help of an American agency, if they can untangle the red tape of federal immigration laws and state and international adoption requirements. A home study, foreign dossier, immigration documents, and an application to a reputable agency or orphanage are required. According to the National Council For Adoption, your local state department of public welfare or social services can help you find an agency to do the required home study. You will need a reputable agency or legal counsel knowledgeable about foreign adoption.

Couples considering international adoption must be careful to contact people with excellent references. Warns the National Council For Adoption: "Do not work with agencies or individuals who suggest that agencies or national groups such as the National Council For Adoption should not be contacted for recommendations. Don't evade established procedures, pay 'finders fees,' or become involved in 'black market' adoption." Says one adoption attorney: "If a couple go abroad and pick up a child, they had better know who they are dealing with."

Says the National Council: "Do your homework first. Buy and read sound books on adopting. Obtain the materials from the Immigration and Naturalization Service and the Department of State dealing with foreign adoption. Do investigate thoroughly at each step of the process. Adoption is a major step for the child and for you. International adoption adds extra complexities, and you should not proceed unless you are comfortable with each step in the process."

Support groups consisting of adoptive parents of foreign-born children are willing to share their experiences with interested couples. One such organization, called Adoptive Families of America, publishes a bimonthly magazine called *Adoptive Families* dedicated to both domestic and foreign adoption. The address is: 3333 Highway 100 North, Minneapolis, MN 55422 ([612] 535-4829).

The Gladney Center now has international adoption programs in China, Paraguay, Russia, Guatemala, and Honduras. Staff members can assist would-be parents with all aspects of foreign adoption. Says Gladney's president: "We have children waiting for international adoption whose lives will be less than wonderful if they remain in an institution or a difficult environment in their country. In Russia, for example, nonminority toddlers are waiting for homes. Many have correctable or non-correctable medical problems. In China, you generally can adopt a baby girl in three or four months. We have helped some wonderful couples adopt these children."

The National Council For Adoption (NCFA) recommends several books to help couples interested in adopting children from other countries. A publications list is available from the NCFA. Just send a stamped self-addressed envelope.

Private Placement
(Independent Adoption)

Some couples finally find their child through independent adoption, with the aid of an attorney or another intermediary rather than through an established state-licensed adoption agency such as Gladney. In recent years the number of independent adoptions has increased to the point that probably 40 percent of all adoptions are handled by private placement. Many people have successfully started their family this way, but prospective adoptive parents considering this option should be aware that they could get hurt.

In most states, birth parents have the right to place their child with anyone they wish, although the court need not approve the adoption of a child who has been placed in an inadequate home. Obviously, when a child is placed directly by a biological parent, any hope of confidentiality is destroyed. For this reason, one of the key emotional questions prospective adoptive parents and birth parents considering private adoption must ask themselves is whether they can handle such an "open" adoption arrangement.

Intrastate placements can be accomplished without the preliminary involvement of a licensed agency, although in many states an investigator, often a licensed agency, will eventually have to prepare a social study before consummation of the adoption. In addition, some states, such as Texas, require the placing agency or birth parent to complete and furnish to the prospective adoptive couple a report containing the genetic, social, health, and educational (if applicable) history of the child, including relevant information about the child's biological parents and extended family. To comply with the law, this report must be furnished to the adoptive parents at or prior to the time of placement.

Some states, such as Texas, prohibit attorneys, doctors, clergymen, or other persons from placing children for adoption as the intermediary

or "go-between" linking the birth mother and the adoptive parents—
that is, unless the lawyer or other acting intermediary is licensed by the
state as a child-placing agency. To obtain such a license, state requirements for adoption agencies must be met. Violation of these laws can
result in both civil and criminal penalties. These agencies, many of which
are attorney-driven, are subject to the same minimum standards applicable to other licensed agencies.

The mere fact that an intermediary such as a lawyer has an agency
license doesn't necessarily mean that the agency employs the kind of
highly experienced people on its staff that an established agency such
as Gladney does. Attorney-driven agencies are supposed to have a minimum staff. The intermediary is supposed to be concerned with the
welfare of the child; the agency is not supposed to place the youngster
with unfit adoptive parents. Before placement such an agency is supposed
to study the child's needs and the home of the prospective parents. If
such standards aren't followed, the potential for emotional damage to
the child and the adoptive parents is enormous. Often the pain of an
improperly handled adoption can never be rectified.

Interstate placement of children for adoptive purposes is an entirely
different situation from adoption within a state. Be forewarned that a
prospective adoptive couple should be extremely cautious about accepting a child from another state. Almost all states have enacted varying
forms of a law known as the Interstate Compact on the Placement of
Children (ICPC). It prescribes certain procedures that must be met
before a child is sent or received for adoption.

Assuming that all requirements have been legally satisfied, additional
considerations have to be addressed before the adopting parents can
breathe a sigh of relief. Depending on the state in which the adoption
is transacted, the birth parents may sign consent, relinquishment, or
surrender papers, either before or after the actual placement of the
child. If the placement occurs before the consent is executed, the placement is riskier than if consent documents are signed before or at the
time of placement. Each state has its own laws governing the timing of
the signing of adoption consent documents, including laws that state
when and under what circumstances birth parents may revoke or otherwise negate the legal effect of signing such papers.

In Texas, the birth mother signs the relinquishment, and on the basis
of that relinquishment, the hospital releases the child to the adoptive
couple, because custody has already been transferred. In other words,
the placement generally is preceded by the execution of the document,
rather than followed by it. Ordinarily the adoption is finalized later. In
some states, the birth mother has the right to seek the return of the

baby for a limited amount of time after placement. Again, make sure you understand your state's adoption laws.

As mentioned earlier, an adoptive couple also must learn how their particular state's law treats the rights of the putative birth father. Many couples become so excited that the birth mother intends to release the baby that they completely ignore the rights, or potential rights, of the child's biological father. Failure to address this issue can lead to legal, emotional, and financial disaster if a postplacement legal confrontation occurs.

If you are considering independent adoption, it is extremely important to choose an attorney, an intermediary, or a "go-between" with absolutely impeccable credentials. State laws vary and are complicated and confusing! You need and deserve an independent legal counsel to help you with the complicated legal ramifications of adoption procedures. The person must be well versed in the laws of every state having a connection with the adoption, and in federal adoption laws as well. Some adoptive-parent groups will furnish the names of possible "go-betweens," but you will still be responsible for checking their credentials and seeking further references. Resolve, Inc., 1310 Broadway, Somerville, MA 02144-1731, counsels infertile couples and is a possible source of help. The American Academy of Adoption Attorneys, P.O. Box 33053, Washington, D.C. 20033-0053 is another resource for information.

Some adoption experts worry that the "go-between" might lack the time and experience to counsel the biological mother, or to match the adoptive parents to the baby. Another concern is that some intermediaries may not take the time to gather medical information about the birth parents, particularly the father. In addition to lack of time and experience, the "go-between" may have a definite conflict of interest. Whom does he represent? Does his loyalty lie with the adoptive couple or with the birth parent? If he claims to be loyal to both, with whom will he side if a conflict develops? As a rule, the adoptive parents should have their own attorney, and the lawyer for the birth parents should be independent.

A possible problem that anxious parents involved in private placements may overlook is the destiny of a child born with a physical or mental handicap. This also is a problem the birth mother should consider. The adoptive couple may not be financially or emotionally able to care for such a child. If the "go-between," although licensed, isn't equipped to provide care or alternative placement, what happens to the baby? Established agencies are in a much better position to provide for the medical needs of a handicapped child. They have greater resources with which to locate placements for children with special needs.

During independent adoption, the birth mother may receive little, if any, counseling services that help her make an informed decision. Says a Gladney representative: "The young pregnant woman often is vulnerable and fragile. At the very least, she deserves an opportunity to review and discuss all her options. We want her to make a decision that she can live with the rest of her life. An established agency gives a young woman considering adoption time to study the relinquishment papers so that she is aware of the finality they bring." (From a legal point of view, once the agency has been appointed by the court as the managing conservator of the child, that appointment will be withdrawn only under exceptional circumstances.)

Although independent adoption can be successful, it may leave the door open to heartache. One of my friends adopted through a lawyer; during the six-month waiting period before the adoption was final, the biological mother demanded to have the baby back. She hadn't received any counseling before placing her child for adoption. A bitter lawsuit followed. Aware of cases such as this, I recommend that couples adopt through one of the many fine established adoption agencies such as Gladney.

Gladney's Designated Adoption Program

Gladney's designated adoption program is designed to assist couples and singles through the private adoption maze. Says Gladney: "This program is directed by the couples, who, upon completion of the application and home study process, work at their own pace in locating a birth mother. Our staff members assist adoptive parents in their search by providing support, suggestions, and information about advertising and networking. Once a prospective family has located their birth mother, our agency initiates the legal process." This is a flexible program with no age limit for the would-be parents and no limit to the number of children in the family. Gladney has no requirement concerning the degree of openness or confidentiality of the adoption.

Avoiding "Gray-Market" and "Black-Market" Adoption

Sometimes the children have been kidnapped or taken from their parents by fraud. Other times, there is no

*baby and couples are left with both an empty wallet and
an empty bassinet.*
> E. KEERDOJA, "Adoption: New Frustrations,
> New Hope," *Newsweek*

Since many infertile couples seeking to adopt are willing to pay any price for a child, unethical or illegal adoption practices do occur. There is, indeed, a "gray market" and a "black market" in babies.

Reprehensible tactics followed by black-marketeers include charging high fees, pressuring the birth mother to relinquish her baby, using faulty forms, falsifying the baby's age and medical records, hiring a prostitute to become pregnant in order to provide the baby, offering the same baby to two or more couples and selecting the family who will pay the highest price, and even blackmailing adoptive parents by threatening to take the child back. It obviously pays to know your intermediary before adopting!

If handled properly, however, either through a state-licensed agency or through a reputable "go-between," adoption can be successful. It may be the answer to an infertile couple's prayers. Bringing home an adopted child can end a husband and wife's longing for a baby and their struggle to start a family.

Says Mark G. Allen in an article from *Home Life* entitled "Advice from an Adoptive Dad": "Could there be any greater thrill than following God's example and adopting a child into one's own family? Take it from an adoptive dad, the answer is no."

The National Council For Adoption will send you an adoption publications list of recommended reading. The Gladney Center has a list of books for adopted children and adult adoptees. Write The Gladney Center, Post-Adoption Department, 2300 Hemphill, Fort Worth, TX 76110.

Glossary

acrosome—The caplike head of a sperm, containing enzymes.

adenomyosis—A disease in which some of the glands and cells of the endometrium are found within the muscle wall of the uterus.

adhesions—Rubbery bands of scar tissue linking two abdominal structures such as a fallopian tube and an ovary.

*adrenaline—A hormone of the adrenal medulla that acts as a powerful stimulant in times of fear or arousal and has many physiological effects, including increasing breathing, heart, and metabolic rates to provide quick energy, constricting blood vessels, and strengthening muscle contraction; also called "epinephrine."

agglutination—Occurs when sperm clump or stick together, as when either the husband or wife develops immunity to sperm. Also used to describe fallopian tubes in which the inner tubal walls stick together.

AID—Artificial insemination by donor.

AIH—Artificial insemination by husband.

amenorrhea—Medical term for absence of menstruation.

*An asterisk preceding an entry indicates the definition is from *Medical Dictionary for the Non-Professional*, Charles Chapman © 1984, Barron's Educational Series, Inc., Hauppauge, N.Y.

*amniocentesis—The taking of amniotic fluid by needle puncture through the abdominal wall of the pregnant woman to aid in the diagnosis of fetal abnormalities.

ampulla—Widened part of the fallopian tube, where fertilization usually occurs.

androgen—Hormones responsible for producing secondary masculine sex characteristics.

anomalies—Malformations, as in an inherited defect.

anovulation—Lack of ovulation.

*anoxia—An abnormally low amount of oxygen in the body.

*antibody—A complex molecule that is produced by lymph tissue in response to the presence of an antigen and that neutralizes the effect of that foreign substance.

Asherman's syndrome—Adhesions inside the cavity of the uterus.

asthenospermia—A condition in which the sperm swim slower than normal or not at all.

*atrophy—A decrease in size of a part or organ, resulting from a wasting away of tissue, as may occur, for example, in disease or from lack of use.

autoantibodies—Antibodies against one's own cells. Some men have autoantibodies against their own sperm.

azoospermia—Absence of sperm in the semen; may be caused by blockage or impairment in sperm production.

*basal body temperature (BBT)—Temperature of the body taken in the morning, before rising or moving about or eating or drinking anything. Reflecting progesterone production by the ovaries, the BBT rises after ovulation. It usually takes about six hours of sleep to arrive at a BBT.

Beta-hCG—Beta-human chorionic gonadotropin; a subunit or portion of human chorionic gonadotropin—a hormone of pregnancy secreted by the placenta that is detected by a positive pregnancy test (see hCG).

bicornuate uterus—A uterine anomaly or malformation present at birth in which the uterus has two horns.

biphasic—Having two phases, as pertaining to a normal ovulation chart.

*cannula—A flexible tube inserted into a cavity for transferring fluids or other materials into or out of it.

capacitation—The process whereby the enzyme inhibitor is removed from the sperm head, rendering the sperm capable of fertilizing the egg.

*carcinoma—A malignant growth of cells that arises in the coverings and linings of the body parts and in glands.

cervix—The mouth of the womb or uterus, which extends into the vagina, through which the menses exit the body and the sperm enter the uterus.

chlamydia—The most common sexually transmitted disease, caused by the *Chlamydium trachomatis* bacterium. Can lead to infertility; frequently destroys the inside of the fallopian tubes with no warning symptoms.

chocolate cyst—Endometrioma or benign ovarian tumor filled with old blood and misplaced menstrual tissue.

chorionic-villus sampling—A prenatal genetic screening test in which a small sample of the chorionic villi (the fingerlike projections of the outermost fetal membrane) is aspirated vaginally and analyzed.

*chromosomes—Threadlike structures in every cell nucleus that carry the inheritance factors.

*cilia—Hairlike projections from a cell.

*cleavage—The process of dividing, as of the fertilized egg into successive multiples of cells from the single cell.

Clomid—Trade name for clomiphene citrate, the drug most commonly used to induce ovulation.

clomiphene citrate—A drug with a chemical structure similar to estrogen that is taken orally to induce ovulation; marketed as Clomid and Serophene.

cornual tubal end—The portion of the fallopian tube that enters the uterus.

corpus luteum—An orange-yellow gland that forms in the dominant ovarian follicle after ovulation. The corpus luteum produces hormones, the most important of which is the female sex hormone progesterone.

*cortisol—The adrenal-cortex hormone hydrocortisone, used in the treatment of rheumatoid arthritis and other inflammatory conditions.

cryopreservation—Preservation of cells by dehydration and freezing.

cryptorchidism—Occurs when a testis is not in its normal position in the scrotum. An undescended testicle, it may be in the groin or abdomen.

danazol—A drug used to treat endometriosis.

*D&C—Dilatation and curettage: dilatation of the cervix of the uterus and scraping of the endometrium (lining) of the uterus.

DHEA-S—Conjugated adrenal androgen measured to determine adrenal-androgen activity.

dysmenorrhea—Pain related to menstruation.

dyspareunia—Pain with intercourse.

ectopic pregnancy—A misplaced pregnancy outside of the uterus, usually in the fallopian tubes.

EIA—Enzyme immunoassay; a test used to diagnose chlamydia.

ejaculation—The ejaculatory process involves two distinct events: (1) emission (the deposition of seminal fluid components from the vas deferens, seminal vesicles, and prostate gland into the posterior urethra) and (2) ejaculation (passage of this fluid through the urethra and expulsion from the urethral opening).

*electrosurgery—Surgery performed using electrical devices.

*embryo—The early developing organism, from the zygote to the fetal stage; in humans, from about week 3 to week 8 after conception, at which time the main organ systems have formed, at least in their early stages.

*endocrine system—The network of endocrine glands that produce and secrete hormones directly into the bloodstream for transport to specific target organs where they exert their effect.

*endocrinologist—A physician who specializes in the diagnosis and treatment of diseases affecting the endocrine system.

endometrioma—Benign ovarian tumor filled with old blood and lined with endometrial glands and stroma; also called a "chocolate cyst."

endometriosis—A condition in which misplaced menstrual tissue grows outside the uterus, often in the pelvis. Endometriosis is associated with infertility.

*endometrium—The mucous-membrane lining of the uterus, which, under hormonal control, changes in thickness and complexity during the menstrual cycle and if pregnancy does not occur is mostly shed during menstruation.

*enzyme—A protein produced in cells that acts as a catalyst, speeding up the rate of biological reactions without itself being used up.

epididymis—The long, coiled canal located behind and attached to each testis, where sperm mature and are stored.

epiphysis—The end portion of a long bone, separated by cartilage from the shaft until the bone stops growing, at which time the shaft and head unite. (Plural: epiphyses.)

*epithelium—The cell layers covering the outside body surfaces as well as forming the lining of hollow organs and the passages of the respiratory, digestive, and urinary tracts.

*estradiol—The most active naturally occurring estrogen; a female hormone.

estrogen—Female hormones secreted mainly by the ovaries in women. Estrogen is also produced in small quantities in men and women by the adrenals and in men by the testes.

*etiology—The study of the causes of disease.

fallopian tubes—Uterine tubes or oviducts that act as secretory conduits between the ovaries and the uterus, through which the sperm and egg travel.

fertilization—The moment of conception when the sperm enters and unites with the egg.

fibroid—A benign smooth-muscle tumor of the uterus associated with infertility and spontaneous abortion.

*fimbriae—The petallike fingers of the fallopian tube that whisk the egg from the surface of the ovary into the oviduct.

follicle—A small fluid-filled sac in the ovary that contains an egg.

FSH—Follicle-stimulating hormone. A hormone secreted by the pituitary. In women, FSH stimulates maturation of the follicle in the ovary. In men, FSH stimulates the formation of the sperm in the testes.

galactorrhea—Milky discharge from the breasts.

gamete—A biological term for an egg or a sperm.

*general anesthesia—An agent, usually given by inhalation or intravenous injection, that produces unconsciousness and complete loss of sensation throughout the body.

GIFT—An acronym for "gamete intrafallopian transfer," a procedure in which sperm and eggs are placed directly in the ends of the fallopian tubes through a lighted endoscopic instrument called a "laparoscope."

GnRH—Gonadotropin-releasing hormone; a hormone secreted by the hypothalamus that stimulates the release of follicle-stimulating hormone and luteinizing hormone from the pituitary gland, both of which then stimulate the ovaries in women or the testes in men. GnRH also is known as "LH-RH."

*gonad—A gland that produces sex cells (gametes); in males the gonads are the testes; in females, the ovaries.

gonadotropin—A hormone that stimulates the gonads or sex glands.

gonorrhea—A common venereal (sexually transmitted) disease caused by the bacteria *Neisseria gonorrhoeae*. A gonorrheal infection can destroy the fallopian tubes.

Graafian follicle—The dominant ovarian follicle, which usually contains an egg and fluid rich in the female hormone estrogen. Normally one dominant follicle matures each menstrual cycle.

gram stain—A type of Pap smear allowing immediate diagnosis and treatment; used to classify bacteria.

*gynecomastia—Abnormal development of one or both breasts in males, usually the result of hormonal imbalance, liver malfunction, or treatment with steroid compounds.

*habitual abortion—[Traditionally] the reported spontaneous expulsion of the products of conception in three or more pregnancies, often for no known cause. The cause of abortion should be sought before the third pregnancy loss.

hCG—Human chorionic gonadotropin, marketed as Profasi *HP*; a hormone of pregnancy secreted by the placenta. HCG causes the corpus luteum to continue to produce progesterone during pregnancy. In females, hCG is sometimes given by injection to trigger final maturation and release of an egg. In males, hCG is used to stimulate production of the male hormone testosterone by the testicles.

hirsutism—Excessive hair growth due to genetic causes or increased androgen activity.

hMG—Human menopausal gonadotropin; see Pergonal.

hypoglycemia—Low levels of glucose in the blood.

hypothalamus—Lower brain, which regulates many bodily functions, some of which are hunger, thirst, temperature, sleep, growth, and reproduction.

hypothyroidism—Decreased thyroid-hormone production by the thyroid gland, caused by thyroid disease or pituitary dysfunction.

hysterosalpingogram (HSG)—An X-ray of the uterus and fallopian tubes or uterine tubes.

hysteroscopy—A lighted endoscopic instrument introduced through the vagina and cervix to view the cavity of the uterus.

immunological infertility—Infertility attributed to antisperm antibodies.

implantation—The process by which the pre-embryo attaches itself to the endometrium (the tissue lining the inside of the uterus).

incompetent cervix—A condition in which the cervix, or mouth of the uterus, becomes dilated, causing loss of the fetus.

*incomplete abortion—Termination of pregnancy in which some of the products of conception are not expelled but, rather, are retained in the uterus.

IUD—Intrauterine device. A contraceptive device put in the uterus via the vagina to prevent pregnancy.

IVF—*In-vitro* fertilization or "test-tube" fertilization. During *in-vitro* fertilization, the ovas (eggs) and the sperm are mixed in a laboratory dish to create pre-embryos, which are later returned to the uterus.

karyotyping—A test studying the chromosomal makeup of cells.

*keloids—Overgrowth of collagenous scar tissue at the site of a wound on the skin. Sometimes found in operative incisions.

*Klinefelter's syndrome—A defect in which at least one extra "X" chromosome is present in a male, characterized by small testes, enlarged breasts, long legs, decreased or absent sperm production, and mental retardation.

laparoscope—A fiber-optically lighted endoscope or telescopic instrument used to look within the abdomen.

laparotomy—Major surgery in which an incision is made through the abdomen.

leiomyomas—Benign muscular tumors of the uterus that are commonly called "fibroids."

Leydig cells—Cells in the testes that secrete the major male hormone testosterone.

LH—Luteinizing hormone. A sex hormone secreted by the pituitary. In women, the LH surge precedes ovulation. During the menstrual cycle, LH causes the corpus luteum to make the female hormone progesterone. In men, LH stimulates production of the male hormone testosterone by the Leydig cells in the testes.

*local anesthetic—An agent that reduces or eliminates sensation, especially pain, in a limited area of the body by blocking the transmission of nerve impulses in the area.

Lupron—Trade name for leuprolide acetate, one of the LH-RH agonists; an injectible medication that inhibits the ability of the pituitary to produce the pituitary hormones FSH and LH.

*luteal phase—The second half of the menstrual cycle, during which the corpus luteum secretes the hormone progesterone, which, in turn, causes the endometrium to become rich and developed for implantation of a fertilized egg.

lymphocyte—a white blood cell that increases in the presence of a viral infection.

menarche—The first menstrual period, which usually occurs between the ages of nine and sixteen.

*menopause—The stoppage of the menstruation, usually occurring naturally between the ages of forty-five and fifty-five.

*microsurgery—That branch of surgery performed using special operating microscopes and miniaturized precision instruments to perform delicate and intricate procedures on very small structures and structures not previously accessible to surgery.

miscarriage—A spontaneous abortion or pregnancy loss before viability.

morphology of sperm—Refers to the form or shape of the sperm.

motility of sperm—Refers to the percent of sperm demonstrating any type of movement. (Fertile men tend to have more motile sperm than those with lower fertility ratings.) Forward progression is the quality of movement demonstrated by the majority of motile sperm.

myometrium—The muscle wall of the uterus.

*nidation—Implantation of the conceptus in the endometrial layer of the uterus.

occluded—Blocked; as in an occluded fallopian tube.

oligospermia—Abnormally low number of sperm in the semen.

oocyte—A cell that can develop into a mature ovum (egg).

*oral contraceptive (OC)—A pill containing a combination of estrogen and progestin preparations that inhibits ovulation and thus prevents conception.

*orchiopexy—A surgical procedure to bring an undescended testis into the scrotum and attach it so that it will not retract.

*osteoporosis—Abnormal loss of bony tissue causing fragile bones that fracture easily; pain, especially in the back; and loss of stature.

oviducts—Fallopian or uterine tubes.

ovulation—The release of a mature ovum (egg) from the ovary.

ovum—The female egg or gamete.

palpate—Examine by touch.

*Pap smear test—Papanicolaou test; a method of examining stained cells shed by mucous membranes.

patent—Open, as in an open fallopian tube.

*pathologic—Pertaining to or arising from disease.

*Pergonal—Trade name for a preparation of gonadotropins (FSH and LH), originally extracted from the urine of menopausal women and used to induce ovulation in some cases of infertility. Known to doctors as "human menopausal gonadoptropin" or "hMG."

peritoneum—The smooth membrane lining the organs and walls of the pelvis and abdomen.

peritonitis—An inflammation of the peritoneum causing abdominal pain.

*pituitary gland—A small endocrine gland attached to the hypothalamus that releases many hormones controlling many body activities and influencing the activity of many other endocrine glands.

*PMS—Premenstrual syndrome, also called "premenstrual tension" (PMT). A poorly understood syndrome of tension, irritability, edema, headache, mastalgia, bloating, appetite changes, and changes in muscular coordination occurring several days before the onset of the menstrual flow. Sometimes PMS lasts from ovulation until menstruation.

polycystic ovarian disease (PCO)—Also called Stein-Leventhal syndrome or sclerocystic ovarian disease, PCO is a complicated endocrine disorder characterized by enlarged cystic ovaries, excess male hormone, irregular or lack of menstruation, and infertility. Chronic excess adrenal and ovarian androgen is associated with weight gain, acne, and male-pattern hair growth.

polyps—Small benign growths.

pre-embryo—A product of gametic union from fertilization to the appearance of the embryonic axis. The pre-embryonic stage is considered to last until fourteen days after fertilization. This definition is not intended to imply a moral evaluation of the pre-embryo. (The Ethics Committee of the American Fertility Society.)

premature ovarian failure—Early menopause; early cessation of female hormones from the ovary.

*progesterone—The hormone produced by the corpus luteum of the ovary, the placenta during pregnancy, and in small amounts by the adrenal cortex; it prepares the uterus for a fertilized egg.

prolactin—A pituitary hormone whose primary action is to stimulate and sustain lactation in nursing mothers. Serum prolactin can also be elevated for other reasons.

prostaglandins—Hormonelike fatty acids with a wide range of effects. Prostaglandins can cause smooth muscles such as the uterus to contract or relax. They can change the blood supply to the ovary and can cause uterine spasm, both of which can affect fertility.

prostate—A chestnut-sized gland in males that surrounds the urethra, near the bladder. The prostate produces a portion of the seminal fluid.

retrograde ejaculation—A neurologic problem sometimes seen in diabetics in which the seminal fluid flows backward into the bladder instead of forward through the urethra.

retroverted uterus—A womb that is tilted backward. May be a normal anatomic variation or may be caused by a pathologic condition such as endometriosis.

salpingitis—An inflammation of the fallopian tubes.

salpingitis isthmica nodosa (SIN)—A condition in which the end of the fallopian tube near the uterus is thickened with irregularly shaped nodules. Sometimes causes tubal blockage, with increased incidence of ectopic pregnancy.

semen or seminal fluid—A thick white liquid composed of elements formed by the testes (sperm) and the male accessory glands (the prostate gland and the seminal vesicles). Only a small part of the visible ejaculate (semen) comes from the testicle.

*seminal vesicle—Either of a pair of accessory male sex glands that produce most of the fluid portion of semen, secreting it into the vas deferens before it joins the urethra.

*seminiferous tubule—Any of the numerous long and convoluted tubes found in the testis; they are the sites of spermatozoa maturation.

septate uterus—An anomaly or malformation of the uterus present at birth in which the uterus is either partially or completely divided by a septum or wall. Women with a uterine septum have a high incidence of pregnancy loss. The septum can often be removed with minor surgery through the hysteroscope.

Serophene—A brand name for clomiphene citrate, a drug used to induce ovulation.

Sertoli cells—Cells found in the seminiferous tubules of the testis that nourish developing sperm.

SIN—See "salpingitis isthmica nodosa."

*spermatogenesis—The process of spermatozoa development, from early stages of spermatogonia through other stages, leading to spermatids and finally mature spermatozoa.

spermatogonia—Sperm-cell generators; the sperm-producing mother cells.

sperm count—Concentration (density) of sperm per cubic centimeter of fluid.

*spontaneous abortion—Noninduced, natural loss of the products of conception.

stenotic—Abnormally narrowed, as in a stenotic cervix.

teratogen—An agent that can cause a congenital defect in the embryo.

testicular failure—Occurs when the testes do not produce a normal number of mature sperm and when the hormones needed for normal sperm production (LH, FSH) are abnormally elevated.

testosterone—The primary male sex hormone, secreted mainly by the testes, which is responsible in part for a man's masculine appearance.

thermogenic—Heat-producing, as in the upward shift in basal body temperature after ovulation produced by the female hormone progesterone.

*thyroid gland—A large endocrine gland situated at the base of the neck.

totipotential—Cells having the ability to develop in any direction, to become any part of the body.

*trichomoniasis—An infection of the vagina caused by the *Trichomonas vaginalis* protozoon and characterized by a foul-smelling, pale-yellowish vaginal discharge, burning, and itching.

Turner's syndrome—A rare genetic abnormality found in women in which one of the sex chromosomes is missing. It is marked by short stature and associated with infertility.

*ultrasonography—The process by which the reflection of high-frequency sound waves is used to develop an image of a structure.

unexplained infertility—Infertility in a couple for whom a doctor has performed exhaustive studies to determine the cause(s) of the couple's inability to conceive without finding an identifiable reason.

ureters—Tubes that carry urine from the kidneys to the bladder.

*urogenital—Pertaining to the urinary and reproductive systems.

uterosacral ligament—A fan-shaped ligament that connects the uterus to the sacrum. The uterosacral ligament is one of several ligaments that support the uterus and contain primary nerves to the uterus.

uterotubal spasm—Sudden involuntary contraction of the tubes and uterus.

vaginitis—An inflammation of the vagina often caused by an infection such as moniliasis or candidiasis, gardnerella or hemophilus vaginitis (HV), and trichomoniasis.

varicocele—A collection of varicose veins in the scrotum that elevates testicular temperature and may decrease sperm motility.

vasa deferentia—The two spermatic cords, which are severed during a vasectomy to make a man sterile.

vasography—An X-ray picture produced when a dyelike substance is injected into a spermatic cord to determine if there is a blockage.

viscosity—The thickness of the semen.

zona pellucida—Relatively thick membrane enclosing the egg that keeps more than one sperm from penetrating and fertilizing the egg.

*zygote—The fertilized ovum.

Index

Note: Italicized page numbers refer to illustrations.